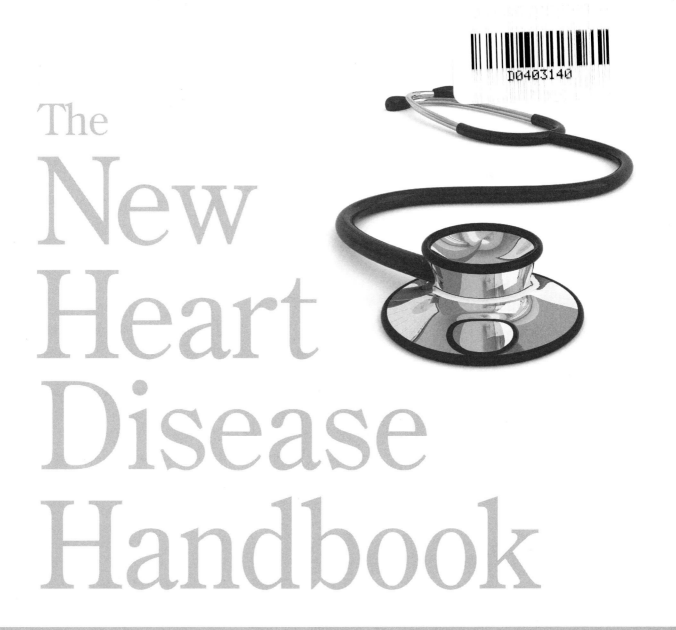

The New Heart Disease Handbook

EVERYTHING YOU NEED TO KNOW TO EFFECTIVELY
REVERSE AND MANAGE HEART DISEASE

Christopher P. Cannon, M.D.

with Elizabeth Vierck, M.S.

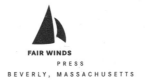

FAIR WINDS
PRESS
BEVERLY, MASSACHUSETTS

CONTENTS

INTRODUCTION

Maybe you've had chest pain or palpitations. Maybe you have a child who was born with a congenital heart defect, such as a ventricular septal defect or a patent ductus arteriosus. Or perhaps you have an elderly parent who has congestive heart failure. Whatever the reason, we understand that you picked up this handbook because you want to do everything you can to improve your health and the health of your loved ones. To help you accomplish that, we have created this highly informative, accessible, and up-to-date handbook about the heart.

THE PRESCRIPTION

This is how we begin each chapter—with the prescription you or your family member has likely received from your doctor. In the chapters of Part I, we explain the treatments for illnesses ranging from angina to stroke, covering the major diseases that strike the cardiovascular system. We provide information about diagnostic tests and detailed explanations of the specific illnesses, in language you'll understand.

Most of the prescriptions begin with healthy lifestyle changes such as quitting smoking, eating heart-healthy foods, and exercising (a lot). The prescriptions emphasize the facts that, except for congenital conditions, heart disease and its complications are often preventable, and managing heart disease is a partnership between you and your medical team.

Depending on your circumstances, your doctors will prescribe medications and/or arrange for surgery, which we describe in detail in each chapter. But it is up to you to take medications as prescribed, to let your doctor know about any new and uncomfortable symptoms or side effects, to follow a heart-healthy diet and make the other vitally important lifestyle changes that can save your heart, and to participate fully in a cardiac rehabilitation program. This collaborative effort is the key to preventing and managing heart disease.

Part II of this handbook begins with a tour of the intricate and fascinating heart, and goes on to provide you with tools to accomplish your end of the partnership. The chapters will help you determine your risk for heart disease, lower your cholesterol, manage diabetes, and make other positive changes that will lead to a longer, healthier life. We have also included a special chapter on heart disease in women.

WHAT'S NEW

Developments in heart-saving devices, medicines, and procedures are offering new hope to those currently suffering from heart disease and those at risk. In this book, we have highlighted the newest developments in every area of heart disease. In the epilogue, we look into the crystal ball at emerging treatments such as the increasing use and refinement of mechanical heart pumps called ventricular assist devices (VADs) and the stunning potential that stem cell research has for rejuvenating diseased hearts.

In the spirit of providing you with all the information you'll need to learn about and manage heart disease, we have also included four important appendixes and a glossary of cardiology terms. The appendixes provide information on how to save a life (correct and incorrect procedures for cardiopulmonary resuscitation), comprehensive reviews of the major tests used to determine the various types of heart disease, the major medications and other treatments used for heart disease, and common heart-saving procedures such as catheterization and heart bypass surgery.

We will also keep you updated through our blog, www.newhearthandbook.com, where we highlight ongoing developments in the prevention and treatment of heart disease, and give you the opportunity to ask Dr.Cannon questions about everything from the newest surgical procedures to the value of adding omega-3 essential fatty acids to your diet. We'd like to hear your thoughts about the handbook; let us know what has been useful to you and what we can add to the next edition!

PART I:

THE MOST EFFECTIVE TREATMENTS FOR MAJOR DISEASES THAT STRIKE THE HEART

chapter 1:

CHEST PAIN AND ANGINA

ANGINA

R_x THE PRESCRIPTION

Your treatment plan for angina has two important goals:

➡ Control angina symptoms (allowing you to do the things that are important to you).

➡ Prevent worsening of heart disease or heart attack.

It is important to keep both of these goals in mind when approaching your treatment. Interestingly, some of the treatments (such as beta blockers) are used for both purposes. Achieving these goals requires a multifaceted approach, not the least of which is making positive and permanent changes to your lifestyle (see chapter 14).

In addition, your doctor is likely to prescribe medicines that will reduce your symptoms and/or help prevent heart attacks. When appropriate, he may suggest an interventional or surgical procedure such as stenting or bypass surgery.

THE DISCOMFORT OF ANGINA

You have chest pain caused by angina. Your symptoms may feel like pressure or squeezing in your chest and may also strike in your shoulders, arms, neck, jaw, or back. During an angina attack, you may feel like you ate too many tacos (causing indigestion, nausea, and/or a sensation that you have heartburn); that you smoked too many cigarettes (shortness of breath); or that you are overheated (sweating).

The discomfort of angina is as specific to each of us as eye color or facial expressions. Some people have angina when they exercise vigorously. Other people experience symptoms when they are in cold temperatures, and still others when they feel angry or emotional or are under extreme stress. Many people have symptoms at all of these times. If you have angina, you will likely be able to predict the activities that bring on your symptoms, which should last only a few minutes.

Angina can also occur while resting. This is a potentially serious problem indicating that you have unstable angina, which could lead to a heart attack. (Unstable angina is a medical emergency. Read about this condition in the "Angina Explained" section at the end of this chapter.) Angina is the first indication of trouble for about half of all people with heart disease, and people who have it are at greater risk of having a heart attack. It is important to understand how to treat your condition so that you can stop it from getting worse and leading to a heart attack.

Atypical Symptoms

Many people have symptoms of chest pain—or other pain—that does not come from the heart. Check with your doctor to see whether the pain or symptoms you are feeling are thought to come from

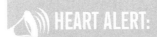

HEART ALERT:

Angina

- Nearly seven million people in the United States suffer from angina.

- About 400,000 patients go to their doctors with new cases of angina every year.

- Angina occurs equally in men and women.

- Women with angina are less likely to have chest pain than men with the condition.

Source: American Heart Association (AHA) and American College of Cardiology (ACC)

the heart. Some atypical descriptions of chest pain reduce the likelihood that symptoms represent a lack of blood flow to the heart (myocardial ischemia) or injury.

The following pain descriptions are *not* characteristic of angina, according to the ACC/AHA guidelines for heart disease:

- Sharp or knifelike pain brought on by breathing or coughing
- Discomfort primarily in the middle or lower abdominal region
- Pain that may be localized at the tip of one finger, particularly over the left breast
- Pain reproduced with movement or palpation of the chest wall or arms
- Constant pain that lasts for many hours
- Very brief episodes of pain that last a few seconds or less
- Pain that radiates into the lower extremities

TREATING ANGINA WITH MEDICINE

Most people with angina benefit from drug treatment to relieve symptoms. The medicines work in one of two ways: by increasing blood flow through the arteries or by reducing the work that the heart has to do (and thus reducing the amount of blood and oxygen needed by the heart muscle).

Nitrates Dilate Blood Vessels

Commonly known as *nitro*, nitrates are the mainstay of treatments for angina, and are ubiquitous in the pockets and purses of people with the condition. Nitrates widen (dilate) blood vessels, allowing more room for blood to get past blockages. Nitrates also can decrease blood pressure and the pressure in the heart, thereby decreasing demands on the heart. Taking nitrates to relieve symptoms, as well as taking them before activities that bring on attacks, can help you live as normally as possible.

Learning how to use nitroglycerin effectively is important to living well with angina. Prescription nitroglycerin is available in several forms including patches and sprays, and is offered through many trade names. For information on how to sort through these options and effectively take nitroglycerin to manage angina, see appendix III.

Beta Blockers Resist Adrenaline

By blocking the effects of the stimulating hormone adrenaline on your body's beta receptors, beta blockers slow the heart rate and help it beat less hard. The result is a reduction in blood pressure. Beta blockers also help blood vessels open up to improve blood flow. By reducing the workload on the heart, beta blockers help relieve symptoms of angina.

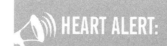 HEART ALERT:

Nitrates and Viagra

If you are taking nitrate medication such as nitroglycerin, do not take Viagra. Taking Viagra with a nitrate medicine can cause a serious decrease in blood pressure, potentially leading to fainting, stroke, or heart attack.

Also, if you have taken Viagra, Cialis, or Levitra in the 24 to 48 hours before you experience chest pain, do not take nitro or let any emergency responders give other treatments to you.

Commonly used beta blockers include the following:

- Atenolol (Tenormin)
- Bisoprolol (Zebeta)
- Carvedilol (Coreg)
- Metoprolol (Lopressor, Toprol XL)
- Timolol (Blockadren)

Potential side effects of beta blockers include slowing the heart rate excessively, worsening heart failure, and rarely, confusion, depression, and impotence (erectile dysfunction) can occur.

Calcium-Channel Blockers Improve Blood Flow

Calcium-channel blockers reduce the amount of calcium inside the muscle cells of the heart and the arteries. By blocking calcium channels, these medicines allow the heart muscle cells to function normally. The medicines also help dilate the arteries, thereby lowering blood pressure. Calcium-channel blockers include the following:

- Amlodipine (Norvasc)
- Felodipine (Plendil)
- Isradipine (DynaCirc)
- Nicardipine (Cardene)
- Nisoldipine (Sular)

Calcium-channel blockers can have side effects and are used with caution in patients with pulmonary arterial hypertension and congestive heart failure. Many calcium-channel blockers cause constipation and swelling in the ankles and feet.

Treatment to Reduce the Risk of a Heart Attack

A second goal of treating angina is to slow the development of fatty deposits in the heart arteries and if they have already developed, to prevent the blockages from breaking open and leading to a heart attack.

All of the therapies are outlined in appendix III, but for now here is a brief description of each:

- Statins reduce cholesterol (see chapter 11) and decrease inflammation in the heart arteries, thereby preventing the buildup of fatty deposits in the heart arteries; they

⋀⋀— WHAT'S NEW:

Ranolazine Improves Angina

Ranolazine is a new addition to the arsenal of drugs used for the treatment of chronic, stable angina. Ranolazine is sold under the trade name Ranexa.

How does it work? Although scientists are not yet sure exactly how it works, ranolazine is believed to affect the sodium levels in the cells of the (sodium-dependent) calcium channels, indirectly preventing calcium overload and improving blood flow to the heart. Ranolazine is used to treat chronic angina when other medications have not helped. Ranolazine may prevent episodes of angina, but it does not relieve episodes that have already begun.

What are the risks? Side effects of ranolazine include nausea, constipation, and dizziness. You should not take ranolazine if you have liver disease or a personal or family history of Long QT syndrome, a heart rhythm disorder. Before you take ranolazine, tell your doctor about all other medications you are using. You should not take ranolazine with certain medicines to treat heart rhythm disorders, malaria, infections, HIV or AIDS, seizures, mental illness, pain, cancer, or stomach disorders. In addition, do not take ranolazine during an acute (emergency) attack of angina.

How should I take ranolazine? Do not crush, chew, or break ranolazine tablets. They are extended-release tablets specially made to release medicine slowly into the body. Breaking the pill would cause too much of the drug to be released at one time.

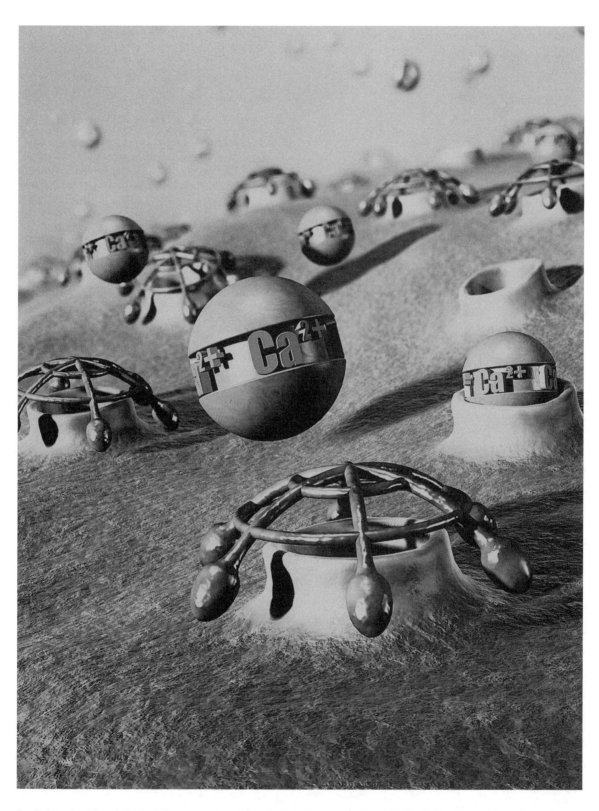

Depiction of calcium ions, which are being kept away from calcium channels by drugs. By blocking calcium channels, these medicines allow the heart muscle cells to function normally.

also prevent deposits from breaking open and leading to a heart attack.

- Aspirin is an anticlotting drug that can prevent blood clots from forming in the heart arteries, again reducing the chance of developing a heart attack.
- Blood-pressure-reducing medications such as angiotensin-converting enzyme inhibitors or calcium-channel blockers can also be used to help prevent future heart attacks.

INTERVENTIONS TO TREAT ANGINA

Interventional procedures are treatments that open (or in the case of surgery, bypass) blockages in heart arteries. The main goal, paradoxically, is to reduce the symptoms of chest pain, not necessarily to reduce the risk of another heart attack. In patients with angina, having angioplasty or bypass surgery has not been shown to reduce the risk of dying or having another heart attack. (The exceptions to this rule are if you have unstable angina or recently had a heart attack—then interventions can help prevent another attack; see appendix IV.)

Cardiac Catheterization for Balloon Angioplasty and Stenting

Interventional procedures begin with cardiac catheterization, which involves the insertion of a long, narrow tube called a *catheter* into a blood vessel in your leg or arm. The catheter is gently run through the blood vessel to your coronary arteries. Once the catheter is in place, a doctor performs a procedure such as balloon angioplasty or stenting to open the artery.

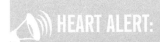

HEART ALERT:

Stopping Your Medication

Stopping your prescription heart medicines too quickly can worsen angina symptoms. Always talk to your doctor before stopping your medications, even if you think you have a good reason, such as that you are feeling better or economizing. Make sure your prescription is always filled so that you don't run out. If you do run out, call your doctor's office for a refill—don't wait for your next appointment.

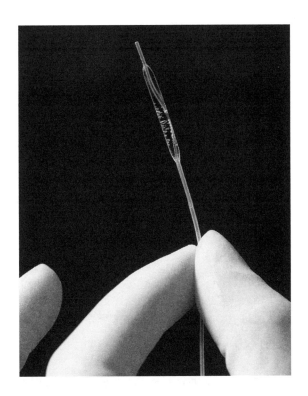

Angioplasty balloon shown expanded. These devices are used to open clogged arteries.

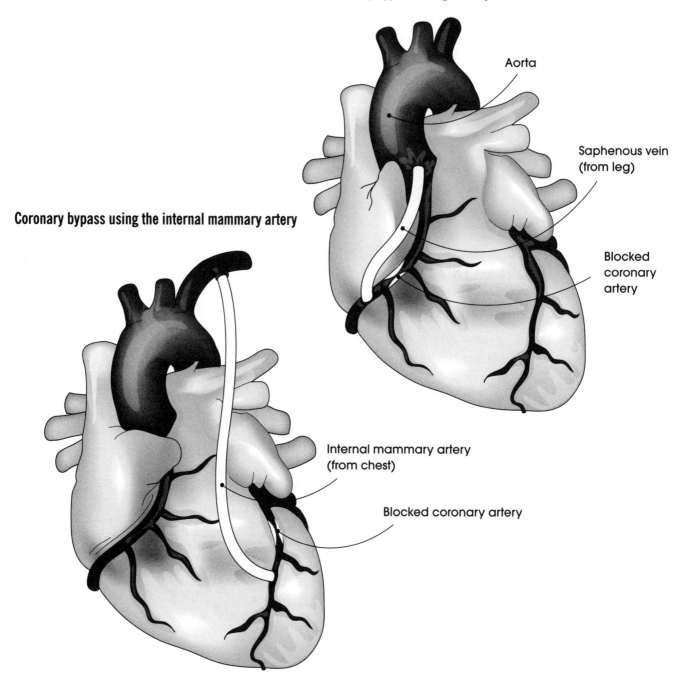

Coronary bypass using the sephenous vein

Aorta

Saphenous vein (from leg)

Blocked coronary artery

Coronary bypass using the internal mammary artery

Internal mammary artery (from chest)

Blocked coronary artery

A depiction of a coronary artery bypass graft (CABG), which is used to treat severe coronary artery disease (CAD). Part of a vein or artery (called a graft) from another part of the body is used to bypass a blockage in one or more of the coronary arteries. The graft is attached above and below the blocked area so that blood actually flows around it and to the area of the heart below the blockage.

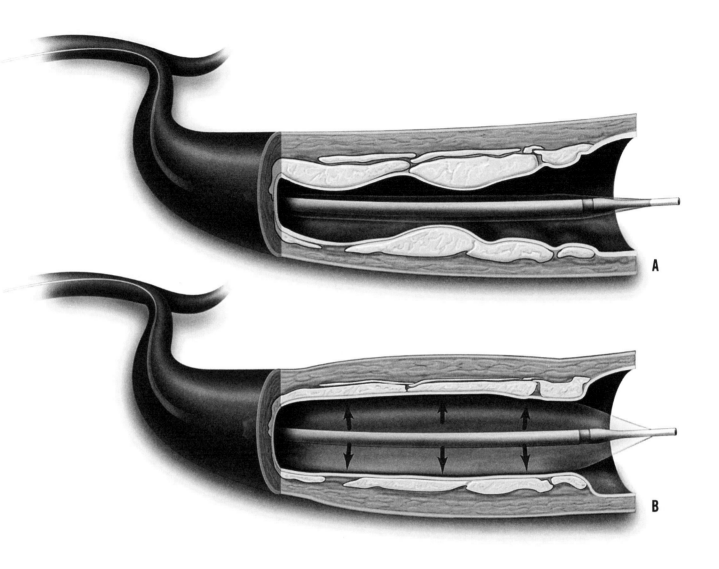

Cross section of an artery showing how angioplasty balloons are inserted **(A)** and inflated to open clogged arteries **(B)**.

Coronary Artery Bypass Graft

Bypass surgery lives up to its name. This technique provides a new route (a bypass) for blood and oxygen to reach your heart. The surgeon uses a blood vessel from your leg or chest and grafts it to your heart. The procedure is quite invasive—your chest will be opened, your heart will be stopped, and a heart-lung machine will circulate your blood while the surgeon performs the graft.

TESTS AND DIAGNOSIS OF ANGINA

Whether you're in a physician's office or a hospital, the first thing the medical staff will do is ask you to describe your angina symptoms and if possible, your medical history. If you have kept a heart diary (see page 25), this will be very helpful.

Typically, you will next have an electrocardiogram (ECG), which is explained shortly. A doctor will then perform a physical examination to look for any injury to your heart's outer muscle and other indications of artery disease. The exam will also include measurement of your vital signs, such as listening to your heart and lungs, and a look at the jugular vein in your neck to see whether it shows signs of elevated pressure, which can indicate heart distress. The doctor will also check your ankles for any swelling and may check the pulses in your feet. If you haven't had blood work recently, the doctor may have blood drawn to be sent to a lab for analysis of cholesterol levels, a kidney test, and cardiac markers. (The name of one such marker is a mouthful: *creatine kinase MB isoenzyme troponins T.* A relatively new test, called C-reactive protein [CRP], looks for increased inflammation.)

ECG

If you have chest pain or other distressing signs of heart trouble, an ECG can help determine whether your heart is the cause. This painless and fast test records the electrical activity of the heart. Many of us have had one as part of a routine evaluation—it involves sticking electrodes to the skin while a machine measures the heart's electrical activity. However, if you are not having symptoms, or your heart is not experiencing arrhythmia at that time, the ECG cannot show what your heart did in the past or what it might do in the future.

Depending on the results of the ECG, your doctor may order other tests, some of which are less invasive than others; in other words, some require surgery and some do not. For more information about these tests, see appendix II.

Exercise Stress Testing

During an exercise stress test, an ECG records the activity of your heart while you walk on a treadmill (or sometimes a drug is used to make your heart beat faster). The test identifies signs of inadequate blood flow to your heart. Your doctor will also monitor you for symptoms such as low blood pressure and chest pain. If symptoms become too uncomfortable, the test is stopped.

Thallium or Methoxyisobutyl Isonitrile (MIBI) Stress Test

In a thallium or MIBI stress test, a small amount of radioactive material is injected into the blood stream, which enables a camera to show how the blood is flowing to all parts of the heart muscle. If there is a blockage, less blood flows to that part of the muscle during exercise or stress.

CT Angiogram

A computed tomography (CT) angiogram uses X-rays to make detailed pictures of blood vessels.

Calcium Score

Cardiac calcium scoring uses CT to check for the buildup of calcium in plaque on the walls of coronary arteries.

Angiography (Cardiac Catheterization)

Angiography is an X-ray examination of the coronary arteries. Under a local anesthetic, a catheter is inserted into a main artery in your wrist, arm, or groin, and then passed gently through your blood vessels until it reaches your coronary arteries. Dye is inserted to fill the arteries, allowing doctors to see any blockages.

ANGINA EXPLAINED

Angina is a symptom of heart disease, not a disease itself. Coronary artery disease (CAD), a specific type of heart disease, is most often the culprit behind the symptoms. CAD is the buildup of plaque (fatty deposits) within the inner walls of your coronary arteries. These important vessels supply your heart with the blood and oxygen it needs to pump blood throughout your body. When plaque builds up in arteries, the condition is called *atherosclerosis*.

Although CAD is the major cause of angina, other conditions can cause symptoms resembling angina, such as spasms of the coronary arteries or problems with the linings of the arteries (the *endothelium*). This is why when you are evaluated for angina symptoms your doctor and other medical professionals will take an extensive history and will probably order a lot of tests to rule out other conditions and pinpoint your particular problem.

HEART HELP:

Angina and Daily Living

From carrying groceries into the house to arguing with a neighbor, any activity that makes demands on your heart can bring on an angina attack. Many of these activities are unavoidable parts of daily life. But you can adjust your schedule and corresponding exertions so that you don't reach the threshold where angina symptoms kick in. Generally, if angina develops with only strenuous activity (such as running) it can be avoided by reducing the activity. However, if angina comes during routine life activities such as carrying groceries or washing dishes, it could be a sign that the heart artery blockage is severe.

Try breaking big jobs into smaller tasks. If climbing three flights of stairs kicks off symptoms, stop when you need to and rest before continuing. If your house needs cleaning, dust and mop one room on Monday and another on Tuesday, not both on the same day. If food shopping always wears you out and brings on symptoms, make sure you take your medication before you start filling your grocery cart.

For more tips on how to adjust your daily life to live successfully with angina and other heart diseases, see chapter 14.

Plaque in coronary artery

Plaque in coronary artery

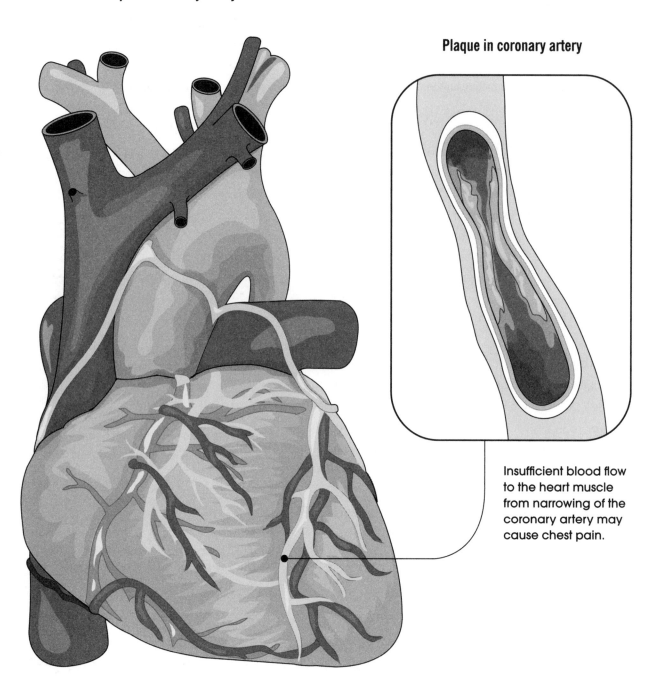

Insufficient blood flow to the heart muscle from narrowing of the coronary artery may cause chest pain.

Plaque accumulated in a coronary artery, blocking blood flow and damaging heart muscle.

Some of these problems may be serious. Get immediate medical care if you have chest pain that does not go away, crushing pain or pressure in the chest, or chest pain along with nausea, sweating, dizziness, or shortness of breath. Treatment will depend on the cause of the pain.

Stable Angina

Stable angina is the most common form of the condition. Angina is considered stable when symptoms have stayed the same for months. Stable angina is usually brought on by physical activity, strong emotions (such as anger, frustration, or excitement), eating a heavy meal, or cold weather. Chest discomfort while exercising in cold weather, while walking uphill, or after a heavy meal is a classic sign of stable angina.

The pain of stable angina occurs most frequently behind or to the left of the *sternum* (the long, narrow bone in the middle of the chest). It can also radiate to other parts of the body. During an attack, people often look pale and/or gray and become quiet.

People with stable angina usually describe their symptoms as "discomfort" or "pressure." Most people with the condition have symptoms in a crescendo pattern which builds up over a few minutes and vanishes if the exertion or other precipitating factor is stopped. The discomfort usually lasts only a couple of minutes.

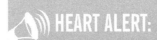 **HEART ALERT:**

Symptoms That Last More Than Five Minutes

If you have angina symptoms that last longer than five minutes, despite taking one or two *sublingual* (under the tongue) nitroglycerin tablets or the equivalent, call 9-1-1 or get to an emergency room as quickly as possible!

 HEART ALERT:

Unstable Angina—A Medical Emergency!

Unstable angina means angina symptoms are spiraling out of control. It is a warning that a heart attack may strike soon. (If you have a history of angina, and symptoms occur when you are resting and won't go away, call 9-1-1!) Unstable angina occurs when a coronary artery is constricted because a blood clot has formed on the plaque in its walls.

Unstable angina symptoms have the following characteristics:

- They are more severe than usual.
- They occur while you are resting.
- They last longer than twenty minutes.
- They are accompanied by weakness, nausea, or fainting.
- They do not improve after you take two or three nitroglycerin tablets.

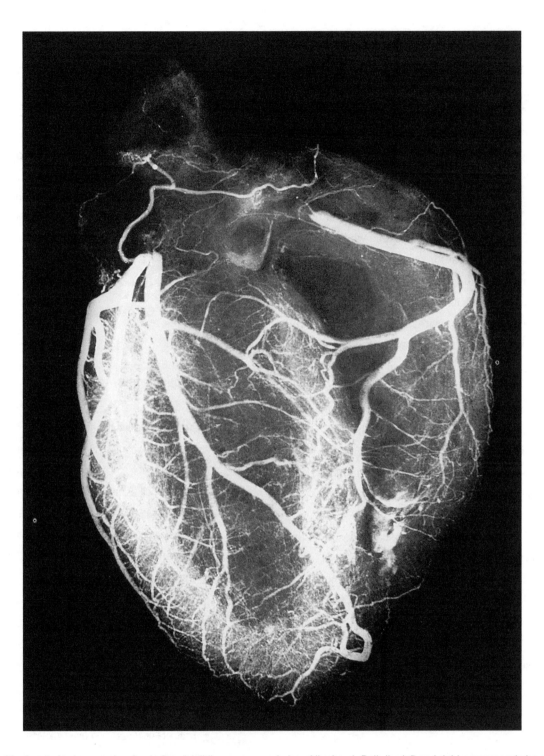

Healthy heart. Angiogram showing in fine detail the coronary arteries of the heart. Both the left and right coronary arteries are visible here, branching to supply blood to the heart muscle. These arteries follow the rounded shape of the heart. An angiogram, or arteriogram, is made by injecting the blood vessels of the patient with an X-ray opaque dye and then taking an X-ray. Blood vessels show up clearly, allowing conditions such as coronary artery disease to be diagnosed. Blockages in either of these arteries that may lead to a heart attack may also be identified.

Record Your Angina Pattern in a Heart Diary

It is important to know the pattern of your angina attacks so that you can tell when you are about to have (or are having) an episode—and can take action to thwart it. Maintaining a heart diary is a great way to pinpoint and keep track of your symptoms. By comparing your pattern day by day, you will be able to determine when a change occurs.

The types of questions to answer in your heart diary include the following:

- What brings on the symptoms—exercise, anger, eating heavy meals?
- How often do your symptoms strike—once a week, every day?
- What do your symptoms feel like—uncomfortable, strangling?
- Where do the symptoms occur—your chest, back, where else?
- How long do your symptoms last—five minutes, ten minutes?
- What relieves the symptoms—nitroglycerin, rest, both?

If your angina pattern changes, it could signal that your condition is getting worse and/or you need to change your treatment.

Tell your doctor if any of the following occurs:

- Factors such as climbing stairs or feeling stressed are causing symptoms and they didn't in the past.
- Your symptoms are occurring more often—for example, once a day when they were once a week.
- Your symptoms feel different from how they felt in the past. Perhaps they were previously mild but now give you a strangling sensation; or a recent attack felt like a very large object was sitting on your rib cage, whereas in the past you felt only a dull ache behind your breastbone.
- Your symptoms have changed. Have they moved from your chest down your arm? Do they now occur in both your chest and your arm?
- Your symptoms are lasting longer than they did previously. How long do they last now as compared to the past?
- Your symptoms are occurring when you are not exercising, feeling strong emotions, or eating heavy meals.
- Your symptoms are not improving as quickly with rest or when taking nitroglycerin or other prescribed medications.

Q. & A. with Dr. Cannon

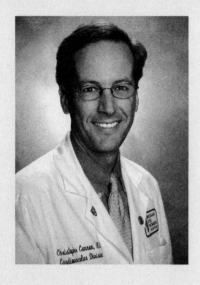

Q. My doctor always asks me whether I have chest pain, but what I feel isn't pain. It feels more like pressure in my chest. Should I say "yes" or "no" to this question?

A. You should say "yes." What you describe is potentially coming from the heart. In fact, it is a big misnomer that we always ask about chest pain, because most people will feel a vaguer, uneasy feeling. It varies a lot from patient to patient. A key thing we look for is the pattern. Does this feeling come on with exercise (when the heart has to do more work) and get better with rest? If so, that pattern would fit for potentially being from the heart.

Q. I just had a stress test and it was fine. Does that mean I won't have a heart attack?

A. This is not necessarily true. The stress test tells you whether enough blood is flowing to the heart muscle during exercise. From that, we can deduce whether there are or aren't severe blockages in the heart's arteries. However, there may still be mild blockages in the artery. These are best treated by lowering cholesterol and blood pressure, controlling other cardiac risk factors, and exercising regularly.

Q. I have angina. When should I call my doctor?

A. It is important to call your doctor if the number of attacks you experience in a given week increases, or if you start having pain when you are at rest (i.e., not doing any activity). It is best to call the doctor's office even if the change is only slight. If you have pain at rest that doesn't go away after five or ten minutes, call 9-1-1!

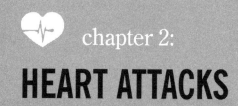

chapter 2:

HEART ATTACKS

HEART ATTACK

Rx THE PRESCRIPTION

If you think you are having a heart attack, call 9-1-1 so that you can be brought to the emergency room (ER) as quickly as possible. If the medical team at the hospital determines that you are having a ST elevation myocardial infraction (STEMI), the priority will be to restore the blood supply to your heart. You will have thrombolysis (the breakdown of blood clots using medicines) and/ or primary percutaneous coronary intervention (PCI). Your medical team will want to start these treatments as quickly as possible. For smaller heart attacks, you will be admitted to the hospital and given several anticlotting medications, and a cardiac catheterization or stress test will be set up for the coming days.

GET HELP FAST

"Time is muscle." "Act in time." Heart advocates use these common mantras to stress the importance of getting help *fast* when the symptoms of a heart attack strike and with good reason: Treatment is most effective when started *within one hour* of the beginning of symptoms. Delay can lead to disability or death. Of the people who die from heart attacks, about half die within an hour of the first symptoms, before they reach the hospital.

The good news is that if you or a loved one acts in time to get medical assistance, the odds of living and recovering after a heart attack have greatly improved over the past two decades.

There are two major kinds of heart attacks: one in which the heart artery is 100 percent blocked and needs to be opened as soon as possible, and a lesser one in which the artery is more often 80 percent to 90 percent blocked and a smaller amount of heart damage occurs.

The more serious heart attacks are called *ST elevation myocardial infarctions (STEMIs)* because of the findings on the graph created by the electrocardiogram (ECG). ECGs have five points on their graphs, all of which represent different levels of electrical activity. The ST segment connects two points on the graph, called the *QRS complex* and the *T wave*. ST segment elevation on the graph may indicate a heart attack.

The smaller heart attacks are called *non-STEMIs (or NSTEMIs)*. Both need immediate treatment in the hospital, but the STEMI needs treatment with angioplasty to open the artery within minutes to hours. NSTEMI patients also usually need angioplasty, but that can be done within one or two days.

SIGNS OF A HEART ATTACK

The symptoms of a heart attack often strike suddenly and last for more than twenty minutes, although occasionally symptoms "come and go." According to the American College of Cardiology (ACC), the following symptoms might signal a heart attack:

- Chest pain or pressure
- Chest tightness
- Chest pain, pressure, or tightness that extends from the chest to the neck, throat, jaw, shoulder, and/or arm
- Chest discomfort just below the breastbone
- Chest burning, similar to heartburn or indigestion
- Shortness of breath

Other symptoms that might occur are nausea, lightheadedness, fainting, or profuse sweating.

If You Think You Are Having a Heart Attack

If you or a loved one is experiencing the signs of a heart attack, the first thing to do is call 9-1-1 or the emergency services in your community. Be sure to mention your location, particularly if you are calling from a cell phone. (Locations cannot be traced easily from cell phones.) Leave the phone off the hook so that if you pass out, emergency services can trace your call.

If you have been prescribed nitroglycerin tablets, take one at a time, up to three pills, under the tongue every five minutes if your symptoms continue.

If your doctor has prescribed aspirin, take it right away if you are having signs of a heart attack. If you are unsure whether to chew a baby aspirin, wait until paramedics arrive.

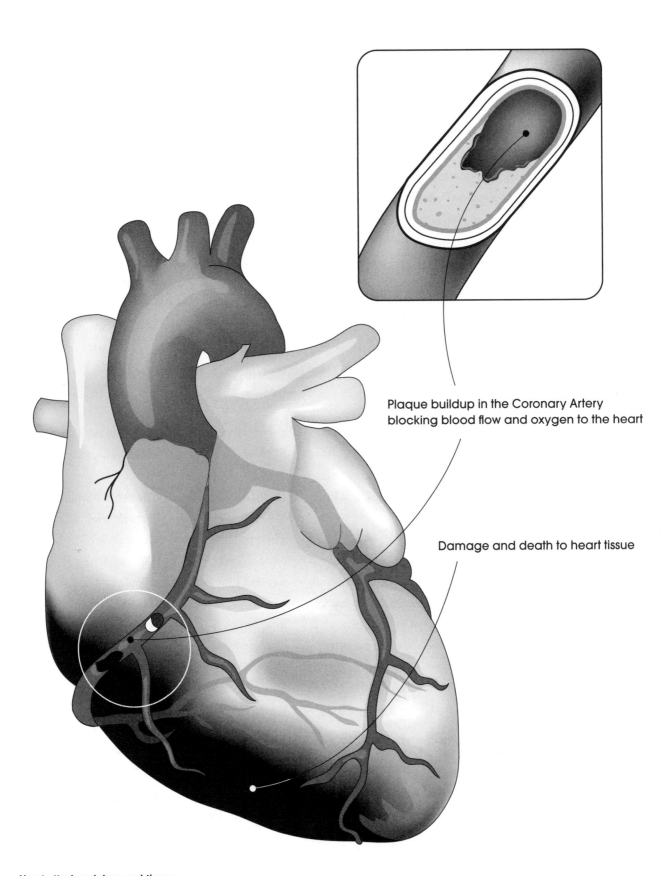

Plaque buildup in the Coronary Artery
blocking blood flow and oxygen to the heart

Damage and death to heart tissue

Heart attack and damaged tissue

Do not drive yourself to the hospital. The emergency personnel who arrive with the ambulance are trained to begin lifesaving procedures at your location and in the ambulance so that precious minutes won't be lost before blood is restored to your heart's muscle. You will also get much faster attention at the hospital if you arrive by ambulance.

If you are by yourself, unlock the door to your main entrance so that the paramedics can get in. If you have been keeping a heart diary (see page 23), have it with you if you can locate it easily and without stressing your heart. Sit or lie down until the ambulance arrives.

OPENING A BLOCKED ARTERY IN STEMI PATIENTS

There are two ways to open a blocked artery, and both need to be done as soon as possible (within thirty to ninety minutes): administering thrombolytic drugs and performing Percutaneous Coronary Intervention (PCI).

Thrombolytic Clot Busters

Thrombolytic drugs are clot-buster drugs that involve using a fibrinolytic medication such as streptokinase or tissue plasminogen activator (tPA) to break up blood clots. (Thrombolytics are also used to treat blood clots that cause strokes.)

You cannot take fibrinolytic medications if you are at high risk for bleeding complications. A bleeding ulcer or recent surgery might also mean you shouldn't use this therapy. These drugs work best if given within twelve hours of the start of a heart attack (or within three hours of the start of a stroke). Your doctor will ask you in the ER whether you have any of these bleeding risk factors.

Because fibrinolytic drugs can cause bleeding, especially in the brain, extreme caution is applied before deciding to use them. The following fibrinolytic drugs are approved for use in patients with a heart attack:

- Alteplase (tPA, Activase)
- Reteplase (Retavase)
- Streptokinase (Streptase)
- Tenecteplase (TNKase)

Streptokinase is the least expensive of the fibrinolytic drugs, but studies have shown that it is less effective at restoring blood flow than tPA. Tenecteplase has fewer bleeding complications and is used most often.

 HELP ONLINE:
Heart Attacks and Related Diseases

The American Heart Association (AHA) aims to reduce the number of deaths due to heart disease.
www.americanheart.org

The National Heart, Lung, and Blood Institute provides information for the public on heart attacks and other diseases of the heart, blood vessels, lungs, and blood.
www.nhlbi.nih.gov

American College of Cardiology patient website.
www.cardiosmart.org

Percutaneous Coronary Intervention (PCI)

PCI is an invasive procedure in which a slender tube called a *catheter* is threaded through an artery in the groin to a blocked artery of the heart, and a balloon-tipped wire is placed into the heart artery where the blockage is. (PCI is also called *coronary angioplasty* or *angioplasty*.) The balloon is then inflated, compressing the plaque and widening the narrowed coronary artery so that blood can flow normally. Most often, a wire mesh tube called a *stent* is inserted to keep the artery open. (For more information about PCI, see appendix III.)

Emergency PCI is the most effective treatment to restore blood flow and is usually the first choice for heart attack victims. It has fewer unfavorable events, lower risk of death, and better clinical outcomes than fibrinolytic therapy. However, PCI is not always an option. The hospital you are in must have a catheterization laboratory and a skilled PCI medical team on-site, and many hospitals do not have these facilities.

ANTICLOTTING TREATMENTS

A cornerstone of treatment for all heart attack patients is antithrombotic therapy, which has two components: antiplatelet therapy and anticoagulant therapy. This therapy is used with the aforementioned reperfusion treatments (thrombolysis or primary PCI) for STEMI, and in all patients with NSTEMI or unstable angina. Antiplatelet therapy reduces platelet formation and aggregation. (*Platelets* are colorless bodies that are present in blood and have a sticky surface that causes them, along with other substances, to form blood clots.) Anticoagulant therapy targets the clotting cascade to prevent the accumulation of fibrin in the clot. (*Fibrin* is a protein involved in the clotting of blood.) Both therapies are given as soon as possible after the patient is seen in the ER.

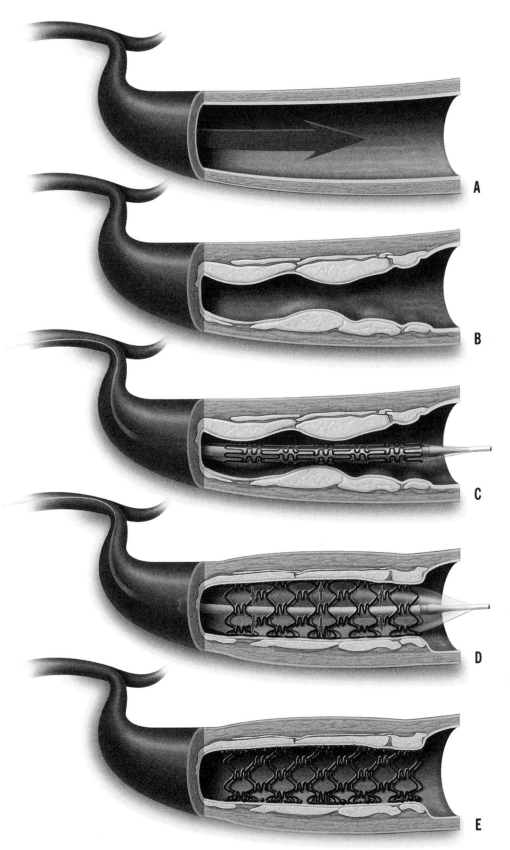

A normal coronary artery **(A)**, a coronary artery displaying atherosclerosis **(B)**, and treatment with angioplasty **(C)**. Image **(D)** shows the insertion of a balloon catheter and stent (small mesh tube), which is then expanded to reopen and strengthen the weakened artery. The balloon is then deflated and removed, leaving behind the stent **(E)**, which is lined with a drug that prevents the vessel from narrowing again in the future.

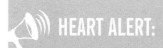
Aspirin

Aspirin is given to all heart attack patients as soon as possible—usually chewed in the ER. A full aspirin (325 mg) is usually given at first, and maintained for a few months after stents are inserted. At discharge, patients are frequently switched to low-dose aspirin (e.g. 81 mg) because of a lower risk of bleeding.

Clopidogrel

Clopidogrel is another antiplatelet agent that has been shown to reduce the risk of a second heart attack or death. It is given at "a loading" dose of 300 mg and then 75 mg per day. Sometimes 600 mg loading doses are given.

GP IIb/IIIa Inhibitors

GP IIb/IIIa inhibitors are also antiplatelet agents but are stronger and are given intravenously. They are usually used for patients undergoing PCI, and they help prevent clotting complications and heart attacks during the procedure. They are associated with a higher risk of bleeding, and so they are targeted to higher risk patients.

Anticoagulants

Anticoagulants, or blood thinners, are medications that make it more difficult for blood to clot. Anticoagulants interfere with the proteins in the blood that are needed for clotting. There are now four different anticoagulant medications; your doctor will choose which of these agents is best for you. Current guidelines say that any of the four is okay but that you should only receive one of them:

- Heparin is the most widely used anticoagulant. It is given intravenously, and then adjusted with the blood test APTT (activated partial thromboplastin time) to target the right level of thinning of the blood.
- Low-molecular-weight heparin is a modified version of heparin and is given *subcutaneously* (in the skin) twice per day.
- Fondaparinux is a once-daily anticoagulant that blocks factor Xa. It works a bit differently than heparin but accomplishes the same thinning of the blood. If you need to have PCI though, the doctors will give you a different anticoagulant for the procedure.
- Bivalirudin (a member of the direct thrombin inhibitor class) is the fourth choice. It is used often for patients who have PCI.

Anti-Ischemic Medications

In addition to reperfusion therapy, anti-ischemic medications will play essential roles in your overall treatment if you have had a heart attack. We discuss these medications in the following subsections.

Beta Blockers

Beta blockers reduce your risk of death after a heart attack and help prevent a repeat heart attack. The drugs reduce blood pressure by blocking the effects of the hormone epinephrine (also called adrenaline). Beta blockers also slow the heart rate. Beta blockers can be administered intravenously or orally.

ACE Inhibitors/ARBs

Angiotensin-converting enzyme (ACE) inhibitors can reduce the risks of a future heart attack or stroke. ACE inhibitors prevent an enzyme in your body from producing angiotensin II, a substance that causes narrowing of your blood vessels, which can cause high blood pressure and force your heart to work harder. Angiotensin receptor blockers are an alternative to ACE inhibitors that act in a similar way.

Nitrates or Nitroglycerin

Doctors prescribe nitrates to alleviate chest pain by widening the blood vessels, resulting in improved blood flow to the heart. Although this class of drugs helps with pain, it will not help prevent a heart attack. You might experience headaches if you take this medicine, but they usually wear off after the first few times you take it.

As we mentioned in chapter 1, if you are taking nitrate medication such as nitroglycerin, do not take Viagra. Taking Viagra with a nitrate medicine can cause a serious decrease in blood pressure, potentially leading to fainting, stroke, or heart attack. Conversely, if you have taken Viagra or a related medication in

WHAT'S NEW:

Prasugrel (Effient)

How does prasugrel work? Prasugrel is similar to clopidogrel, but the body processes it more strongly and more rapidly so that it can inhibit platelets more rapidly. It also works by blocking the ADP receptor found on the outside of platelets.

When is prasugrel used? Prasugrel does not have the same wide array of uses as clopidogrel, but it has been tested in one of the more common circumstances: patients who have had a heart attack or new chest pain, and undergo PCI with angioplasty or stenting. It is given with aspirin. Of note, patients who have had strokes or a *transient ischemic attack* (a near stroke) should *not* take prasugrel due to a higher risk of bleeding in the brain.

What are the side effects of prasugrel? Prasugrel increases the risk of bleeding compared to clopidogrel and is avoided in patients at higher risk for bleeding.

the past 24–48 hours, *do not* take nitroglycerin if you have chest pain. Call 9-1-1 and rest.

Calcium-Channel Blockers

Calcium-channel blockers prevent calcium from entering cells of the heart and blood vessel walls, resulting in lower blood pressure. They are used to treat high blood pressure, angina, and abnormal heart rhythms such as supraventricular tachycardia.

Cardiac Catheterization and PCI

For NSTEMI and unstable angina patients, it is not critical that the artery be opened within minutes or hours, but cardiac catheterization and PCI are frequently needed over the first day or two. Doctors will look at the ECG and do blood tests, as well as review your history to see whether you have factors that put you at high risk for a recurrent heart attack. If so, a cardiac catheterization will be set up for that day or the following few days to locate the blockages, and angioplasty or stenting will be done to open any blockages. If there are no high-risk factors, medical treatment will be the key approach and a stress test will be arranged to make sure you don't have more chest pain after starting all the medications.

Coronary Artery Bypass Grafting

Coronary artery bypass grafting (CABG) is a surgical technique that can improve blood flow to the heart in people with severe coronary artery disease (CAD). During CABG, a healthy artery or vein from another part of the body (usually the leg) is grafted to the blocked coronary artery. The grafted vessel becomes a new pathway for blood to travel through to the heart muscle.

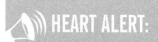 HEART ALERT:

Know the Signs of Sudden Cardiac Arrest!

Sudden cardiac arrest (SCA) occurs when the heart stops pumping blood. Usually, the condition is caused by an electrical problem in the heart. Patients who have a heart attack are at high risk for SCA.

The following are signs of SCA:

- Loss of consciousness

- Loss of respiration

- Loss of heartbeat (or pulse)

These symptoms always constitute a medical emergency. Call 9-1-1 right away!

More than 500,000 CABG surgeries are performed every year. Most of these surgeries successfully restore blood flow to the heart of the patient. However, early complications are more serious for CABG than for PCI. The surgery may be an option for you if you have diffuse coronary disease (*three-vessel disease*), coronary vessels that are not appropriate for stenting (due to size, twisting, or characteristics of the lesions), or disease of the left main coronary artery.

Noncardiac Chest Pain

Many health conditions have symptoms that are similar to those of heart attacks. For example, chest pain and difficulty breathing are symptoms of both panic attacks and heart attacks, so it is easy to mistake one for the other. Chest pain can also be caused

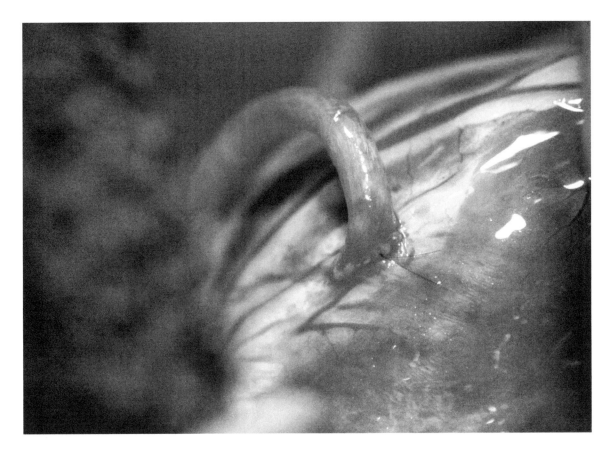

A heart with a vein grafted to it by coronary artery bypass surgery. The vein bypasses a blocked coronary artery, which could have caused a heart attack.

by problems with your digestive system, such as heartburn, ulcers, gallbladder disease, gallstones, esophageal spasm, or gastroesophageal reflux. Even indigestion can cause chest pain.

Other conditions that can cause symptoms resembling a heart attack include the following:

- Anxiety and stress
- Fibromyositis (muscle inflammation)
- Injury of the ribs and/or surrounding muscles and tendons
- Pleurisy (inflammation of the lining around the lung)

- Pneumonia
- Pneumothorax (a collapsed lung)
- Pulmonary embolism (a blood clot to the lung)

The chest pain associated with these conditions can be similar to heart attack pain, so it is important to see a doctor for them. If you have acute symptoms that are ongoing after five minutes, call 9-1-1!

PREVENTING FUTURE HEART ATTACKS

Second and third heart attacks following an initial heart attack are alarmingly common. However, many heart patients have cardiac rehabilitation programs available to them, usually through their hospital, which can help prevent future heart attacks. Several major studies have demonstrated significantly lower rates of recurring heart problems for patients with Acute Coronary Syndrome (ACS) who attended cardiac rehabilitation programs. One analysis found a 25 percent lower risk of death by all causes in patients who were enrolled in cardiac rehabilitation programs as compared with those who were not.

Whether you attend a cardiac rehabilitation program or not, you can take a number of measures to help prevent cardiovascular events after a heart attack. These include lifestyle modifications such as quitting smoking, exercising, taking antihypertensive medications, managing diabetes, taking statins and other therapies for high cholesterol and related problems, taking antiplatelet medications, and treating depression. These recommendations were established by the 2006 American College of Cardiology/American Heart Association guidelines.

Lifestyle Modifications

A healthy lifestyle is the key to your survival and quality of life after ACS. If you are not already leading a heart-healthy life, modifications to make include quitting smoking, exercising regularly, maintaining a healthy diet, and maintaining a healthy weight. For information on how to make these modifications, see chapter 14.

Antihypertensive Drugs

Certain classes of antihypertensive drugs can help reduce the risk of another heart attack. They include adrenergic blockers, ACE inhibitors, and aldosterone receptor antagonists. Cardiologists often prescribe adrenergic blockers for patients even if they do not have hypertension, because of the drug's benefits in preventing future heart attacks.

Managing Diabetes

Heart disease and stroke account for about 65 percent of deaths in people with diabetes, and adults with diabetes have heart disease death rates about two to four times higher than adults without diabetes. Studies have shown that for people with diabetes, managing their disease plays an important role in preventing further heart attacks. For information on diabetes and heart disease, see chapter 13.

Treating Dyslipidemia

Studies have demonstrated that the risk for heart attacks and other cardiovascular events is directly proportional to increasing levels of LDL-C (the bad cholesterol) and decreasing levels of HDL-C (the good cholesterol), a condition called *dyslipidemia*. Despite exercise training, dietary modifications, and weight loss, a significant number of patients will need pharmacologic therapy for dyslipidemia after a heart attack.

Statins such as Simvastatin and Atorvastatin are the drugs of choice among the lipid-lowering medications. New agents are now in development to increase HDL-C. One agent is now available, niacin, but it is often associated with side effects that limit its use.

Antiplatelet Therapy

Antiplatelet drugs inhibit the formation of blood clots. Aspirin and clopidogrel are the most widely used antiplatelet agents and are often given in combination to prevent recurrent heart attacks.

Treating Depression

Depression is common after a heart attack. Depression and heart disease are a chicken-and-egg issue, and there is an ongoing debate about whether the disease worsens depression or depression worsens the disease. Either way, if you or a loved one is depressed for more than two weeks following a heart attack, it is important to get help before the depression spirals out of control. As we mention in chapter 10, depression can make your recovery longer and harder. It can cause physical problems such as an irregular heart rhythm, chest pain, reduced exercise capacity, a decrease in energy, and an increase in fatigue, and it may even increase your risk of death. It can also affect your relationships, your family, and your marriage and can keep you from returning to work. In addition, depression can limit your ability to make important lifestyle modifications, follow medication schedules, and carry out rehabilitation programs.

TESTS AND DIAGNOSIS OF HEART ATTACK

When you arrive at the hospital, the first thing the facility's medical staff will do is ask you to describe your symptoms and, if possible, give your medical history. If you are able to talk to the staff and supply information about your symptoms, it will help with your diagnosis and treatment. Your medical team might ask you the following questions:

- What are your symptoms? For example, men may have chest pain or shortness of breath and women may have extreme fatigue.
- When did the symptoms first appear, and what were you doing at the time?

- Are the symptoms getting worse? When have they been the most intense?
- On a scale of 1 to 10, what is your pain level?
- What medicines have you taken recently?

After your initial conversation with your medical team, you will have an ECG and blood tests to look for heart damage. ECGs record the electrical activity of the heart and are painless and fast. Depending on the results of the ECG, your doctor will order other tests. Here is a brief description of the types of tests frequently used. For more information about these tests, see appendix II.

Exercise Stress Testing

During an exercise stress test, an ECG records the activity of your heart under stress—either while you walk on a treadmill or as your body responds to a drug that makes your heart beat faster. The test identifies signs of inadequate blood flow to your heart.

Thallium Test or Methoxyisobutyl Isonitrile (MIBI) Test

In a thallium or MIBI stress test, a small amount of radioactive material is injected into the blood stream, which enables a camera to show how the blood is flowing to all parts of the heart muscle. If there is a blockage, less blood flows to that part of the muscle during exercise or stress.

Echocardiography

The echocardiogram provides detailed images of the heart using ultrasound. The ultrasound probe generates sound waves that collide with the heart and surrounding structures.

A Focus on Inflammation

Why is inflammation a red flag? Cardiologists and researchers are focusing on inflammation as a key factor in the biological cascade that causes ACS and heart attacks. Until recently, the conventional wisdom has been that heart attacks are primarily caused by the build up of plaque in coronary arteries. (The accumulation of plaque narrows the artery so that blood can't get through, or the artery becomes clogged by a blood clot, cutting off blood supply to the heart.) But studies have shown that not all heart attack victims have arteries that are severely narrowed by plaque. What they do have is soft plaque *within their artery walls*, which is covered by a thin barrier.

How does inflammation lead to a heart attack? Inflammation causes irritation to the lining of the blood vessel that can weaken the covering over the artery and plaques. This occurs when inflammatory cells such as monocytes (see diagram) get into the lining of the artery and plaque. They can also release cytokines that can degrade the lining of the artery as well. If there is a stressor on the artery, a tear can develop in the artery wall, and the inside of the plaque (cholesterol and cells) is exposed to the blood, and a blood clot can form, leading to a heart attack.

Who is at risk for inflammation? Patients with soft plaque within their artery walls usually don't have symptoms or warning signs. However, cardiologists have found that by measuring a marker for inflammation in the blood, called C-reactive protein (CRP), they can predict a patient's risk of heart attack or stroke.

What tests can be done? The blood test used for detecting CRP is called the high-sensitivity CRP (hs-CRP) assay test. Many cardiologists test hs-CRP levels along with cholesterol to determine their patients' risk of heart disease.

The AHA and U.S. Centers for Disease Control and Prevention have defined the following risk groups for heart disease based on the high-sensitivity CRP assay:

- Levels of hs-CRP that are lower than 1 mg per liter, or mg/L, indicate low risk.

- Levels between 1 mg/L and 3 mg/L indicate average risk.

- Levels of hs-CRP that are higher than 3 mg/L indicate high risk.

Note: High CRP can be due to diseases and events other than heart disease, such as rheumatoid arthritis, cancer, burns, and surgery. In these situations, CRP is not predictive for heart disease.

How inflammation leads to a heart attack

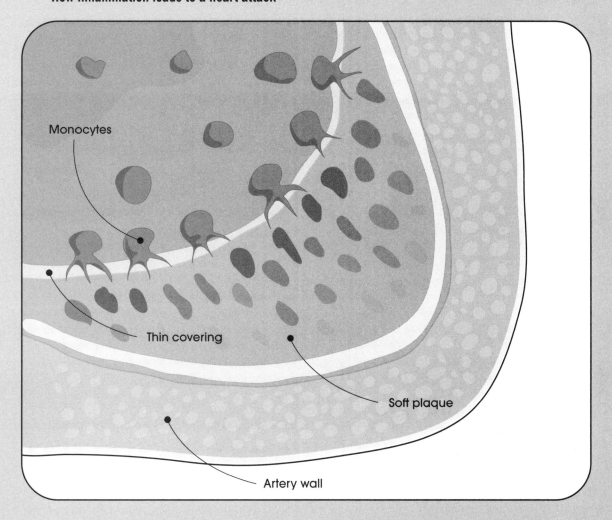

Monocytes

Thin covering

Soft plaque

Artery wall

A depiction of the inflammatory process in an artery.

HEART ATTACK EXPLAINED

A heart attack is often referred to as a *myocardial infarction*. Both terms describe damage to an area of the heart muscle caused by a blockage of a coronary artery that has choked off the blood supply to that area. Such a blockage is a classic outcome of Coronary Artery Disease (CAD), resulting from ruptured plaque and the fast formation of a blood clot, or *thrombus*. (The blood clot blocks blood from moving through the artery.) The longer the blockage is, the greater the loss of heart muscle. When such a blockage occurs, speedy *reperfusion* (reestablishing blood flow through the blocked artery) is the key to limiting injury of the heart.

The following sections describe in more detail the disease process behind a heart attack.

CAD

Your heart pumps blood through your cardiovascular system to all of the organs and tissues in your body, supplying them with the oxygen, sugar, and other nutrients they need to survive, thrive, and function (see chapter 8 for a full tour of the heart). This intricate and elegant process includes delivering blood through the vessels that feed your heart muscle. These vessels, called coronary arteries, are on the outside of the heart muscle.

CAD is a condition in which the coronary arteries are narrowed by plaque. The plaque consists of cholesterol and fats, and their build up in arteries is often referred to as atherosclerosis. CAD can cause a condition called *ischemia*, a lack of adequate blood supply available to an area of heart muscle. If you have this condition, you may have chest pain (and angina; see chapter 1).

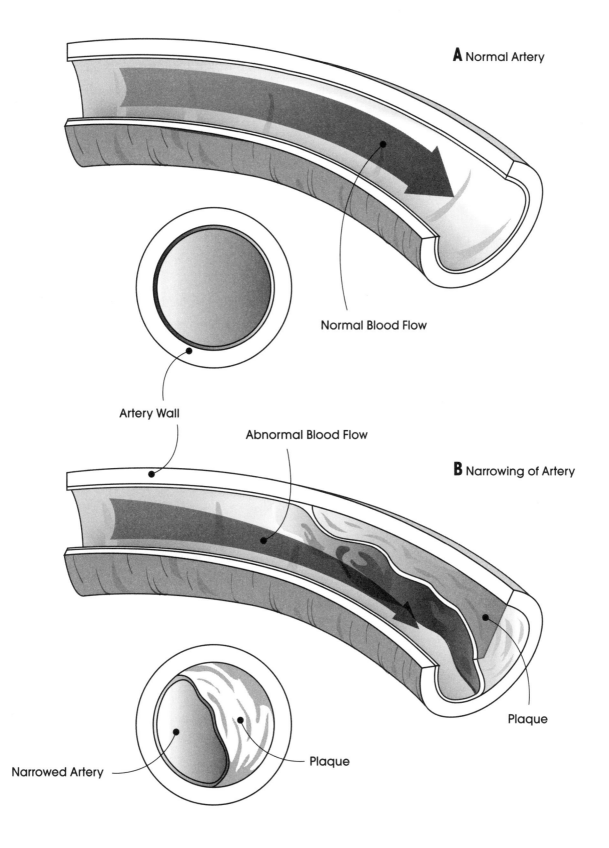

A Normal Artery

Normal Blood Flow

Artery Wall

Abnormal Blood Flow

B Narrowing of Artery

Plaque

Narrowed Artery

Plaque

An illustration showing coronary artery disease (CAD), a condition in which the coronary arteries are narrowed by plaque. The top artery is healthy and free of plaque **(A)**. The bottom artery has been narrowed by the buildup of plaque **(B)**.

Plaque Rupture and Clot Formation

Plaque in a coronary artery can burst or rupture; your body will respond to this event as it would any injury—by causing a blood clot to form. However, in a quirk of nature, the blood clot does not help but it hinders, and it partially or completely blocks the coronary artery. The resultant lack of blood supply can cause damage to the heart muscle. If such damage occurs, the heart will not have enough oxygen, sugar, and other nutrients it needs to do its important job of circulating blood through your body. And if the blockage causes damage to the heart muscle, the result is a heart attack.

Cardiologists don't yet know the cause of atherosclerosis. It may begin with damage to the inner layers of arteries, which sets in motion a natural healing process that backfires. This process may cause plaque to build up where the arteries are damaged. Over time, the plaque may crack and causes blood clots to form in the arteries.

According to the ACC, the damage in arteries may be the result of such factors as smoking, high levels of fats and cholesterol in the blood, high blood pressure, or high amounts of sugar in the blood caused by diabetes. In other words, lifestyle plays an extremely important role in the disease process.

Scientists are studying why atherosclerosis develops. According to the ACC, they are searching for answers to such questions as the following:

- Why and how do the arteries become damaged?
- How does plaque develop and change over time?
- Why does plaque break open and lead to clots?

Acute Coronary Syndrome (ACS)

Heart attacks are a type of CAD called acute coronary syndrome (ACS). ACS is always a medical emergency. ACS describes the following conditions, which are caused by the rupture of plaque inside coronary arteries:

- Unstable angina
- A small heart attack called an NSTEMI
- A large heart attack called a STEMI

We covered unstable angina in chapter 1. The information in this chapter applies to the two types of heart attacks: STEMI and NSTEMI.

NSTEMI: This type of heart attack is sneaky; NSTEMIs do not cause identifiable changes on an ECG. However, markers that indicate that the heart muscle has been damaged show up in blood tests. NSTEMI, gratefully, often results in smaller amounts of damage.

STEMI: This is the serious type of heart attack. STEMIs are caused by an extended period of blockage to a large area of the heart muscle. STEMIs cause characteristic changes on the ECG, and markers that are signs of damage to the heart muscle show up in blood tests.

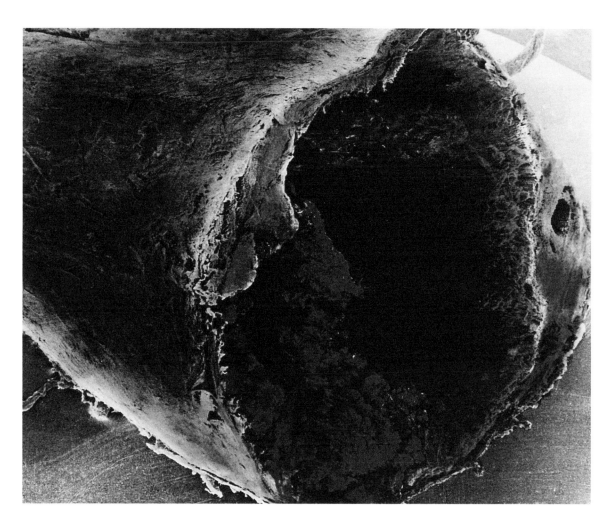

A blood clot inside a coronary artery. The artery has been cross-sectioned, showing its wall and inner lumen. The blood clot is blocking about 30 percent of the width of the artery.

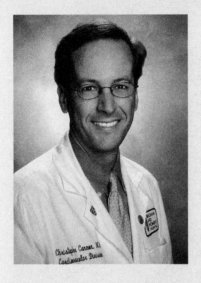

Q. I just was in the hospital with chest pain, and they said I didn't have a heart attack, but they did have to place a stent in one artery. I spent only a day and a half in the hospital. Was it a "heart attack?"

A. You had what we call unstable angina—worsening chest pain due to a blockage in the artery. Although the prognosis is better than if you had a heart attack, it still is a very serious event. Unstable angina is part of acute coronary syndrome—a change in the heart arteries that requires new treatments. The cause is a cholesterol blockage in the artery, which broke open. A blood clot formed and led to a severe blockage in the artery, limiting blood flow to your heart. The stent opened it up, but the prevention work is actually from the medication and lifestyle changes. This is a key warning sign; the risk of a heart attack is high, and clearly we want to prevent one from occuring.

Q. I had a stent placed—one of the new drug-coated stents—and the doctor said I need to take clopidogrel (Plavix) for at least one year. I had planned to have a knee replacement next month; can I stop the clopidogrel prior to the surgery?

A. *No.* This is a key issue. Multiple studies show that the risk of a blood clot abruptly forming inside the stent (stent thrombosis) is very high if patients stop their clopidogrel. For the drug-eluting stents, it is strongly recommended that you continue uninterrupted for one year. After that, many physicians still recommend a second or third year. However, if you need elective surgery, it is recommended that you do it after a full year of clopidogrel. You should discuss all of this carefully with your cardiologist.

Q. We live far outside a city and have only a small community hospital near us. If my husband or I have a heart attack, is it better to go to the small hospital nearby, or to ask to be taken into the city to the large hospital?

A. It is always critical to get to the nearest hospital. Thus, when you call 9-1-1, they will take you to the community hospital. The key is that if you are having a heart attack in which the artery is 100 percent blocked (STEMI), time is muscle and the treatment to open the artery must begin as soon as possible. If your condition warrants, they might transfer you to a tertiary care hospital (a facility with the full complement of cardiac services). Many states and national programs are trying to establish rapid transfer systems. The American Heart Association's Mission Lifeline is one such program.

chapter 3:

DISEASES OF OTHER ARTERIES

PERIPHERAL ARTERY DISEASE (PAD)

℞ THE PRESCRIPTION

Your treatment plan for PAD has two important goals:

➡ Control symptoms such as leg pain to improve functioning and quality of life.

➡ Stop the progression of atherosclerosis (blockage of blood vessels by fatty deposits on the vessel walls) throughout your body, which will lower your risk of having a heart attack and stroke.

To achieve these goals, your doctor may recommend lifestyle changes such as regular exercise and quitting smoking, which are imperative if you want to avoid surgery. In many cases, your doctor will also prescribe medicines to prevent blood clots and control your blood pressure, diabetes, and cholesterol.

If you have incapacitating symptoms that do not respond to these measures or if you experience pain at rest, your doctor might suggest having a surgical procedure to open or bypass the blockages in the arteries of your legs.

The effects of heart disease extend beyond the heart muscle to the legs, aorta, and lungs. In this chapter, you'll find information about peripheral artery disease (PAD), diseases of the aorta, and pulmonary embolism.

PERIPHERAL ARTERY DISEASE (PAD)

You may experience cramping, pain, or discomfort in your calves, thighs, or buttocks when you walk or exercise. The discomfort goes away when you rest. The doctor says you have peripheral artery disease (PAD), a common circulation problem of clogged or narrowed arteries in the extremities.

The return of leg pain with exercise—and relief with rest—is called *intermittent claudication*. Claudication comes from a Latin word meaning "to limp" and is the most common complaint in people with PAD. However, many people with this condition experience no symptoms whatsoever.

In severe cases, you may experience a burning or aching pain in your foot or toes while resting or have a sore on your leg or foot that does not heal. In extreme cases, tissue death or gangrene develops, requiring amputation of a leg, foot, or toes.

))) HEART ALERT:

PAD Increases Risk of Heart Attack

Although the word *peripheral* might sound unimportant, if you have PAD, you are at a higher risk of having a heart attack and stroke, which can be life-threatening.

Treating PAD with Lifestyle Changes

Stop Smoking

This is the single most important thing you can do to halt the progression of PAD. For advice on how to stay away from cigarettes, see chapter 14.

Exercise

Regular exercise is the cornerstone of treatment for PAD, even though you might fear worsening leg pain. In study after study, patients who have taken part in a regular exercise program (most commonly, using a motorized treadmill) for at least three months have seen substantial increases in the distances they are able to walk without experiencing painful symptoms. Some studies have suggested that patients who participate in a supervised exercise program do better than those who exercise unsupervised. Consult your physician before undertaking any exercise program.

Control Cholesterol, Hypertension, and Diabetes

Aggressive treatment of these three risk factors is important not only to reduce the symptoms and complications of PAD but also to counteract the increased risk of heart attack and stroke. For more information on how to manage your cholesterol, blood pressure, and sugar see chapters 11, 12, and 13.

Treating PAD with Medicine

Several medications are available to treat your symptoms. Consult your doctor to see whether you are a candidate for the following drugs.

Antiplatelet Therapy

Antiplatelet medicines lower your risk of developing blood clots in the arteries of the legs, in much the same way they do in the arteries of the heart. They

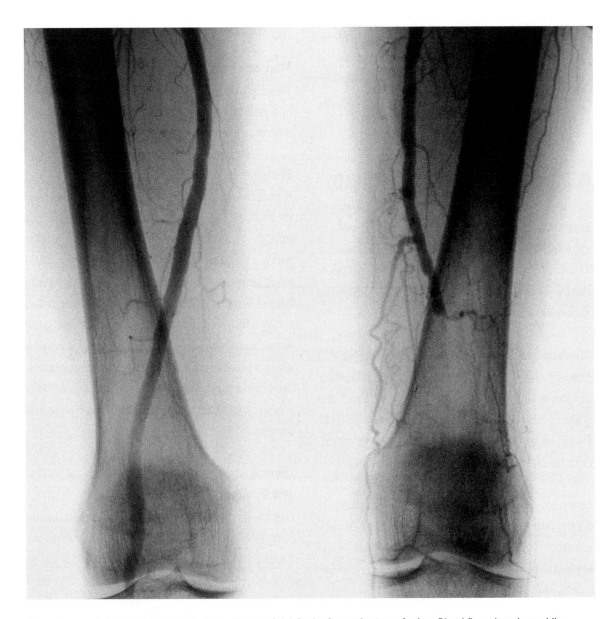

An angiogram (arterial X-ray) of a blockage (center, right) in the femoral artery of a leg. Blood flow stops toward the bottom of the femur (thigh bone). This may be caused by thrombosis, abnormal blood clotting, or an embolism. The blockage of the artery may cause pain and/or tissue death.

reduce your chances of requiring vascular surgery or of having a heart attack or a stroke. The most widely prescribed of these drugs is aspirin, followed by clopidogrel (Plavix). For more information about these medications, see appendix III.

Cilostazol (Pletal)

Cilostazol works by widening blood vessels in your legs, and blocking certain blood cells—called platelets—from forming harmful blood clots. It improves the blood flow and oxygen to your legs and helps to increase your walking distance. Cilostazol is particularly effective when combined with exercise. Your symptoms may improve in two to four weeks, but it may take up to twelve weeks to notice improvement. Take this medication twice daily by mouth at least thirty minutes before (or two hours after) breakfast and dinner or as directed by your doctor. Common side effects include headache, diarrhea, and dizziness. Avoid eating lots of grapefruit or drinking more than a quart a day of grapefruit juice, as doing so can increase the concentration of the medication in your blood. Do not use cilostazol if you have congestive heart failure.

Pentoxifylline (Trental)

Pentoxifylline decreases the stickiness (viscosity) of your blood, thereby improving blood flow and oxygen delivery to your legs. It is less proven than cilostazol in reducing symptoms. Take this medication at doses directed by your doctor. Common side effects include lightheadedness, drowsiness, belly pain, nausea, and vomiting. Do not take this drug if you are sensitive to caffeine.

HEART HELP:

Improve Quality of Life and Prevent Complications

- Quit smoking.

- Walk at least thirty minutes, five times per week.

- Maintain an appropriate body weight.

- Control your blood pressure and cholesterol.

- Aggressively manage your diabetes.

- Exercise proper foot care. Wash your feet daily, wear dry socks and shoes that fit well, and carefully trim your nails. Do not walk barefoot; treat athlete's foot quickly, and see your doctor at the first sign of a sore or injury to your skin. Seek medical attention if you have foot pain at night or discomfort in the calves upon walking a short distance.

Treating PAD by Restoring Blood Flow

Percutaneous Intervention

In surgery, *percutaneous* refers to procedures that access the body's interior through a needle puncture, as opposed to an "open" approach, usually with a scalpel.

Similar to the heart, arteries in the legs can be opened via angioplasty using balloon-tipped catheters (thin, flexible tubes inserted through an artery in the groin, wrist, or arm and guided to the blocked blood vessel). In some cases, a stent—a small, wire-mesh tube—is used to hold the artery open. The procedure involves far fewer risks than surgery, and the recovery time is much faster.

Surgery

Sometimes an artery cannot be successfully opened by percutaneous intervention and surgery may be the only option. Surgery involves using a graft (either an artificial graft or a vein or artery taken from elsewhere in the body) to bypass the narrowed or blocked area of the blood vessel and restore blood flow.

Tests and Diagnosis of PAD

Your doctor will ask several questions about your symptoms and medical history. These questions will help your doctor identify symptoms of intermittent claudication and other related medical conditions.

The doctor will then perform a physical examination, check blood pressure and pulses in the arms and legs, and examine for *bruits* (whooshing sounds heard with a stethoscope), which may indicate restricted blood flow caused by narrowed arteries. He or she will look for absence of hair on the legs, which can occur if the blood flow to these cells is inadequate.

Routine blood tests such as tests for cholesterol level and diabetes will then be ordered. If your doctor suspects PAD, he or she will do one or more of the following tests to confirm the diagnosis.

WHAT'S NEW:

Computed Tomography Angiography (CTA)

CTA is a type of X-ray that examines blood flow in arteries when they are filled with a contrast material (a substance that makes the blood vessels show up on the test). The test is often used to detect atherosclerosis (narrowing of the arteries) or an aneurysm (ballooning of a section of a blood vessel), which could lead to a heart attack or stroke.

How is the test performed? Most CTA scans are fast and painless, with the insertion of an IV. The CT scanner looks like a large box with a tunnel in it. You lie down on a narrow table that slides into and out of the tunnel. The machine takes X-rays from many different views, producing detailed, two-dimensional images that can then be combined by a computer to form three-dimensional views. The result is a detailed, multidimensional view of the body's interior. A CTA is done to help doctors identify diseased, narrowed, enlarged, and blocked blood vessels and locate where internal bleeding may be occurring.

Will I be able to move? It's important to stay still during the scan. The technologist may ask you to hold your breath for ten to twenty-five seconds to ensure that the images are not blurred by any movement. It takes only seconds to record all the images needed.

Ankle/Brachial Index (ABI)

Often the first test, an ABI involves comparing the blood pressure in your arms and legs and arriving at a ratio that gives a good indication of whether your peripheral arteries are narrowing.

Ultrasound

A painless, noninvasive procedure, ultrasound sends high-frequency sound waves into your arteries. As the sound waves bounce back, the images can be analyzed to measure real-time blood flow and detect blockages in your arteries.

Magnetic Resonance Angiography (MRA)

MRA uses a powerful magnet and radio waves to produce a detailed, three-dimensional view of your arteries. This noninvasive test can identify narrowed and blocked arteries. If you have a metal device in your body (e.g., a pacemaker) you cannot have this test.

Arteriography

An arteriogram is a "road map" of your arteries used to pinpoint the exact location of blockage in a limb. It involves injecting dye through a needle or catheter into the artery, and then taking an X-ray. If a blockage or narrowing is discovered, it occasionally can be treated with a balloon or stent, often during the same procedure.

PAD Explained

The arteries outside your heart, such as those supplying your arm and leg muscles and the organs inside your abdomen, get clogged in the same fashion as the arteries of your heart. Fatty deposits build up in the inner linings of the artery walls, restricting blood flow and causing problems. The most common arteries involved are those of the legs.

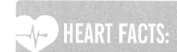

HEART FACTS:

PAD

- PAD affects eight million people in the United States.

- Older people are more susceptible; 12 percent to 20 percent of people over the age of sixty-five suffer from the disease.

- Many people mistake the symptoms of PAD for something else, such as hip arthritis, a herniated disc, spinal stenosis, or a normal sign of aging.

- Public awareness of the disease is alarmingly low. It often goes undiagnosed by health care professionals. At least half of the people who have PAD do not have any symptoms or signs, making the diagnosis difficult.

- The disease is under-recognized in women, who are more likely than men to have the condition without experiencing symptoms.

The risk factors for developing PAD are the same as those for coronary artery disease (which causes heart attacks): smoking, diabetes, high blood pressure, and high cholesterol. Cigarette smokers have a particularly strong risk of developing the disease.

AORTIC DISSECTION

℞ THE PRESCRIPTION

Emergency treatment will aim to relieve pain and reduce blood pressure, prevent extension of the dissection, and avoid rupture of the aorta. Your doctor will admit you to an intensive care unit (ICU), where your pulse, blood pressure, and breathing rate will be closely monitored.

Soon after drug therapy begins, your doctor must decide whether to continue with medicine or recommend surgery. This will depend on whether the dissection involves the ascending aorta (type A dissections) or the descending aorta only (type B dissections).

Surgery aims to prevent extension by replacing the segment of the aorta that is susceptible to rupture, reestablishing blood flow in the extremities and inner organs. Uncomplicated type B dissections and chronic dissections (more than two weeks old) are usually managed medically. Type A and complicated type B dissections are usually managed surgically.

DISEASES OF THE AORTA

The aorta is the largest artery in the body. It carries oxygen-rich blood from your heart to all your limbs and organs, except the lungs. The aorta arises from the left side of your heart and moves upward (ascending aorta), curves like a candy cane (aortic arch), and then heads down (descending aorta), carrying blood to the lower parts of your body. The descending aorta branches into the thoracic aorta (above the diaphragm) and the abdominal aorta (below the diaphragm). (The diaphragm is the layer of muscle that acts as a partition between your chest and abdomen.)

A healthy aorta has strong and flexible walls, allowing it to accommodate regular thrusts of large volumes of blood with each heartbeat. Various conditions, however, can cause the aorta to malfunction, which can lead to serious consequences. We discuss two of these, aortic dissection and abdominal aortic aneurysm, at length on the following pages.

Aortic Dissection

Perhaps you were born with a bicuspid aortic valve—a defect of the aortic valve in which there are only two flaps that open and close instead of the usual three. The only other medical condition that you have is high blood pressure, which has been difficult to control over the years. You are lifting heavy weights when all of a sudden you develop severe, tearing pain in the chest that goes to your back, between your shoulder blades.

You might have developed a tear in the wall of your aorta that causes blood to force apart and flow between the layers of the aorta wall, a condition called *aortic dissection.*

Treating Aortic Dissection with Medicine

Beta Blockers Lower Pressure and Heart Rate

These drugs are the initial treatment of choice to lower your blood pressure and heart rate, minimizing stress on the aortic wall. The beta blockers used most often in this setting are intravenous propranolol, labetalol, and esmolol.

Sodium Nitroprusside Is Delivered Intravenously

If your blood pressure remains high despite maximal beta-blocker therapy, intravenous nitroprusside will be added. Your doctor might place a catheter in one of the arteries in your arm to continuously monitor your blood pressure and titrate therapy.

Strong Medications Relieve Pain

You will be given strong pain medications such as intravenous morphine sulfate to relieve your pain.

Repairing Aortic Dissection with Surgery

A highly skilled surgeon will perform this open-heart procedure since the potential for complications is very high. The surgeon will remove part of the aorta where the tear is found and then rebuild it with a synthetic graft. If your aortic valve is leaking, the surgeon will either repair or replace it. The entire surgical procedure usually takes three to six hours, and the hospital stay is usually seven to ten days.

Tests and Diagnosis of Aortic Dissection

After hearing about your symptoms and brief medical history, your doctor will perform a physical examination to check your blood pressure and pulses in your arms and legs and listen to your heart and

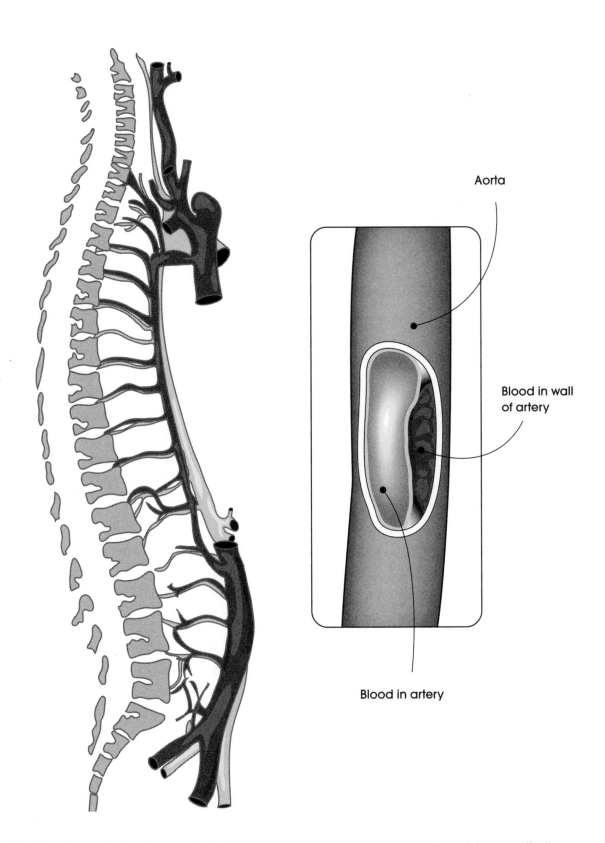

Aorta

Blood in wall of artery

Blood in artery

A depiction of an aortic dissection showing blood in the wall of an artery. The inner lining of the aorta has torn, allowing blood to surge through and separate (dissect) the layers of the aorta, creating a false channel for blood.

Endovascular Stent Graft

The surgeon might be able to repair an aortic dissection using an endovascular stent graft. The term *endovascular* means "inside blood vessels." An endovascular stent graft is a tube composed of fabric supported by a metal mesh, or stent, which is used to reinforce a weak spot in an artery.

What is the procedure? Endovascular procedures require only a small incision or puncture in an artery or vein.

Through this puncture, a vascular surgeon inserts a catheter, which carries the stent through your blood vessels to reline and strengthen your artery at the point of injury. Generally, endovascular treatments allow you to leave the hospital sooner and recover more quickly—with less pain and lower risk of complications than traditional surgery—because the incisions are smaller.

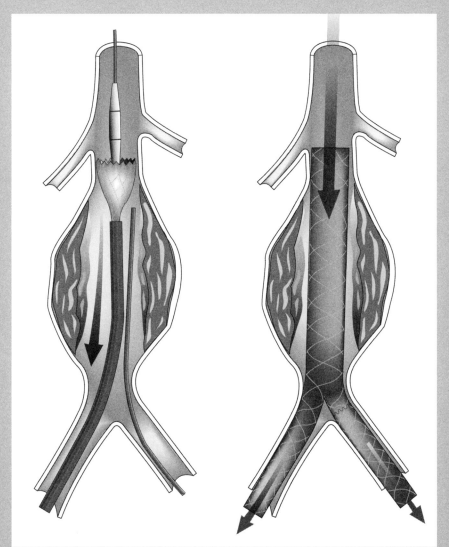

A depiction of an endovascular repair. In endovascular repair, the aneurysm isn't removed. Instead, a graft is inserted into the aorta to strengthen it. This type of surgery does not require surgically opening the chest or abdomen. In the first figure a catheter is inserted into an artery in the groin. The catheter is threaded to the abdominal aorta, and the stent graft is released from the catheter. In the second figure the stent graft allows blood to flow through the aneurysm.

Act Fast!

Acute aortic dissection is one of those conditions you wouldn't wish on even your worst enemy. If you experience symptoms such as those described, call 9-1-1 immediately. If an aortic dissection is detected early and treated promptly, your chance of survival greatly improves.

HEART HELP:

Reduce Your Risk of Aortic Dissection

- Control your blood pressure. If you have high blood pressure, get a portable blood-pressure-measuring device to help you monitor and control it.

- Keep your doctor informed. If you have a family history of aortic dissection, discuss this with your doctor.

- Take safety precautions to prevent injuries that can cause traumatic aortic dissections (e.g., wear your seat belt while driving).

- If you are a smoker, stop smoking.

- If you have survived aortic dissection, you will need to take blood-pressure-lowering medication for the rest of your life. In addition, you will need a follow-up CTA or MRA every six to twelve months to monitor your condition.

lungs. The initial tests for chest pain—blood tests, an electrocardiogram (ECG), and a chest X-ray—are then usually done. Following that, certain imaging procedures are done to help the doctor diagnose and visualize your dissection to distinguish it from other more common causes of chest pain, such as heart attack.

CTA

CTA is the preferred method for diagnosis of aortic dissection due to its speed and wide availability. A contrast dye is injected into your vein that allows the doctor to visualize your heart, aorta, and other blood vessels.

Transesophageal Echocardiogram (TEE)

In a TEE, the doctor puts an ultrasound probe through your mouth into your esophagus (food pipe) to identify potential problems with your heart, heart valves, and aorta. This test provides a clearer picture of your heart and its structures than a regular ECG does.

MRA

MRA takes longer to perform and is not as widely available as CTA. Similar to CTA, it uses contrast material to enhance the pictures.

Aortography

Aortography involves placement of a catheter through the groin and into the aorta and injection of a radiopaque substance (an opaque dye) to visualize aortic dissection. It is rarely done now with the advent of the imaging technologies mentioned above, as it is invasive, takes longer to perform, and is less accurate.

Aortic Dissection Explained

Think about a small tear in the lining of an old coat. One day, while putting on the coat, your hand gets caught in the torn edge of the lining and rips it apart from the outer portion of the coat. Aortic dissection is a condition in which the inner lining of the aorta suddenly tears; allowing blood to surge through and separate (dissect) the layers of the aorta, creating a false channel for blood.

The length of the false channel grows over time and can encroach upon points at which one or more arteries branch off from the aorta, blocking blood flow. This can lead to a heart attack, stroke, abdominal pain, back pain, and paralysis. Blood may leak from the dissection and collect in the chest and around the heart, a condition that can rapidly become fatal.

 HEART FACTS:

Aortic Dissection

- Uncontrolled high blood pressure (hypertension) is the strongest risk factor for aortic dissection and is observed in at least two-thirds of all cases.

- Aortic dissections are two to three times more common among men than women, more common among African Americans, and less common among Asians.

- About three-quarters of aortic dissections occur in people ages forty to seventy.

- Certain hereditary connective-tissue disorders, especially Marfan syndrome and Ehlers-Danlos syndrome, can increase the risk of aortic dissection, as can certain birth defects of the heart and blood vessels such as coarctation compression of the aorta and bicuspid aortic valve.

- Cocaine use has been implicated as a risk factor for aortic dissection.

- Infrequently, aortic dissections occur in otherwise healthy women during the third trimester of pregnancy.

ABDOMINAL AORTIC ANEURYSM (AAA)

R℞ THE PRESCRIPTION

The goals of treatment for AAA are to do the following:

➡ Prevent the aneurysm from growing.

➡ Repair the AAA in a timely fashion before it ruptures.

➡ Preserve your quality of life.

➡ If the aneurysm ruptures, do the best you can to permit survival.

Treatment recommendations for AAA are based on the size of the aneurysm, the rate of expansion, and the presence of symptoms, if any.

ABDOMINAL AORTIC ANEURYSM (AAA)

Consider Sam, a construction worker who injured his back while lifting something heavy and now has shooting pain down his left leg that has not gone away in two weeks. Suspecting a prolapsed disk, his doctor recommends magnetic resonance imaging (MRI).

At a meeting to discuss the MRI results, Sam discovers that he does have disk prolapse, which is causing his symptoms, but his doctor is more worried about something else. A section of Sam's aorta has started to bulge and he might need surgery in the future. Sam is surprised because he hasn't felt anything. Although he has been a chain smoker, he is otherwise healthy.

Sam's doctor gives him a handout to read and Sam learns that he has the condition called abdominal aortic aneurysm or AAA, often pronounced "Triple A." He now understands the look on his doctor's face. Sometimes, usually in men who smoke, the aorta swells up like a balloon, and if it continues to grow and isn't surgically repaired, it eventually bursts and kills you. Sam decides never to smoke cigarettes again.

Watchful Waiting

Small aneurysms found early can be treated with watchful waiting, which means ongoing surveillance of the AAA, usually every six months, to detect any changes in size or appearance. This strategy is safe if your AAA is larger than 1.6 inches (4 cm) but smaller than 2.2 inches (5.6 cm) in diameter, since early surgery has not been shown to increase your chances of long-term survival.

If you have high blood pressure, your physician may prescribe medication to lower it to decrease stress on the weakened area of the aneurysm. If you smoke, you should try to quit. An aneurysm will not go away by itself and it is extremely important to continue to follow up with your physician as directed.

Surgical Intervention for AAA

If your AAA is larger than 2.2 inches (5.5 cm) in diameter, is expanding rapidly (more than 0.2 inches [0.5 cm] in a six-month period), or is causing symptoms such as abdominal pain, your doctor will recommend surgery, as the risk of rupture is quite high. Two surgical options are available for the repair of AAA: open repair and endovascular repair.

Open Repair

Open repair involves a major incision in the abdomen. The aneurysm is removed and the section of aorta is replaced with a synthetic graft made of material such as Dacron, a polyester fiber. Following surgery, you will be in the ICU usually for up to three days, and in the hospital for an average of five to ten days. Recovery time for the return to full activity is around two to three months. The good news is that more than 90 percent of open aneurysm repairs are successful in the long term.

Because heart disease is common in people who have AAA, your doctor may recommend an evaluation of the heart prior to considering aneurysm surgery. This evaluation may range from a simple exercise stress test to heart catheterization.

Endovascular Repair

With endovascular repair, the surgeon will make a small incision in your groin area and use live X-ray pictures to guide a catheter containing an endovas-

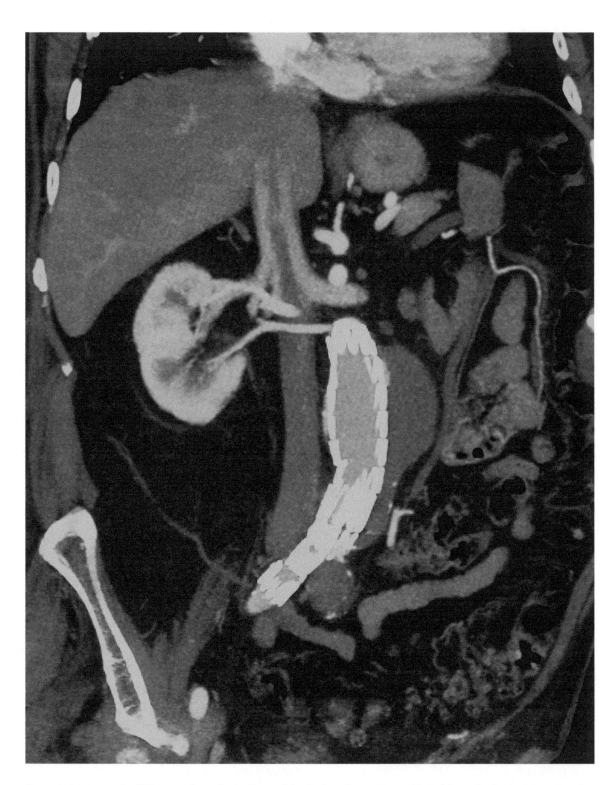

Computed tomography (CT) scan of a patient with an abdominal aortic aneurysm. Part of the aorta, the body's main artery is at center; the widest part is the aneurysm. The patient has previously had a stent placed in the aorta to treat an aneurysm. If left untreated, the aneurysm could rupture.

cular stent graft to the site of the aneurysm. The graft is then expanded inside the aorta and fastened in place to strengthen it. Recovery time is usually much shorter than for open surgery; your hospital stay may be reduced to two to three days.

Although endovascular repair may be an option for patients who cannot tolerate open surgery due to age or concurrent medical conditions, open surgical repair may be the best way to cure AAA. Your vascular surgeon will help you determine the best method of treatment for your particular situation.

Tests and Diagnosis of AAA

Often producing no symptoms, AAA is frequently detected by chance (in three out of four cases) during an X-ray, ultrasound, or CT scan performed for another reason, such as abdominal or back pain. Sometimes your physician may feel a large pulsating mass in your abdomen on a routine physical examination.

If your physician suspects that you have AAA, he may recommend one of the following tests to confirm the diagnosis and evaluate the aneurysm further.

Ultrasound

Simple and painless, an ultrasound uses high-frequency sound waves to create an image of your abdominal aorta. It shows the size of an aneurysm, if one is detected.

CT Scan

A CT scan provides computer-generated X-ray images of the internal organs. A liquid dye is injected into an arm vein to line the aorta. The size and shape of an aneurysm can be determined more accurately with CT scan images than with an ultrasound.

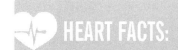

MRI

MRI uses a combination of large magnets and radiofrequencies to produce detailed images of organs and structures within the body. It is very accurate in detecting aneurysms and determining their size and exact location.

AAA Explained

An aneurysm occurs when the aortic wall weakens, causing it to balloon like a weak spot in an old, worn-out tire. Smoking, high blood pressure, hardening of the arteries (atherosclerosis), genetic conditions, and normal wear and tear from aging can result in a weakened aortic wall. Although an aneurysm can develop anywhere along the aorta, the large majority occur in the belly area (abdominal aorta).

Although most AAAs do not cause symptoms, sometimes they can cause pain from pressure on nearby organs or nerves. Occasionally, debris (emboli) contained within the aneurysm can break off and travel to the legs or vital organs, blocking the flow of blood to these tissues.

The weakened part of an aorta progressively bulges outward, becoming large, thin, and fragile, and may eventually rupture like a balloon that bursts from overinflation. Ruptured AAAs cause massive amounts of blood to be pumped inside the belly, which leads to excruciating pain and death within minutes of or shortly after arrival at the hospital in up to 90 percent of cases.

PULMONARY EMBOLISM (PE)

℞ THE PRESCRIPTION

The main goals of a treatment plan for pulmonary embolism are as follows:

➡ Stop the blood clot from getting bigger.

➡ Prevent new blood clots from forming.

These goals are usually accomplished by medicines that thin your blood and slow its ability to form clots. The medicines won't break up blood clots that have already formed. The body dissolves most clots with time.

PULMONARY EMBOLISM (PE)

Soon after a long airplane flight, you develop pain in your chest and have difficulty breathing. You should rush to the emergency room because you might have developed a blood clot in the lungs, called pulmonary embolism or PE. A large blood clot, or sometimes many repeated smaller ones, can be fatal in a short period of time.

Other symptoms that you might experience are coughing or spitting up blood, feeling lightheaded or fainting, rapid breathing, feelings of anxiety or dread, sweating, and a rapid heartbeat.

In some cases, the symptoms are related to *deep vein thrombosis (DVT)*, which is formation of a blood clot (thrombus) deep within the veins of your legs or pelvis. Symptoms of DVT include swelling, pain or tenderness, a feeling of increased warmth, and red or discolored skin on the affected leg. The clot can sometimes break off and travel as a free-moving thrombus (embolus) in the bloodstream, before finally lodging in the lungs to cause pulmonary embolism. The term *venous thromboembolism* includes both DVT and pulmonary embolism.

It is possible to have a blood clot in the deep veins or the lungs and not have any symptoms or signs.

Anticoagulants

Anticoagulants are blood-thinning medicines that decrease your blood's ability to clot. The regimen often begins with intravenous drugs such as heparin, or injections such as enoxaparin (Lovenox), followed by three to twelve months of the oral drug warfarin (Coumadin). If you have had blood clots before, you may need a longer period of treatment.

Emergency Treatment for Pulmonary Embolism

If your symptoms are life-threatening, your doctor may administer medicines (thrombolytics) to quickly dissolve a blood clot. Because they can cause serious bleeding, these clot-dissolving drugs are used only in emergency situations. Rarely, the doctor may use a catheter or surgery to remove the blood clot (embolectomy).

Inferior Vena Cava Filter Catches Clots

If you can't take medicines to thin your blood (most commonly because you have experienced bleeding) or when you're taking blood thinners but continue to develop clots anyway, your doctor may insert a mechanical filter in your inferior vena cava (the large vein in your abdomen that carries blood from the lower body back to the heart). This device catches

HEART ALERT:

Watch for Bleeding!

Bleeding is the most common side effect of anticoagulants. The bleeding can be internal and sometimes life-threatening. Your doctor will order regular blood tests that measure your blood's ability to clot, called PT/INR/PTT; these stand for prothrombin time, international normalized ratio, and partial thromboplastin time. By checking these numbers on a periodic basis, your doctor is able to adjust your medicine to keep your blood at a certain *viscosity level* (relative thickness or thinness). Call your doctor right away if you have easy bruising or bleeding or if you feel dizzy or pass out.

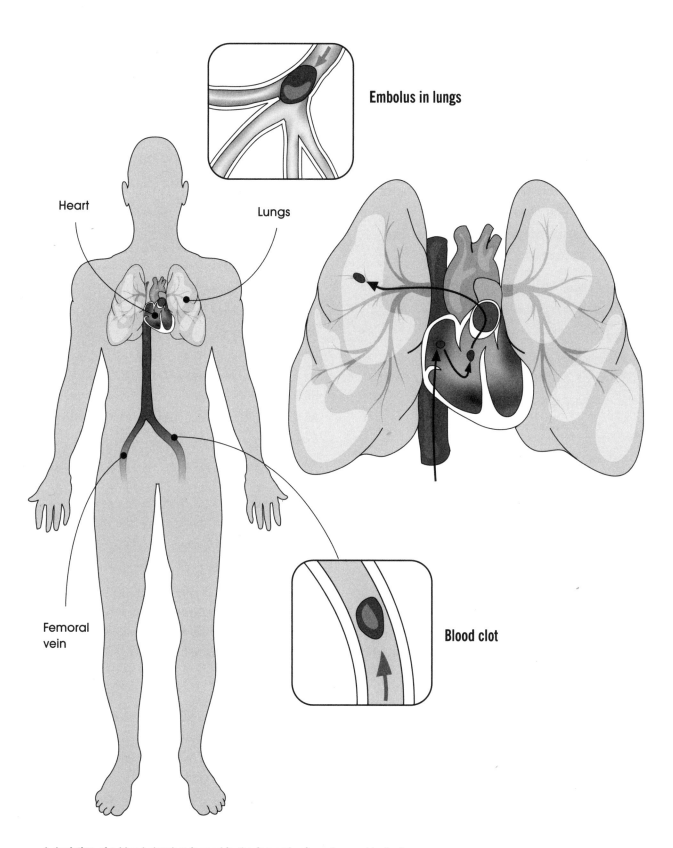

Embolus in lungs

Heart

Lungs

Femoral
vein

Blood clot

A depiction of a blood clot that formed in the femoral vein and moved to the lungs.

HEART FACTS:

Venous Thromboembolism (Including Pulmonary Embolism)

- More than 200,000 new cases of venous thromboembolism occur annually in the United States. This includes DVT (about two-thirds of cases) and pulmonary embolism (about one-third of cases).

- Of these, 30 percent of patients die within thirty days and about 30 percent develop recurrent venous thromboembolism within ten years.

- Caucasians and African Americans have a significantly higher incidence of venous thromboembolism than Hispanics and Asians or Pacific Islanders.

- Accurate diagnosis followed by effective therapy with anticoagulants (blood thinners), decreases the mortality rate from venous thrombo-embolism from 30 percent to as low as 2 percent.

blood clots before they reach the heart and lungs. It doesn't, however, stop the blood clots from forming elsewhere.

Tests and Diagnosis of Pulmonary Embolism

First, your doctor will ask you questions about your symptoms and medical history to identify your risk factors for venous thromboembolism, determine how likely it is that you have a blood clot, and rule out other possible causes for your symptoms. Your doctor will then perform a physical exam to check your blood pressure, heart, lungs, and legs for signs of DVT.

Depending on the initial impression, your doctor will order more tests to confirm or exclude the diagnosis of pulmonary embolism. We discuss some of these tests in the following subsections.

Chest X-Ray (CXR)

You are probably familiar with a chest X-ray—the procedure involves briefly exposing the chest to radiation to produce images of the organs and structures inside.

ECG

An ECG measures your heart's electrical activity. (See chapter 5 for an explanation of the heart's electrical system.)

Blood Tests

Blood tests include the D-dimer test (high levels mean there may be a blood clot; if your test is normal and you have few risk factors, pulmonary embolism is unlikely), arterial blood gas (to measure the amount of oxygen and carbon dioxide in your blood), and other blood tests to look for inherited disorders that can cause blood clots.

Ultrasound

An ultrasound uses high-frequency sound waves to look for blood clots in your legs.

Spiral CT Scan or CTA

Spiral CT scans or CTAs generate X-ray images of the blood vessels in your lungs to look for any blood clots.

Ventilation/Perfusion Lung Scan (V/Q Scan)

A V/Q scan uses radioactive material to determine how well oxygen and blood are flowing to all areas of your lungs.

Pulmonary Angiogram

In a pulmonary angiogram, a catheter is inserted through the groin and into the blood vessels of your lungs; then dye is injected, and X-ray pictures are taken to visualize the blood flow. If a clot is discovered, the doctor may use a catheter to extract it or deliver medicine to dissolve it.

Echocardiogram

An echocardiogram uses sound waves to check heart function and detect the presence of blood clots inside the heart.

Pulmonary Embolism Explained

Pulmonary embolism is a condition that occurs when one or more arteries in your lungs become blocked. In most cases, the blockage is caused by one or several blood clots that form in the deep veins of your body (DVT). The most common sites for blood clots to form are the deep veins of your legs, followed by the veins of your pelvis or arms. The clots can break free, travel through your bloodstream, and lodge in your lungs. Certain inherited conditions (e.g., factor V Leiden or prothrombin gene mutation) or acquired conditions (e.g., cancer) increase your chances of forming a blood clot.

Normally, blood flows from the right side of your heart to your lungs, where it picks up oxygen. The left side of your heart then pumps this oxygen-rich blood through a network of blood vessels called arteries. After oxygen has been delivered to all parts of your body, blood enters another network of blood vessels called veins, which carry this oxygen-poor blood back to the heart.

If your lung arteries become blocked by a blood clot, you may experience high blood pressure in your lungs. As a result, your heart pumps harder than usual, may enlarge, and eventually fails to perform. Your fate depends on the location and size of the blood clot, and any prior heart or lung disease that you may have.

HEART HELP:

Prevention is Better Than Cure

- To prevent pulmonary embolisms, walk or exercise your leg muscles every hour during long car trips and airplane rides.

- Drink plenty of fluids to prevent dehydration, which can increase blood's tendency to clot.

- Get out of bed and move around as soon as possible after having surgery or being ill. During such periods of limited mobility, your doctor may direct you to take medicines or wear sleevelike devices on your legs to prevent blood clots.

- If you have had previous episodes of blood clots, wear elastic compression stockings to prevent blood from pooling in your veins.

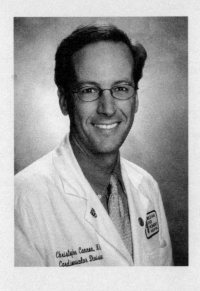

Christophr Cannon, M.D.
Cardiovascular Division

Q. Is it true that walking up and down the aisle is important on long plane rides?

A. Yes! This is not just an old wives' tale. Walking will help move blood through the veins of your legs, and thus prevent blood clots from forming. This in turn prevents deep vein thrombosis and pulmonary embolism.

Q. Abdominal aortic aneurysms have been reported to be deadly. How can I get checked for them?

A. There is a simple test: the ultrasound. This would be an abdominal ultrasound (similar to what is done to check for gallstones). Your doctor would have to order it. It is not currently recommended as routine screening, but for patients at high risk, such as those who smoke, it is something to consider.

Q. If I have peripheral artery disease (PAD), am I at increased risk for a heart attack?

A. Yes! This is a key aspect of PAD—it is not just about pain in the legs when walking. When you have cholesterol blockages in the legs, it is a sign that you may (and most people do) have blockages in the heart arteries too. Thus, the real risk is of a heart attack. That is why it is very important to control all your risk factors, including cholesterol levels.

Q. For my PAD, my doctor said I should walk more. Will that help?

A. Yes! This is one aspect of the treatment that has been very well documented with multiple studies: Regular exercise programs help reduce symptoms of claudication. The key is *regular* exercise. The studies actually show that supervised exercise programs—such as cardiac rehabilitation—will have the best effect in reducing claudication and increasing the distance that patients can walk without developing leg pain. It should be possible to duplicate this at home on your own, but you have to be disciplined and walk regularly for twenty to thirty minutes a day, ideally every day.

chapter 4:

DISEASES OF THE HEART MUSCLE

HEART FAILURE

R︎ THE PRESCRIPTION

Specific treatments for heart failure vary with its severity, but the general goal is to prevent progression from one degree to the next and to keep you feeling well. This is accomplished primarily with medications, and your doctor has many options to choose from. New devices are sometimes used to better synchronize the heart's pumping. Rarely, patients require surgical intervention.

There are four major goals of treatment for heart failure:

➡ Improve your symptoms so that you can get back to life and do the things you enjoy.

➡ Remove fluid that has built up in your body.

➡ Prevent further weakening of the heart muscle.

➡ Avoid hospitalization for heart failure symptoms.

➡ Stem further compromise of heart function or damage to other organs.

➡ Reduce the risk of dying.

Diseases of the heart muscle are also known as *heart failure* or *cardiomyopathy*, and result from a variety of causes that weaken the heart or impair its ability to pump efficiently.

Many of the signs of heart failure are due to the backup of fluid. Your symptoms may include shortness of breath, discomfort when lying flat, waking at night with difficulty breathing, swelling in the legs or abdomen, fatigue and generalized weakness, or even angina (see chapter 1).

TREATING HEART FAILURE WITH LIFESTYLE CHANGES

The first step in treatment of heart failure is to change certain aspects of your lifestyle. This is particularly important with respect to your diet. Patients with heart failure have a difficult time getting rid of salt and fluid. Therefore, it is especially important to limit the amount of salt and fluid that you take in.

Restricting salt and fluid can be very difficult. The feeling of thirst is strong and can be unrelenting. Some people keep their own beverage container, know exactly how much is in it, and therefore know exactly how much they've had to drink each day. Others suck candies, frozen grapes, or ice chips as a way to satiate their thirst. Just remember, what goes in as liquid must come out as urine!

As always, a more active lifestyle (with your doctor's permission) helps the heart. We detail the specifics of these changes in chapter 14. However, many medicines are also used in conjunction with changes to your lifestyle for the treatment of heart failure.

TREATING HEART FAILURE WITH MEDICINE

If you have been diagnosed with heart failure, your doctor may prescribe several medications. Some of these will improve your symptoms by helping to remove fluid. Others will lower your blood pressure and the amount of stress on your heart, which will prevent your heart from getting weaker.

Diuretics Help Drain Fluid

Fluid can accumulate in the legs, abdomen, or lungs. Diuretics help the kidneys produce more urine to eliminate fluid. Here are examples of some typical diuretics used in heart failure:

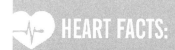

HEART FACTS:

Degrees of Heart Failure

The symptoms of heart failure can range in severity from mild, when they are present only during strenuous exertion, to severe, when you have symptoms while resting. Your doctor may ask you to classify your symptoms by a commonly used scale, as described originally by the New York Heart Association.

Heart failure is classified into four degrees, or classes:

Class 1: You have shortness of breath or fatigue only after exerting yourself to an unusual amount.

Class 2: You have symptoms with daily activities, such as climbing stairs or walking to get the mail.

Class 3: Symptoms come with any activity.

Class 4: Shortness of breath or fatigue occurs while resting.

Source: New York Heart Association

Risk Factors for Heart Failure

The major risk factors for heart failure include the following:

- Coronary artery disease (CAD) and any of its risk factors

- Previous heart attacks requiring bypass surgery or angioplasty (with or without stents)

- Diabetes

- High blood pressure

- High cholesterol

- Smoking

- Some kinds of chemotherapy

- Family members who developed heart failure at a young age

HEART ALERTS:

Diuretics and Electrolytes

Caution! Because diuretics make you urinate a lot, they can also cause you to lose valuable electrolytes—in particular, potassium. Because there is no way to predict how many of these electrolytes a patient might lose, it is very important that you and your doctor follow your laboratory tests carefully, particularly when starting, stopping, or changing diuretic dosing.

- Bumetanide (Bumex)
- Chlorothiazide (Diuril)
- Furosemide (Lasix)
- Hydrochlorothiazide (HydroDiuril, Microzide)
- Metolazone (Zaroxolyn)
- Torsemide (Demadex)

Additionally, your doctor may also prescribe diuretics known as aldosterone blockers They include spironolactone (Aldactone) and eplerenone (Inspra). These diuretics not only increase urine output, but can also slow the progression of heart failure due to their effects on hormones in the body.

MEDICATIONS THAT LOWER BLOOD PRESSURE

One common goal among the many therapies for heart failure is to decrease blood pressure by dilating your body's blood vessels. This is like increasing the size of a straw through which you are trying to drink; the bigger and more dilated (wide) the straw is, the easier the drink will flow through it! Similarly, the more dilated your body's blood vessels are, the lower your blood pressure will be because your heart doesn't have to work as hard to pump blood through them. There are several medications and mechanisms to achieve this.

Angiotensin-Converting Enzyme Inhibitors

Many patients are familiar with angiotensin-converting enzyme (ACE) inhibitors for the treatment of high blood pressure. These medications help dilate blood vessels by blocking an enzyme (ACE) which is part of a chain reaction (called the renin-angiotensin-aldosterone system, or RAAS) initiated by the kidneys, which *constricts* blood vessels. (Aldosterone-blocking diuretics, described previously, block a different part of the same chain of events to give some of the same effects.) Many ACE inhibitors are available, including the following:

- Benazepril (Lotensin)
- Captopril (Capoten)
- Enalapril (Vasotec)
- Fosinopril (Monopril)
- Lisinopril (Prinivil, Zestril)
- Quinapril (Accupril)
- Ramipril (Altace)
- Trandolapril (Mavik)

Not only are these medications excellent therapies for high blood pressure, they also are a key component of the treatment of heart failure. By decreasing the pressure against which your heart must pump, these medications ease the burden of an already weak heart. This increases the heart's efficiency and ability to pump blood to the rest of your body.

Reverse the Damage

Due to their unique mechanism, ACE inhibitors can help the weak heart reshape itself in a productive way. Although scientists have not completely figured out how this occurs, it is clear that effects derived from blocking the RAAS go way beyond simply lowering blood pressure. This system seems to have particular hormonal effects as well—that is, it controls not only the constriction or dilation of blood vessels but can also control how and when cells grow and mature. The self-repair of a weak heart is called *remodeling*, and although your heart may not regain all of its strength and efficiency, it can restructure itself to be more efficient with the muscle that is left and healthy.

Your doctor may not prescribe these medications if your blood pressure is already on the low side.

HEART HELP:

Controlling Fluid Levels

One of the best ways for your doctor to know how to adjust your diuretics is by following your weight. Although your food intake can affect your weight over the long term, significant changes in your weight over several days are more likely a matter of fluid and may require a change in your diuretic dosing. Therefore, remember to weigh yourself at the same time and on the same scale every day, keep a diary, and don't hesitate to inform your doctor if you notice a trend one way or the other!

Additionally, one significant side effect of ACE inhibitors can be a decline in kidney function, particularly when combined with diuretics (see page 71). Therefore, your doctor will monitor you closely. Rarely, patients may also experience a cough or rash from ACE inhibitors.

Angiotensin-Receptor Blockers

Angiotensin-receptor blockers (ARBs) work much like ACE inhibitors. They lower blood pressure by acting on yet another part of the RAAS, and reduce the force with which the heart needs to pump. Here are some examples of ARBs:

- Candesartan (Atacand)
- Irbesartin (Avapro)
- Losartin (Cozaar)
- Telmisartin (Micardis)
- Valsartan (Diovan)

Patients who experience a cough or rash from ACE inhibitors may find these agents more tolerable. However, patients with low blood pressure should not take them, and they can adversely affect kidney function as well.

Hydralazine and Isosorbide Dinitrate

Hydralazine and isosorbide dinitrate are used for high blood pressure and heart failure. For heart failure, they are more commonly used together, often in one pill (BiDil). Both medications act by opening the blood vessels, making it easier for the heart to pump blood, and thus decreasing the workload for a weak heart. They can be more potent blood-pressure-lowering agents than ACE inhibitors or ARBs. However, they lack the benefit of productive remodeling, as they act mainly by dilating blood vessels and do not affect the RAAS.

Side effects of hydralazine and isosorbide dinitrate include flushing or lightheadedness. Also, patients taking these medications should not take certain medicines for erectile dysfunction—specifically, sildenafil (Viagra), tadalafil (Cialis), or vardenafil (Levitra)—as this combination may cause an unsafe drop in blood pressure.

Beta Blockers

Beta blockers are another type of medication used for high blood pressure and heart failure. The main blockers used for heart failure include carvedilol (Coreg) and metoprolol (Lopressor, Toprol XL). These medications block signals to the heart that usually increase the heart rate or strength of contraction. Therefore, they decrease heart rate and also decrease the strength or force with which the heart contracts.

Although this approach might seem counterintuitive for a heart that is already weak, much research has demonstrated its benefit over the long term. The decreased heart rate and force of contraction actu-

WHAT'S NEW:

Racial and Ethnic Factors

Is there a special medication for African Americans? BiDil is the first treatment to be approved by the U.S. Food and Drug Administration (FDA) for the treatment of African Americans with congestive heart failure, implying a physiological difference between black and white Americans, despite research that shows little variation in genetics.

How does it work? BiDil combines two commonly paired generic medicines: hydralazine and isosorbide dinitrate (vasodilators that enlarge veins and arteries). The FDA originally rejected the combined pill in 1997 not because it didn't work, but because the trial was inadequate for approval of a new drug. Two years later, the pharmaceutical company NitroMed purchased the intellectual property rights to BiDil and raised $34 million in venture capital funds for a clinical trial of 1,050 self-identified black people. The combination drug was so effective that the trial was cut short and the FDA granted its approval.

Can it be used by people of other races? BiDil could be equally beneficial to whites and other ethnic groups, but they were not included in the study.

ally decrease the demand placed on a failing heart. They force the failing muscle to take a break. Because it doesn't work as hard, the heart's function is preserved and does not worsen as much over the long term. Indeed, for many patients, heart strength improves after six to twelve months. The effect on blood pressure is similar; through decreasing the force of contraction, the heart generates less pressure in the vessels, thereby reducing overall blood pressure. Instead of providing more room for the pressure (through dilation), it simply lowers pressure at the source by taming the heart.

It is true that occasionally these medications worsen the symptoms of heart failure in the short term. Therefore, your doctor may wait to start them until your symptoms and heart function have been stable for a while. Other potential side effects of beta blockers include slowing the heart rate excessively, and rarely, confusion, depression, and impotence (erectile dysfunction) can occur.

Digoxin Strengthens Heartbeats

Digoxin, or digitalis, is one of the oldest medications used to treat heart failure. It is one of the few oral medications available that actually *increases* (slightly) the strength of each heartbeat. This might seem beneficial for hearts that are weak and have difficulty pumping. However, extensive research has demonstrated that this approach is not a panacea.

Whereas beta blockers relieve a weak heart of its demands, digoxin works in a manner similar to "whipping a feeble horse." Driving a weak heart to pump harder does not prevent it from weakening further, nor does it prolong patients' lives. However, it does reduce the frequency with which some patients require hospitalization, and can relieve their symptoms. It is this subtlety that makes digoxin one of the less-commonly prescribed medications for heart failure. However, if your doctor does prescribe it, be sure to notify him or her of other changes to your entire medical regimen, as blood levels of digoxin can be volatile and can easily reach toxic levels. Side effects of digoxin can include an abnormally low heart rate.

CONTINUOUS INFUSION MEDICATION

The vast majority of patients diagnosed with heart failure are maintained on oral medications as long-term chronic therapy. Under appropriate management with such medicines, as well as dietary and lifestyle changes, longevity is greatly increased.

However, in some patients, heart function continues to decline and their heart failure becomes advanced and severe. They cannot physically move without becoming severely short of breath and fatigued; they may not be thinking right; their kidney function may decline; or they may suffer from severe volume overload. (Severe volume overload occurs when heart function has deteriorated to such an extent that it can no longer pump enough blood to the kidneys for them to produce urine, even with the help of diuretics.) Without urine production, fluid builds up rapidly and can be life-threatening. The following sections on continuous infusion medications, surgical management, and end-of-life care are relevant to these patients.

Rarely, patients with severe heart failure require continuous intravenous infusions of medications to control their symptoms and prevent progressive damage to other organs. Two specific medications are used for this purpose—milrinone and dobutamine—and they are known as inotropes, which are similar to adrenaline, the body's natural stimulant. They

A Little Help Pumping

What's an LVAD? The implantation of an electrical pump to assist the heart, called a left ventricular assist device (LVAD), is one of the latest technologies offered to a select few patients who qualify for it. The LVAD (or VAD) is a kind of mechanical heart. It's placed inside a person's chest, where it helps the heart pump oxygen-rich blood throughout the body.

How is it used? Unlike an artificial heart, the LVAD doesn't replace the heart. It just offers a little help pumping. This can mean the difference between life and death for a person whose heart needs a rest after open-heart surgery, or for a person waiting for a heart transplant.

LVADs also play another role, allowing weakened hearts to recover. In what is called destination therapy, a permanent LVAD is being used in some terminally ill patients whose conditions make them ineligible for heart transplantation.

What are the risks? In studies, therapy with the permanent LVAD device doubled the one-year survival rate of patients with end-stage heart failure, compared with drug treatment alone. However, there are significant risks, including infection, stroke, and bleeding.

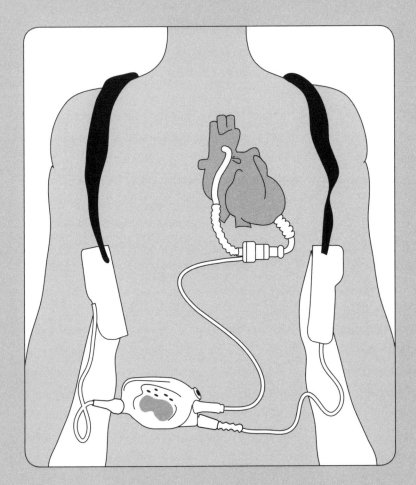

Left Ventricular Assist Device

are also similar to digoxin (yet significantly more potent!) in that they improve how patients feel but can push an already weak heart beyond what it can physically sustain. However, in patients who have constant symptoms and severely depressed heart function, these medications can be used to bridge them to surgical therapy.

Use of intravenous inotropes requires insertion of a long-term IV catheter and very close monitoring both in the hospital and in the less-common scenario in which the patient goes home with them. Multiple right-heart catheterization procedures are needed to ensure proper use, dose adjustment, and response to such medications. Additionally, because of the stimulating effect they have on the heart, they can predispose some patients to dangerous heart arrhythmias (see chapter 5). Thus, some patients may not tolerate them, and most patients who use inotropes have already received a pacemaker or an internal defibrillator.

SURGICAL PROCEDURES FOR HEART FAILURE

Advanced, severe heart failure is a particularly difficult condition to treat and typically requires care at a specialty center by physicians with many different areas of expertise, such as heart failure cardiologists, heart surgeons, nephrologists (kidney doctors to help manage diuretics), and other specialists based on the etiology of the heart failure. Patients who have exhausted therapy with medicines and continue to have symptoms at rest, along with severe, worsening heart function, may be candidates for surgery.

The Rare Heart Transplant

Despite the millions of Americans with heart failure, only a few thousand heart transplants are performed annually. Many factors go into the decision to perform a transplant: Relatively few patients with heart failure progress to such a severe stage as to require a transplant; many patients do not qualify for transplant due to other medical problems or based on their advanced age; and the availability of donor hearts becomes the limiting factor in whether a patient receives a transplant. The road to transplantation is a long one and requires not only advanced care by a multidisciplinary team at a specialized transplant center but also the psychological and emotional support of friends and family to complete a complicated recovery process, as well as help with an extensive medicine regimen afterward.

Internal Cardiac Defibrillators and Dual-Chamber Pacemakers

As the heart muscle becomes more diseased, conduction of electricity declines. The healthy heart uses electrical pulses to contract the heart muscles at close to the same time. When these impulses are severely disturbed, life-threatening arrhythmias can occur. Impulses no longer initiate in any one part of the heart; different parts contract at different times and pumping is lost. This is very dangerous! For this reason, many patients with advanced heart failure receive an implantable cardioverter defibrillator (ICD), which can shock the heart back into correct rhythm should it need to.

This device is surgically implanted in the chest over the heart, with wires through the blood vessels into the heart. It monitors the heart's rhythm, and delivers a shock if it detects a dangerous arrhythmia. It is important to note that this device prevents arrhythmias only; having an ICD will not treat the symptoms

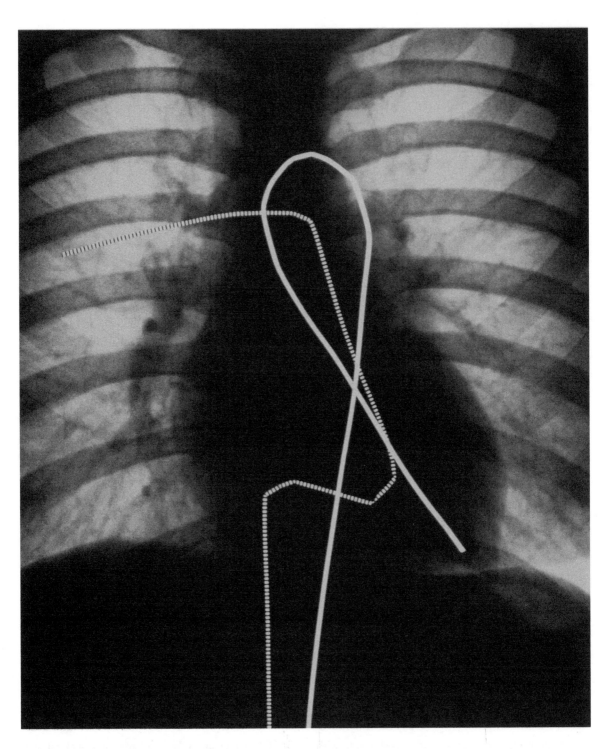

In this chest X-ray showing a cardiac catherization procedure superimposed, two catheters (white line, broken line) trace a path up to the heart from a femoral artery and vein in the leg. The white line catheter traces the arterial route around the aortic arch (at top) and into the left ventricle of the heart. The broken line catheter traces the venous route into the right side of the heart and out to a pulmonary artery of a lung.

of heart failure or prevent progression of the heart's dysfunction.

Additionally, patients with heart failure may have persistent, yet less-severe disturbances of the heart's rhythm. Either they no longer generate regular, evenly spaced impulses (instead, they come at delayed intervals) or there is a constant disruption in the conduction of a normally generated beat to the rest of the heart. In either case, the coordination of the heart's beat is disrupted, and thus the heart loses efficiency. For patients with heart failure, this only makes a bad situation worse, and can significantly increase symptoms. In these patients, a dual-chamber pacemaker can stimulate each part of the heart at the right time and for every beat. (This is called cardiac resynchronization therapy.) Correction of the heart's rhythm can, in fact, improve their symptoms. The heart becomes more efficient at beating and usually beats more slowly than it would without an artificial pacemaker. This is particularly true if the heart failure is the result of a long-standing arrhythmia.

END-OF-LIFE CARE FOR HEART FAILURE

As a result of improved treatment of other heart conditions, such as heart attacks and Coronary Artery Disease (CAD), the number of patients with heart failure has greatly increased over the years.

Yet despite advances in the treatment of heart failure, many patients progress to Class 4, as described by the New York Heart Association (see page 71), experiencing persistent shortness of breath and fatigue even with maximum medical therapy. For many of these patients, the risk of surgical intervention greatly outweighs any potential benefit they might derive; many will not survive surgery.

Therefore, these patients reach end-stage heart failure and become candidates for palliative care, or measures geared mainly toward relieving their symptoms. They are not unlike those with incurable cancer—we despair in the fact that their condition has defied the bounds of modern medicine and seek to keep them as comfortable as possible at the end of their lives. Although they represent only a fraction of those patients diagnosed with heart failure, it is nevertheless a reality for some.

TESTS AND DIAGNOSIS OF HEART FAILURE

Initial evaluation for heart failure always includes a discussion of your symptoms, measurement of your heart rate and blood pressure, and a physical examination to identify any swelling in your legs, extra heart sounds or murmurs, fluid in your lungs, or enlarged veins in your neck. An electrocardiogram (ECG) is also usually performed (see appendix II).

Additionally, your doctor may order other tests to determine whether your symptoms are from somewhere other than the heart. For example, you may undergo X-rays or computed tomography scans to rule out any problems with your lungs, or you may have an ultrasound of the liver. Often, these are not unreasonable, as many symptoms of heart failure can overlap with other diseases.

The Echocardiogram

Not to be confused with the *electro*cardiogram, the echocardiogram (or echo) has become the mainstay of testing for heart failure. An echo is simply a sonogram of the heart. A sonogram, also called an ultrasound, works by measuring how well sound waves penetrate tissues. Sound travels well through water (which shows up black or empty) and poorly

Causes of Heart Failure

Although CAD and high blood pressure are the most common causes of heart failure, the heart may fail for many other reasons:

Common Causes
- CAD, also known as ischemic heart disease (IHD)
- Long-standing high blood pressure

Less Common
- Long-standing alcoholism or cocaine use, producing prolonged stress on the heart, similar to CAD
- Chemotherapy or radiation-induced heart failure—toxic effects of these sometimes lifesaving medications can damage heart muscle
- Acute viral infections of the heart
- Heart failure as a result of long-term heart valve disease
- Heart failure as a result of long-term arrhythmias beating unusually fast over long periods of time
- Unknown or idiopathic (progressive) decline in heart muscle function without a clear cause, though it may be the result of a yet-to-be-identified genetic disorder

Rare
- Nutritional deficiencies—deficiencies in vitamins such as thiamine or selenium—over long periods of time can lead to heart failure.
- Congenital or genetic conditions leading to deposition of minerals in the heart—deposition of copper or iron, as in Wilson's disease or hemochromatosis (respectively), slowly destroys the structure of the heart muscle.
- Rare forms of cancer leading to deposition of protein in the heart—conditions such as multiple myeloma, rare leukemias or lymphomas, and amyloidosis can deposit harmful proteins in the muscle.
- Heart failure related to pregnancy—an unfortunate complication toward the end of pregnancy or shortly after delivery—is thought to be related to disturbances of the mother's immune system from the fetus.
- Heart failure from muscular dystrophy or other neuromuscular disorders: Just as neuromuscular disorders can affect the muscles that move our arms and legs, they can lead to defective heart muscle as well.

through denser structures such as bone or muscle (which is whiter on an ultrasound). Submarines and some sea animals use a similar technique to navigate underwater; it's no coincidence that they call it *sonar*! The same technology is used to look at a fetus inside a pregnant woman. An echo of the heart is a valuable test that can tell your doctor how well your heart is pumping, whether any parts of the heart aren't pumping well, whether the valves are functioning (see chapter 9), and whether your heart has changed shape as a result of heart failure.

An echo can also distinguish between the major types of heart failure: systolic and diastolic (see the next section "Heart Failure Explained"). Your cardiologist can see how well the muscle is contracting and also whether it is relaxing appropriately. One common measurement is the ejection fraction (EF), which indicates how much of the blood that enters the heart is pumped out. This is typically measured by assessing the volume of the heart on echo before and after contraction. It ranges from as low as 15 percent to 20 percent in severe systolic heart failure to as high as 55 percent to 65 percent in healthy individuals and may even be abnormally high (higher than 65 percent) in patients with diastolic heart failure. There is much more to the echo than just the EF. Additional measurements can be equally important, such as the thickness of the heart muscle, the function of the valves, or specific areas of the heart which are not functioning well.

Right-Heart Cardiac Catheterization

Many patients may be familiar with cardiac catheterizations to assess the blood vessels to the heart (the coronary arteries). However, a different type of catheterization (called a right-heart catheterization) can be done to evaluate patients with severe heart failure. The term *right-heart* does not imply a second heart!

It simply means the catheter (thin tube) is inserted into a vein in the neck or the groin and then to the right-sided chambers of the heart—the atrium and ventricle that take blood from the body and pump it back to the lungs (see chapter 8). A right-heart catheterization can provide valuable information in the form of pressure measurements from several parts of the heart. These pressures can help determine the severity of heart failure and how to adjust medicines. Specialized measurements can also be performed to assess how many liters per minute the heart is pumping and how hard the heart has to pump to get blood flowing to the body. Additionally, in patients who have heart failure for an unclear reason, a biopsy or tissue sample of the heart can be taken for analysis under a microscope. This can provide additional clues as to why the heart is not pumping as well as it should.

HEART FAILURE EXPLAINED

The Key Role of Fluid

As muscle disease prevents the heart from doing its job, the rest of the body does not get enough blood flow, depriving it of the oxygen, nutrients, and electrolytes carried in the blood. This can lead to many different problems: Kidney or liver function may become abnormal; thinking may become impaired; other muscles may become weak; and blood may back up because it is not being pumped at an adequate rate.

Systolic and Diastolic Heart Failure

Heart failure, or dysfunction of the heart muscle, is typically the result of another condition that weakens the heart, such as loss of oxygen or high blood pressure. The dysfunction is usually categorized as systolic or diastolic, based on why the heart is having difficulty pumping blood.

Normal   **Systolic Dysfunction**

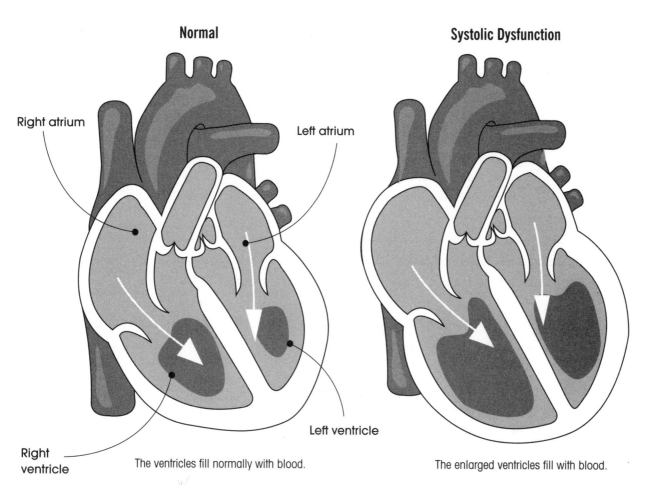

Right atrium   Left atrium

Left ventricle

Right
ventricle

The ventricles fill normally with blood.   The enlarged ventricles fill with blood.

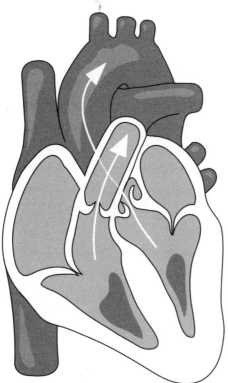

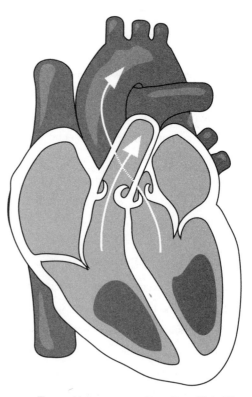

The ventricles pump out   The ventricles pump out less than 40 to 50
about 60 percent of the blood.   percent of the blood.

Diastolic Dysfunction

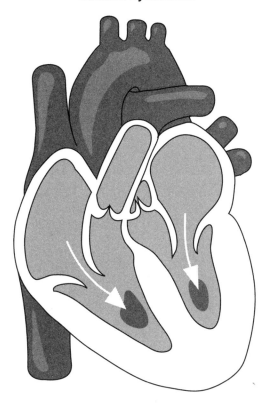

The stiff ventricles fill with less blood than normal.

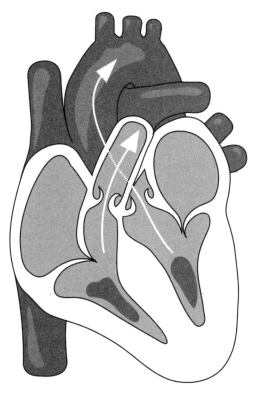

The ventricles pump out 60 percent of the blood, but the amount may be lower than normal.

Weak muscle, or *systolic* heart failure, results when the muscle of the heart is simply too tired and weak to contract strongly enough to move enough blood.

Stiff muscle, known as *diastolic* heart failure, results when the heart muscle becomes so stiff that it cannot relax and expand to allow blood to flow into it. If blood cannot easily get into the ventricles, it cannot efficiently be pumped out (see chapter 8 for a tour of the heart).

Mr. Jones' and Mrs. Edwards' stories (see page 84–85) demonstrate the two major types of diseases of the heart muscle: systolic, caused by weak heart muscle, and diastolic, caused by stiff heart muscle.

Loss of Oxygen

In many patients with heart failure, CAD (see chapters 1 and 2) has caused a decrease in the amount of oxygen supplied by blood to the heart muscle over a long period of time. The muscle may have also experienced times of no blood supply at all (a heart attack), after which a scar forms in the muscle, just as you might see on your skin after an operation. Unfortunately, this scar does not beat like the rest of the muscle, and in fact is "dead" tissue.

Both the acute and chronic loss of oxygen over time weakens the muscle to the extent that the heart cannot pump as well as it used to. This systolic heart failure, when the muscles of the ventricles are no longer strong enough to provide good blood flow, results in the symptoms of heart failure: fatigue, shortness of breath, and fluid accumulation. The heart tries to compensate by enlarging, so some people have "enlarged hearts" when tested by their doctors.

Mr. Jones' Story

Mr. Jones is a seventy-two-year-old grandfather who used to smoke (and still sneaks a cigarette every once in awhile), has had diabetes for several years, and experienced a heart attack at age fifty-nine. Diagnosed with coronary artery disease (which surely existed before the attack), he had bypass surgery at age sixty and felt well after that.

However, over the past several years, he can no longer walk as far as he used to. Climbing more than a flight of stairs elicits fatigue and shortness of breath, and he has noticed that his ankles are a little puffy.

Mr. Jones' doctor orders an echocardiogram, which shows that his heart is not functioning the way it used to. The muscle is not contracting as well as it should. He is diagnosed with systolic heart failure. The doctor starts him on a few new medications—including a diuretic and an ACE inhibitor—and more importantly, educates him on the importance of limiting his salt and fluid intake and taking all of his medications as prescribed.

Several months later, Mr. Jones has lost weight, his ankles are less puffy, and his shortness of breath is reduced. Mr. Jones' doctor has effectively controlled his symptoms. However, it is unlikely that Mr. Jones' heart function will improve greatly. His bypass surgery improved flow to the heart and probably prevented his heart function from being *worse* than it is. Yet the many years of decreased blood flow from CAD, as well as his subsequent heart attack, damaged his heart muscle, which has weakened.

The present goal is to alleviate Mr. Jones' symptoms and prevent his heart from becoming even weaker by treating both his CAD and his heart failure with medications such as aspirin, clopidogrel, a statin for cholesterol, a beta blocker, an ACE inhibitor, and diuretics.

High Blood Pressure

The other common cause of heart failure (and the prototype for diastolic heart failure) is long-standing hypertension, or high blood pressure. Over long periods of time, as the heart pumps against high pressures, it becomes thicker, stiffer, and less efficient. Think of a weightlifter who works out aggressively, lifting more and more weight. His muscle mass increases and he becomes bulkier. Unfortunately, this same phenomenon occurring in the heart does not improve function. It is most often the result of hypertension. Many patients have hypertension as a result of inevitable hardening of the blood vessels as we get older. The vessels do not stretch as much when the heart pumps, and therefore the pressure in them increases. A diet high in salt and fat, as well as a sedentary lifestyle, contribute heavily to the development of hypertension.

When the heart muscle gets bulkier, it does not expand as easily. Expansion occurs when the heart relaxes to fill and is a key component of its pumping cycle—blood must be allowed into the ventricle to then be expelled. The size of the ventricle normally varies greatly to fill and then contract (see chapter 8). As the muscle has more difficulty relaxing and filling with blood, it is less effective at pumping enough blood forward, and the pressure inside builds up and can push back into the lungs, leading to shortness of breath. This dysfunction leads to diastolic heart failure and its symptoms.

TREAT THE UNDERLYING CAUSE

If you have heart failure, it is important to treat the underlying cause. Although your doctor may prescribe some of the medicines detailed in this chapter, you may also be taking medicines to treat the condition that caused the heart failure. For example, patients with CAD may also take aspirin or clopidogrel (Plavix). Patients with high blood pressure should still take medicines to control their blood pressure. Similarly, patients with heart failure from other causes may be candidates for other treatments directed at the underlying disease that led to heart failure.

Myocarditis and Endocarditis: Infections of the Heart Muscle

Heart failure can be precipitated by acute infections of the heart muscle, termed *myocarditis*. This is not to be confused with infections of other parts of the heart, or *endocarditis* (see chapter 6). Myocarditis affects the heart muscle itself, whereas endocarditis is limited to the nonmuscle tissue, such as the valves.

Myocarditis, though uncommon, can strike patients of any age and can range in severity from mild chest pain to severe heart failure requiring a heart transplant. Often, it is caused by a virus and is preceded by a typical illness: fatigue, muscle aches, headache, fever, malaise, or even upper respiratory or gastrointestinal symptoms, then progresses to involve the heart. When a typical viral infection progresses to the heart over a course of several days, symptoms may change to include progressive fatigue, shortness of breath, chest pain, pain on deep breaths, or palpitations (a sensation of the heart pounding). Therapies consist mainly of those used in other types of heart failure. In certain scenarios, however, steroids or other medications to suppress the body's immune system may be warranted. These can be effective because it is often the body's reaction to infection— the subsequent inflammation of the heart's immune cells (similar to when a black eye swells up)—that results in dysfunction of the heart muscle.

Mrs. Edwards' Story

Mrs. Edwards is a sixty-seven-year-old grandmother who had high blood pressure when her kids were born, but she experienced no symptoms for many years. However, over the past several months, she has become fatigued with routine activities; she also has episodes of severe shortness of breath, where she has to sit or lie still for several minutes until she can breathe easier.

Mrs. Edwards visits her doctor during a severe episode; she cannot catch her breath. Her doctor listens to her lungs and orders a chest X-ray. Both tests show that she has extra fluid in her lungs. In addition to several other tests, her doctor orders an echocardiogram. It shows that Mrs. Edwards' heart muscle is thick and is not relaxing enough to fill with blood before contracting.

Mrs. Edwards is diagnosed with diastolic heart failure. Like Mr. Jones' doctor, her physician also prescribes diuretics to help her get rid of the extra fluid. More importantly, her doctor educates her about limiting salt and fluid intake and prescribes medication to control her blood pressure.

Several months later, Mrs. Edwards feels better and has had fewer episodes of shortness of breath, which are also milder in severity. With her medications, she is able to keep the fluid out of her lungs (also by drinking less and urinating more) and control her blood pressure to limit further thickening and stiffening of her heart muscle. However, it unlikely that her heart will return to normal.

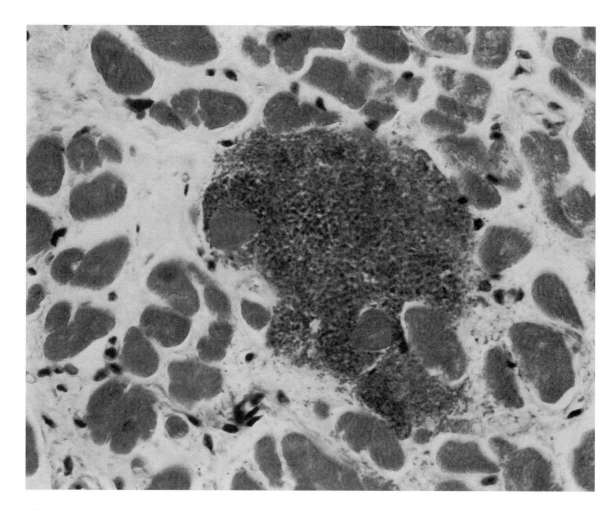

Infected inflamed heart muscle. Light micrograph of heart tissue in myocarditis (heart muscle inflammation). The most common cause is a viral infection. An infected area (center) is seen here. Symptoms may include fever, fatigue, and chest pain, and irregularities in the heartbeat.

Infection of the heart by a specific fungus is the most common cause of heart failure outside the U.S. This condition is called Chagas disease. Specific antibiotics can be used to help cure both the infection and the resultant heart failure, if treated early enough. Chagas disease is an uncommon cause of heart failure in the U.S.

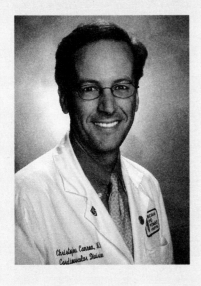

Christoph Cannon, M.
Cardiovascular Division

Q. My doctor said I have congestive heart failure. Does that mean my heart is failing?

A. It depends on which type of heart failure you have. The term *congestive heart failure* describes a syndrome in which the heart is not pumping blood through the body well enough, so the blood begins to back up into the lungs and makes you short of breath. There are two major types. In one type, the heart muscle is weak and it just can't pump enough blood forward. This is called systolic heart failure. The other type occurs when the heart is too strong! But the problem is that the heart muscle is thickened and stiff, so the pressure inside the heart is higher than normal. The heart is sort of "muscle-bound."

The weak heart is "failing," whereas the thickened heart is not.

Q. I have four different medicines for my heart failure. Do I need to take all of them for the rest of my life?

A. Probably yes, but it can depend. Fortunately, the medications for heart failure, such as ACE inhibitors, beta blockers, and diuretics, are very effective and in some cases can reverse the weakness or thickness in the heart muscle (depending on what type of heart failure you have). In that case, you may be able to stop one or two—but don't stop taking any medication without asking your doctor whether it is safe to do so!

Q. My doctor said I should have a special two-sided pacemaker for my heart failure. Should I do this procedure?

A. You should definitely consider it. Biventricular pacemakers are used for patients with severely weakened hearts who have some slowing of the electrical pacing of the heart (measured on the ECG by the QRS duration). These pacemakers get the heart "in sync" so that the weakened heart is well timed and blood moves through the heart smoothly. It is like having your heart engines tuned up. Several large clinical trials have shown that so-called Cardiac Resynchronization Therapy can increase the strength of the heart and improve the ejection fraction, prolonging life span!

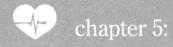 chapter 5:

DISEASES OF THE ELECTRICAL SYSTEM

ARRHYTHMIA

Rx THE PRESCRIPTION

Arrhythmia treatments aim to alleviate symptoms and prevent the occurrence of life-threatening abnormal electrical activity in the heart. This may—or may not—involve correcting the heart's rhythm. Some arrhythmias can be stable for years without significant intervention. In other cases, correcting the arrhythmia is the only way to alleviate symptoms. Maintaining a regular rhythm can help the heart contract in a synchronized, more effective manner.

ARRHYTHMIA

Your doctor has told you that you have an arrhythmia, a disturbance of your heart's electrical system. Your symptoms include dizziness, lightheadedness, pounding of your heart, chest pain, and even passing out and loss of consciousness. These are common symptoms for most arrhythmias.

What causes these symptoms? The muscle of your heart conducts electrical impulses throughout the heart to ensure that all parts beat in a simultaneous, coordinated fashion. This is important—if each muscle cell in the heart marched to the beat of its own drummer, the heart would not contract and there would be no blood flow!

Your heart's electrical system has two main goals:

- The rate of heart contraction is regular and appropriate.
- Each beat is a synchronized contraction that produces blood flow.

If the electrical system goes awry, the result is an arrhythmia.

ᴧᴧ— WHAT'S NEW:

Quicker Fixes for Arrhythmias

Where should I go for treatment? Treatments for patients with arrhythmias have come a long way, with advanced technologies that enable physicians to correct previously untreatable rhythm disturbances in outpatient procedures. At a major hospital's Electrophysiology Lab, for example, a specialized team of electrophysiologists (cardiologists who have additional training in the diagnosis and treatment of abnormal heart rhythms) as well as cardiologists, surgeons, radiologists, and anesthesiologists can perform ablations or implantations of devices on-site.

What is the procedure? During a nonsurgical ablation, a catheter is inserted into a specific area of the heart, and a special machine directs energy through the catheter to small areas of the heart muscle that causes the abnormal heart rhythm. This energy "disconnects" the pathway of the abnormal rhythm. It can also be used to disconnect the electrical pathway between the upper chambers (atria) and the lower chambers (ventricles) of the heart.

Can I just take medicine? The "pill-in-a-pocket" method of medicine delivery is another option. A study conducted in Alberta, Canada, found that patients who popped flecainide or propafenone (antiarrhythmia drugs) on their own had a low rate of rhythm problems and a marked reduction in emergency room visits and hospital admissions.

Lifesaving Defibrillators in Public Places

Arrhythmias of the heart can vary from benign nuisances to life-threatening emergencies. In patients who have severe heart attacks, arrhythmias of the ventricles can cause sudden death. For this reason, many public areas now have automatic external defibrillators available; if someone collapses in public, they can save a life! They are now commonplace on airplanes as well as in airports, stadiums, train stations, public buildings, and even private homes.

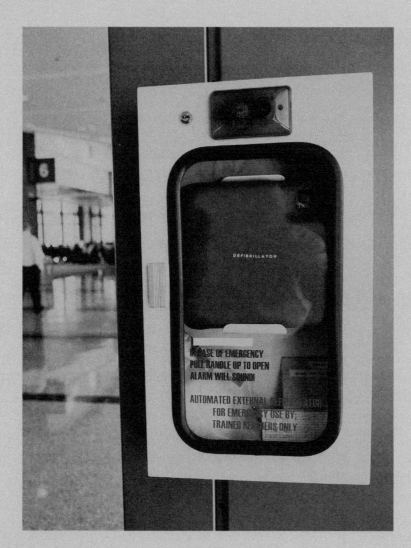

The American Heart Association supports putting automatic electric defibrillators, or AEDs, in targeted public areas such as airports, sports arenas, gated communities, office complexes, doctor's offices, shopping malls, etc. According to the AHA, AEDs are not only accurate, but also easy to use. With a few hours of training, anyone can learn to operate an AED safely.

MEDICATIONS FOR ARRHYTHMIA

The healthy functioning of your heart's electrical system relies on the precise control of different electrolyte levels—specifically, sodium, potassium, and calcium—which move through channels between your cells and your blood. (Electrolytes are minerals that carry an electric charge.) The drugs doctors use to treat electrical problems in the heart affect these different electrolyte channels. We describe the most commonly prescribed antiarrhythmic medications in the following section.

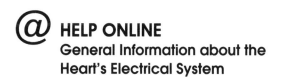

HELP ONLINE
General Information about the Heart's Electrical System

The National Institutes of Health Patient
Education: www.nhlbi.nih.gov/health/dci/

American College of Cardiology:
www.cardiosmart.org

Beta Blockers Resist Adrenaline

Well known to patients with high blood pressure or heart failure, beta blockers are a mainstay of arrhythmia treatment. These medications block certain stimulating signal receptors, called beta-adrenergic receptors, found on cells in the heart, lungs, and blood vessels. The receptors transmit signals that affect heart rate and strength of contraction, airflow to the lungs, and blood flow through vessels. Many of these drugs will block the receptors in most if not all of these locations. They include the following:

- Carvedilol (Coreg)
- Nadolol
- Propranolol
- Timolol (Blockadren)

However, some beta blockers, such as the following, are specific to only the beta-1 receptors found predominantly in the heart:

- Atenolol (Tenormin)
- Bisoprolol (Zebeta)
- Bystolic (Nebivolol)
- Esmolol (Brevibloc)
- Metoprolol (Lopressor, Toprol XL)

These drugs have fewer side effects than drugs that are not as specific: fewer breathing difficulties and less change in blood pressure.

Beta blockers are some of the most popularly used medications to control heart rate. The vast majority of arrhythmias that we treat with medications have to do with the heart beating *too fast*. Beta blockers can easily slow the heart without major side effects, are well tolerated by patients, and are easily available.

Warning: Beta blockers can worsen symptoms of heart failure, especially if they are given at too high a dose and too quickly. Other potential side effects include slowing the heart rate excessively and although rarely, confusion, depression, and impotence (erectile dysfunction) can occur.

Sotalol Blocks Potassium

Sotalol has beta-blocking ability and blocks potassium channels. Your doctor may prescribe sotalol if you have not responded to more commonly used drugs. It is more effective at slowing the heart, but also can carry increased risk of disturbing the heart's natural rhythm. Many patients must be hospitalized for the first few doses to closely monitor how their hearts respond to the medication. People with internal defibrillators may be less likely to receive shocks while taking sotalol.

Amiodarone Decreases Risk

Amiodarone (Cordarone) is a well known and widely used antiarrhythmic drug. It generally decreases the risk of arrhythmias throughout the heart, therefore making it highly versatile. Your doctor may prescribe it if you've previously had a life-threatening arrhythmia, such as ventricular tachycardia or ventricular fibrillation. You may also take it to prevent reoccurrence of atrial fibrillation. Amiodarone can also decrease the number of shocks delivered to patients who have internal defibrillators (described on pages 100–103).

Amiodarone does have some negative side effects. It can cause skin changes, thyroid function abnormality, and more rarely, lung or liver damage. Serious harm is rare, and your doctor will monitor your laboratory and lung function tests carefully while you are on amiodarone.

Flecainide Blocks Sodium Channels

Flecainide blocks the sodium channels in the heart. The result is decreased conductivity of the electrical impulse through the heart tissue. Flecainide is often prescribed for patients who have had life-threatening abnormalities of conduction through the ventricles of their heart.

You can take Flecainide only when you need to—an approach called the pill-in-the-pocket method. This is in sharp contrast to the other medications we cover in this section, which are taken daily to treat and prevent arrhythmias and should not be stopped without your doctor's knowledge.

The pill-in-the-pocket method of taking Flecainide applies to a particular group of patients who always know when they are experiencing an arrhythmia, specifically atrial fibrillation. Flecainide can get some patients' hearts back to a normal rhythm with just one or two doses. However, this approach must be explored with your doctor; inappropriate self-medication could lead to sudden life-threatening arrhythmias or strokes!

Diltiazem and Verapamil Block Calcium Channels

Well known to many patients with high blood pressure, diltiazem and verapamil also are commonly used antiarrhythmic drugs. Both drugs block calcium ion channels in the heart, limiting conduction through the AV node (described later in this chapter) and thus blocking signals from the atria to the ventricles. These drugs are particularly useful in controlling the heart rate in patients with arrhythmias such as atrial fibrillation, atrial flutter, or SVT (described on pages 104–106).

Diltiazem and verapamil are generally well tolerated, with few serious or symptomatic side effects in the vast majority of patients. However, they can decrease blood pressure and heart rate more than desired.

Digoxin (a.k.a. Digitalis)

Digoxin, which is also called digitalis, is usually used to treat heart failure symptoms, and can be useful for arrhythmias as well. Digoxin can decrease the rate of some fast-beating arrhythmias, while at the same time increasing the force of the heart's contraction. However, blood levels of digoxin can fluctuate wildly, reaching toxic levels without warning, particularly when starting or stopping other medications. Therefore, if you are taking digoxin, your doctor should know about all the other medications you take and may follow your blood levels of digoxin occasionally.

Side effects of digoxin can include an abnormally low heart rate, which can cause symptoms of fatigue, lightheadedness, or fainting.

Warfarin Thins the Blood

Although warfarin (Coumadin) is not a drug that affects the heart's electrical system, many patients with irregular rhythms take it. Warfarin is an anticoagulant; it makes the blood thinner and less likely to form a clot. Clots are what stop us from bleeding when we injure ourselves or have surgery; the clot plugs the hole.

Blood clots form in response to certain triggers: injury to a blood vessel, foreign bodies such as prosthetics, intravenous catheters, artificial heart valves, and even when blood is not flowing. This last one is particularly important to patients with arrhythmias. Patients with arrhythmias of the atria, particularly atrial fibrillation, have decreased flow of blood in these chambers of the heart. While the atria are "quivering" as in atrial fibrillation, blood stands still until the ventricles relax and allow them to fill with more blood from the atria. This is in contrast to patients without atrial fibrillation—their atria will contract and eject blood into the ventricles. Thus, because blood is static for a significant period of time in patients with atrial fibrillation, they have an increased risk of forming clots, particularly in the left atrium. If these clots become dislodged from the walls of the atria, they could travel out of the heart and obstruct any of the small blood vessels supplying critical organs—most importantly the brain, where it can cause a stroke. Thus, patients with atrial fibrillation who are not on warfarin have a higher risk of stroke than patients without atrial fibrillation.

This is not to say that every patient with atrial fibrillation should be on warfarin. Several factors deter-

 HEART HELP:

Tips for Patients on Warfarin

- Changes in your diet can affect your blood levels of anticoagulant, and your doctor may need to adjust the doses of warfarin accordingly. Certain foods high in vitamin K, such as green, leafy vegetables, are particularly potent in altering blood levels.

- Many other medicines can interfere with warfarin. It is very important to discuss any medication changes with your doctor.

- Warfarin significantly increases the risk of bleeding. This includes nose bleeds, bleeding when brushing your teeth, bruising from minor bumps, or blood in your stools. Be sure to alert your doctor to any of these symptoms. Furthermore, bleeding may occur during any procedures you have or in places you might not notice right away.

- It is important to tell all people caring for you that you are taking warfarin.

- It may be necessary to stop your warfarin briefly to undergo surgery or certain procedures or tests. This should be coordinated by your doctor to ensure that a plan is formulated for your medicines. Typically, warfarin is stopped three days prior to surgery to allow the effects to wear off, but your doctor will need to determine how long (or if at all) it should be stopped prior to surgery or a procedure.

CHADS2 Score to Predict the Risk of Stroke

Stroke Risk in Patients With Nonvalvular AF Not Treated With Anticoagulation Accordding to the CHADS2 Index

CHADS2 RISK CRITERIA	SCORE
Prior stroke or TIA	2
Age: more than 75 years	1
Hypertension	1
Diabetes mellitus	1
Heart failure	1

PATIENTS (N=1733)	ADJUSTED STROKE RATE (%/Y)* (95% CI)	CHADS$_2$ SCORE
120	1.9 (1.2 to 3.0)	0
463	2.8 (2.0 to 3.8)	1
523	4.0 (3.1 to 5.1)	2
337	5.9 (4.6 to 7.3)	3
220	8.5 (6.3 to 11.1)	4
65	12.5 (8.2 to 17.5)	5
5	18.2 (10.5 to 27.4)	6

*The adjusted stroke rate was derived from multivariate analysis assuming no aspirin usage. Data are from van Walraven WC, Hart RG, Wells GA, et al. A clinical prediction rule to identify patients with atrial fibrillation and a low risk for stroke while taking aspirin. Arch Intern Med 2003;163:936—43 (415); and Gage BF, Waterman AD, Shannon W, et al. Validation of clinical classification schemes for predicting stroke: results from the National Registry of Atrial Fibrillation. JAMA 2001;285:2864—70 (426).

Antithrombotic Thearpy for Patients with Atrial Fibrillation

RISK CATEGORY	RECOMMENDED
No risk factors	Aspirin, 81 to 325 mg daily
One moderate-risk factor	Aspirin, 81 to 325 mg daily, or warfarin (INR 2.0 to 3.0, target 2.5)
Any high-risk factor or more than 1 moderate-risk factor	Warfarin (INR 2.0 to 3.0, target 2.5)

Source: ACC/AHA/ESC 2006 Guidelines for Management of Patients with Nonvalvular AF Not Treated with Antiocoagulation According to the CHADS2 Index (J Am Coll Cariol, 2006; 48:854—906)

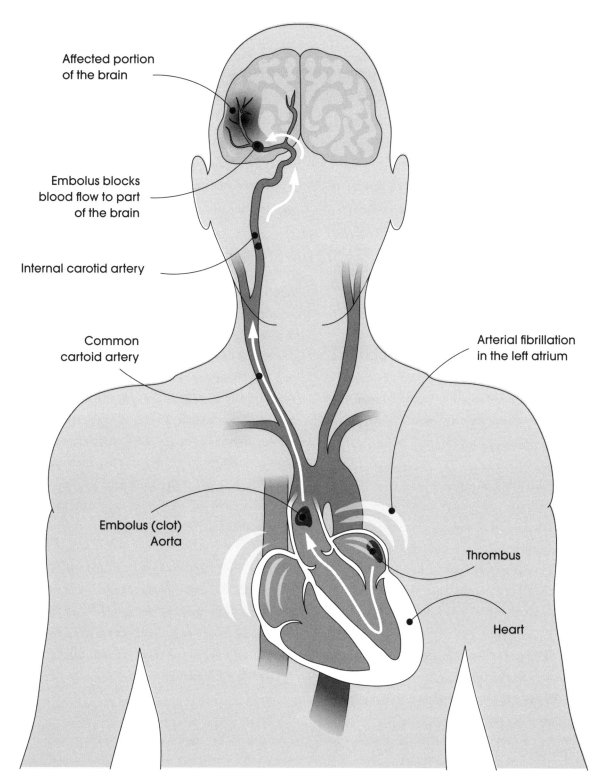

Affected portion
of the brain

Embolus blocks
blood flow to part
of the brain

Internal carotid artery

Common
cartoid artery

Embolus (clot)
Aorta

Arterial fibrillation
in the left atrium

Thrombus

Heart

Aratrial clot leading to stroke

mine your risk of stroke with atrial fibrillation: most importantly, your age, history of high blood pressure, history of heart failure, whether you have diabetes, and whether you have had a stroke in the past. In addition, your doctor will weigh the risk of stroke against the risk of being on warfarin; there is a significant risk of bleeding in patients taking warfarin.

Lastly, because of variable blood levels and the risk of bleeding, patients on warfarin must have their blood levels checked frequently, particularly when just starting on the medication. They may need to be checked as often as several times per week early on and when adjusting doses.

TESTS, DIAGNOSIS, AND PROCEDURES

In addition to hearing about your symptoms and examining you, your doctor has many tests available to evaluate the electrical system of your heart. The first step is an electrocardiogram (ECG or EKG).

Electrocardiogram (ECG)

This is a simple, noninvasive, painless test to assess the heart's electrical conduction in a snapshot. Many of us have had one as part of a routine evaluation—it involves sticking electrodes to the skin, while a machine measures the heart's electrical activity. It can provide your doctor with a lot of information:

- Whether your heart is beating at regular intervals or irregularly and unpredictably
- Whether the heart is beating at the right speed or rate
- The correct beating of both the atria and the ventricles, and the right speed of conduction between the two
- Confirmation of synchronization of left and right ventricular contraction

- Whether the size of your heart's chambers has changed. (Echocardiogram is the best option.)
- Whether you have had a heart attack

However, if you are not having symptoms, or your heart is not experiencing arrhythmia at the time you take the test, the ECG cannot show what your heart did in the past or what it might do in the future. For this reason, your doctor may recommend some related tests, which we discuss in the following sections.

Holter Studies and Event Monitors

Holter studies and event monitors are like security cameras for the heart's rhythm. They record what's happening over a set period of time, in hopes of catching the heart in an arrhythmia. They are ECG recordings that run continuously over days (Holter) or only when you are having symptoms (event monitors). Similar to an ECG, they involve sticking electrodes to your body to measure electrical currents. After you wear the recorder for a certain period of time, you return it to your doctor for analysis. Your doctor then looks at the recording and correlates your symptoms to what your heart rhythm was doing at that time.

Holter studies and event monitors can be particularly helpful for patients who always seem to have symptoms when they are *not* at the doctor! This is not unusual; heart arrhythmias can easily come and go with no sign or warning, making it difficult to catch them "in the act."

Invasive Electrophysiology Studies

Even with Holter studies or event monitors, some patients will not experience symptoms or arrhythmias while their heart is being recorded. Or they will have arrhythmias while on a cardiac monitor in the hospital, without warning or symptoms. These could rep-

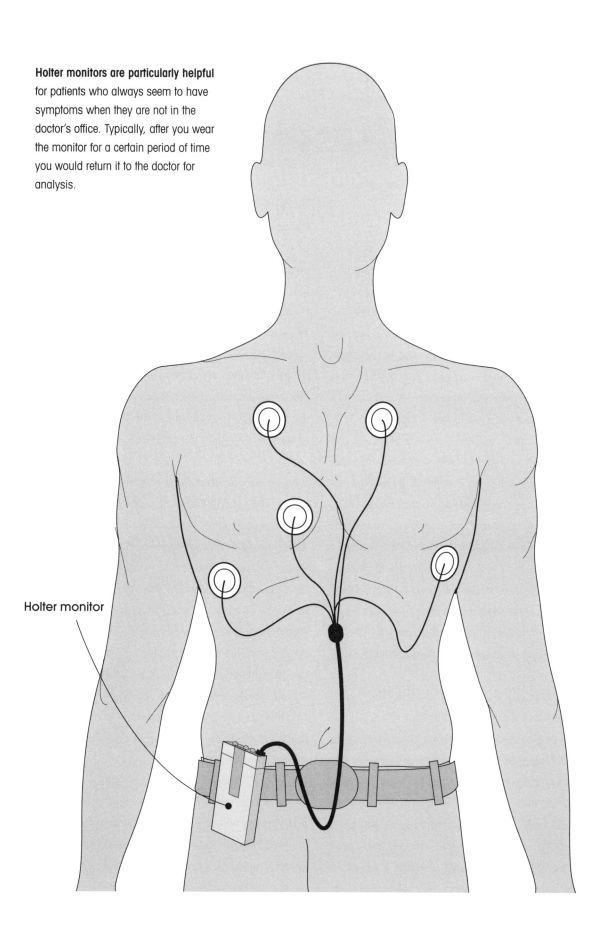

Holter monitors are particularly helpful for patients who always seem to have symptoms when they are not in the doctor's office. Typically, after you wear the monitor for a certain period of time you would return it to the doctor for analysis.

Holter monitor

resent dangerous arrhythmias of the ventricles that need to be addressed, yet come and go without warning. In such scenarios, your doctor may recommend that you undergo a procedure to induce or elicit such arrhythmias to determine where in the heart they are coming from and how they can be prevented.

These procedures are done only by experienced electrophysiologists and their teams of trained medical personnel who know how to handle arrhythmias. Such procedures are similar to cardiac catheterizations, performed for patients with heart attacks or coronary artery disease (CAD). They both involve placing large IVs (intravenous needles) in the groin through which multiple catheters can be threaded up toward the heart. The placement of catheters is verified by X-ray video called *fluoroscopy*.

The electrophysiologist inserts catheters into the heart, which stimulate various parts of the heart to determine where the arrhythmia may have originated. During such a procedure, they can take recordings of the electrical conduction *inside* the heart for a much closer look at the heart's electrical system, and can easily narrow the location of the problem within the system. Based on the results of such tests, the electrophysiologist and your doctor can decide the best course of treatment for your arrhythmia.

Cardiac Defibrillation Shocks the Heart

Defibrillation is the technical term for shocking the heart; it is also commonly known as cardioverting or "undergoing DC cardioversion." It is one of the many ways to convert the heart out of an arrhythmia and is most commonly used in urgent or emergent situations for life-threatening arrhythmias, when the patient is either unconscious or sedated (it is quite uncomfortable). High-voltage electricity is delivered by direct current through two paddles or pads pressed against the chest, stunning the heart back into its natural rhythm. Less commonly, defibrillation is also used for patients with new arrhythmias that are less serious, if drugs have not worked in converting their hearts back to normal rhythm.

Pacemakers and Internal Defibrillators

Pacemakers and implantable cardioverter defibrillators (ICDs) are two devices that are often easily confused and for good reason. Both are little boxes that an electrophysiologist surgically places over the heart to help control the heart's electrical system. Without knowing beforehand, there is actually no way to tell which one (or both!) a patient has. Both devices involve wires that are threaded through blood vessels to the heart and connect to the box under the skin. However, most similarities end there, as they serve very different purposes.

A *pacemaker* ensures that the heart retains a regular, steady beat that is neither too fast nor too slow. To do this, it must know what the heart is doing. Therefore, the pacemaker senses the heart's rhythm at all times, similar to a continuous, internal ECG. When the heart deviates from its proper rhythm the pacemaker steps in to correct it by giving tiny electrical stimulation to cause a contraction. This stimulation is delivered through the implanted wires and can be to either the atria or the ventricles (or both), depending on which needs to beat and when. The electrical stimulation from a pacemaker is much less than that for defibrillation. You cannot even tell when the pacemaker steps in.

There are many reasons to get a pacemaker: for arrhythmias where the heart is beating too slow or too fast; for patients whose arrhythmias have not responded to medicine; or for those who cannot tolerate the medicines because of side effects.

Inner Workings of a Pacemaker

The typical pacemaker has a wire in the right atrium and right ventricle, to sense and pace the rhythms of the heart. Pacing then travels, albeit slowly, to the left. However, some patients with heart failure greatly benefit from having both the left and right ventricles contract at the exact same time. In these patients, a Bi-V or biventricular pacemaker—with wires for both sides of the heart—may be placed to coordinate the precise contraction of both the right and left ventricles simultaneously.

In other circumstances, patients with arrhythmias have an electrical system that is too diseased to repair. In these circumstances, the natural circuits of the heart are disabled, and the patient becomes entirely dependent on the artificial pacemaker to initiate every beat. Without the disturbing arrhythmias of a diseased system, the manmade pacemaker takes over and initiates each contraction the heart makes. This can be somewhat unsettling for some patients, to feel dependent on a manmade device for their heart to beat. However, it is important to remember that many patients have a "backup" rate, at which their ventricles may contract, albeit much more slowly than usual, and the dependability of manmade pacemakers has been superb, with patients undergoing routine checks every six to twelve months to ensure appropriate functionality.

Pacemaker function can be assessed without performing surgery. The pacemaker communicates wirelessly with a specialized computer, which "interrogates" it. The computer can assess many different factors, such as the following:

- Is there sufficient battery life?
- Are the wires still in the correct place?

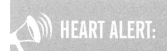

HEART ALERT:

Getting Shocked Hurts!

Many people wonder what it feels like to receive a shock to the heart. It hurts! Patients with ICDs compare the sensation of their ICD firing to that of being punched in the chest, as though the air has been knocked out of them. Therefore, these devices are carefully programmed to recognize only certain arrhythmias that absolutely need to be shocked in life-threatening situations. Should they fire inappropriately, they can be reprogrammed to recognize the correct arrhythmia.

- How many beats has the pacemaker had to "help" with?
- Has the heart rate been abnormally high or low?
- Have there been any arrhythmias, and if so, what did they look like? The pacemaker can record such events and replay them when interrogated.

If the pacemaker has to be adjusted, this can be done without breaking the skin. At some point, however, the battery must be replaced during a procedure similar to the initial implantation. Fortunately, this is necessary only about every five to eight years.

ICD, Just in Case

In contrast to pacemakers, ICDs serve only as defibrillators if hearts go into dangerous life-threatening rhythms. ICDs do not help hearts stay in their proper rhythm. However, should your heart get sidetracked and run away into a dangerous mode, the ICD can deliver a shock of electricity through its wires as a way to "reset" your heart's own pacemaker cells. This is the same effect as a defibrillator placed on a patient's chest to shock the heart out of a dangerous rhythm, only it is always with you. Furthermore, an ICD requires less energy, because it does not have to pass electricity through the skin, as an external defibrillator does.

Many patients get an ICD because their heart previously experienced a life-threatening arrhythmia that either resolved on its own or for which they were externally defibrillated. However, a great majority of patients nowadays receive ICDs because they have moderate or severe heart failure. As described in chapter 4, patients whose hearts have become enlarged are at significantly increased risk for life-threatening arrhythmias of the ventricles. Research has demonstrated that we can prevent deaths by implanting ICDs in these patients, even if they have not yet experienced such an arrhythmia—it might then be too late.

Invasive Surgery for Arrhythmias

Surgery is typically limited for arrhythmias. Atrial fibrillation is the arrhythmia most amenable to surgery because it is often due to the stretching of the atria—a structural change that when reshaped surgically, can sometimes cure the problem (we describe atrial fibrillation further later in this chapter).

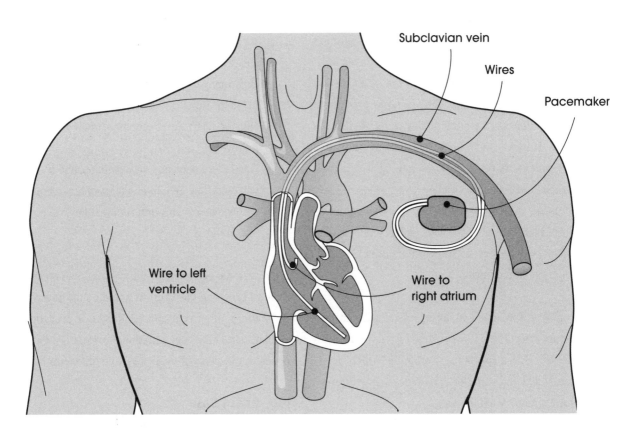

Subclavian vein

Wires

Pacemaker

Wire to left ventricle

Wire to right atrium

A biventricular pacemaker sends wires to both sides of the heart in order to coordinate the precise contraction of both the right and left ventricles simultaneously.

ICD and Pacemaker in One

Occasionally, patients need both an ICD and a pace-maker—but there's room for only one box! A new device combines the action of the ICD (to prevent deadly arrhythmias) and the biventricular pacemaker (to resynchronize failing hearts) to improve the quality of life for patients with heart failure.

How does it work? One such device, the CONTAK RENEWAL 3 AVT Cardiac Resynchronization Defibrillator (CRT-D) from Guidant Corp., consists of an implant-able pulse generator (IPG) consisting of a battery and electronic circuitry connected to three independent leads (insulated wires). The IPG is usually implanted below the collarbone, just beneath the skin. The leads are placed in three different areas:

- One in an upper heart chamber (the right atrium)

- A second lead in a lower heart chamber (the right ventricle)

- A third lead in a vein that overlies the left ventricle

When the device is functioning as an ICD, it senses dangerous abnormal heart rhythms and shocks the heart back into a normal rhythm. The pacemaker portion of the device uses small electrical impulses to coordinate the beating of the left and right ventricles so that they work together more effectively to pump blood throughout the body. An atrial therapy portion of the device detects and treats rapid heart rates in the atrium.

Who needs one? Combination ICD/pacemakers are used in certain patients who have all of the following:

- Symptoms of advanced heart failure despite taking heart failure medication

- A heart rhythm problem that may cause the lower chambers of the heart to beat in an uncoordinated manner

- A history of or the probability of developing heart rhythm problems in the upper chambers of the heart

Combination devices are also indicated for patients with moderate to severe heart failure (NYHA III/IV) who re-main symptomatic despite stable, optimal heart failure drug therapy, and have left ventricular dysfunction.

Are there any downsides? Doctors say the therapy is cost-effective and increases quality of life because of reduced hospital stays. However, at around $20,000, the devices are expensive.

However, heart surgery is a very invasive approach for a condition that can often be managed with medicines; most commonly, surgery is performed only if another operation (such as a bypass or valve replacement) is also planned.

THE HEART'S ELECTRICAL SYSTEM EXPLAINED

How does electricity control the beating heart? The basics of the heart's electrical system involve a node of circuitry in the heart's right atrium that acts as our own natural pacemaker, sparking each beat. This is the sinoatrial (SA) node. Its tissue is special. Its cells beat spontaneously at a certain rhythm, the rate of which is controlled by a host of factors: electrolytes and hormones in the blood, nerve signals from the brain, oxygen supply to the heart, or a change in pressures within or outside the heart.

Electricity from the SA node is then conducted from the right atrium across to the left atrium and they both beat; it then travels down to another special piece of tissue called the atrioventricular (AV) node. The dispersion of current up to this point is relatively slow as it travels through muscle, and that's okay—it's not critical that the atria contract at exactly the same time. However, at the AV node, the current really takes off.

For the heart to pump most efficiently and effectively, the muscle throughout each ventricle must contract at nearly the same time. Unfortunately, if the electrical signals dispersed only through muscle, this would lead to a disorganized contraction of the muscle. Instead, a collection of high-speed fibers called the His-Purkinje system provides a more efficient conduction pathway through the ventricles. From the AV node, the electrical impulse travels much faster down these fibers, and out to the muscle of each ventricle. It is via this system that each ventricle contracts at nearly the same time.

ARRHYTHMIAS EXPLAINED

Disturbances of the heart's electrical system are commonly organized in two different ways:

- By rate, based on whether the heart rate is too fast or too slow
- By location, based on whether the primary disturbance is in the atria or ventricles

Arrhythmias that are too fast are termed tachyarrhythmias, whereas those characterized by heart rates that are too slow are called bradyarrhythmias. These characteristics determine the best treatment and medications to use. The majority of symptomatic, recognized arrhythmias are tachyarrhythmias.

Atrial Fibrillation

Perhaps the most common and well-known arrhythmia is atrial fibrillation—an atrial tachyarrhythmia. Atrial fibrillation is characterized by a quivering or fibrillating of the atria; that is, the atria are not beating in an organized fashion, but merely shaking so fast that they do not contribute meaningfully to moving blood forward. You may wonder how blood flow is maintained in this case. Remember: It is the contraction of the ventricles that is most important to blood flow.

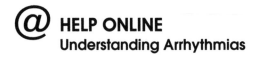

@ HELP ONLINE
Understanding Arrhythmias

The AHA's Arrhythmia Patient Education page: www.hearthub.org/hc-arrhythmia.htm

Heart Rhythm Society: www.hrsonline.org

Although some patients may be symptomatic from atrial fibrillation (they may feel palpitations, lightheaded, or dizzy), blood flow is usually easily maintained.

Atrial fibrillation is often the result of persistent stretching of the atria. As the atria expand, they lose the ability to contract in a coordinated, synchronized, and meaningful way. Thus, they quiver. Patients with long-standing heart failure, CAD, or disease of the heart valves commonly get atrial fibrillation. However, it can occur on its own as well.

Treatment for atrial fibrillation usually involves one of two approaches. Either your doctor will try to control the rhythm of the atria and get them back to their normal contractions, or your doctor will simply try to control the rate at which your ventricles contract in response to the rapid atrial rate. Once the atria have entered fibrillation, it can become difficult to convert them back to their regular rhythm, particularly if the underlying disease (heart failure, CAD, etc.) is still present. However, occasionally, it is worth trying to change the rhythm back, and this can be done with an attempt at external defibrillation (cardioversion), medications, catheter ablation, or if necessary, invasive surgery. The more invasive measures are usually reserved for the minority of patients who cannot tolerate being in atrial fibrillation.

WHAT'S NEW:

Catheter-based Ablations

One of the most significant advances in treating arrhythmias is catheter-based ablation. These procedures are often performed following an invasive electrophysiology study, as detailed earlier. They involve the same catheters and specialized cardiologists and serve as potentially curative procedures for some arrhythmias.

How does it work? Many of the heart's irregular rhythms are the result of abnormal heart tissue—tissue that is overexcitable, misplaced, the result of a scar in the heart, or electrically imbalanced. The technique of ablation commonly involves concentrating radio waves (similar to microwaves) to destroy the specific tissue that is causing such arrhythmias. Computed tomography and magnetic resonance imaging are used to map out complex electrical pathways in the heart prior to such procedures. An alternative technique is to use cryoablation, in which very cold gas and liquid are infused into abnormal tissue, rendering it electrically neutral.

Does it hurt? The ablation itself is painless and cannot be felt.

Further advances in using computer-controlled catheters allow for much more precise ablations of complicated arrhythmias in both the atria and ventricles. This has expanded the role for catheter-based ablations to include many more rhythm disturbances, making it applicable to a broader selection of patients.

More commonly, atrial fibrillation is treated by controlling the ventricular rate. Remember, the ventricles get their cues from the atria. If the atria are quivering too quickly to move blood, they are also sending fast signals to the ventricles. Luckily, these signals must go through the AV node, the gatekeeper of the ventricles. Thus, if we can control the rate at which the ventricles respond to the atria, blood flow is not compromised. Some patients may benefit from anticoagulation with warfarin if they remain in atrial fibrillation over the long term (see the section "Warfarin Thins the Blood," earlier in this chapter).

Atrial Flutter

Atrial flutter is another common atrial tachyarrhythmia. It is closely related to atrial fibrillation. The major difference is that the atria are fluttering at a lower rate than the hummingbird-like quiver that is atrial fibrillation. The treatment approaches are similar, as some patients can even switch back and forth between atrial flutter and fibrillation. Atrial flutter can sometimes be an arrhythmia of young people with otherwise healthy hearts; this may indicate a focal abnormality in heart tissue, where an ablation is more likely to be successful. The overall success at converting atria out of flutter is higher than that for atrial fibrillation.

Supraventricular Tachycardia

Supraventricular tachycardia, or SVT, is a common label for a group of tachyarrhythmias that start above the ventricles, either in the atria or in the AV node. This collection of arrhythmias share a common cause: They typically involve abnormal tissue that creates a circuit of electricity, without exit. Thus, when this circuit is set off, electricity travels around it repeatedly, stimulating various parts of the heart and resulting in faster than normal contractions. SVT is most commonly an arrhythmia

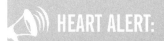

of young patients, born with such circuits. They often experience very distinct episodes of symptoms, where the circuit is acutely activated. SVT arrhythmias can often be cured with catheter-based ablation.

Ventricular Tachycardia

Ventricular tachycardia is a fast arrhythmia of the ventricles. It occurs when the ventricles take off on their own, without cues from the atria, and contract at inappropriately high rates. This can be very dangerous, as the high rates can prevent blood from filling the ventricles, leading them to contract without blood in them, diminishing blood flow to the body. Very rarely, patients with ventricular tachycardia can be stable and asymptomatic; however, the vast majority of occurrences of ventricular tachycardia are medical emergencies due to the potential for compromising blood flow and thus require external defibrillation immediately.

Wolff-Parkinson-White Syndrome

Accessory tract of Wolff-Parkinson-White Syndrome

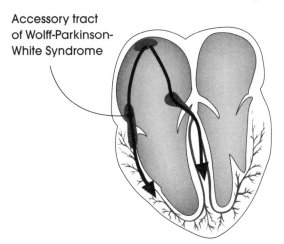

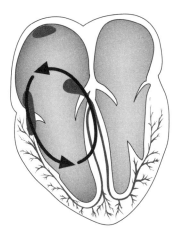

Sinus rhythm

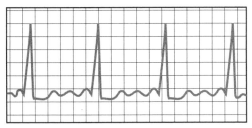

Antidromic tachycardia

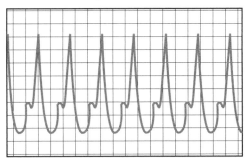

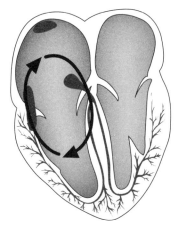

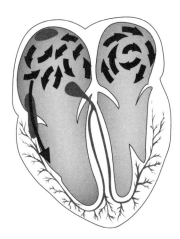

Orthodromic tachycardia

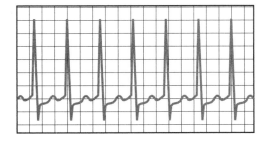

Atrial fibration

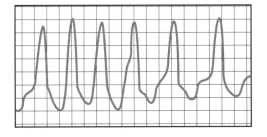

Certain changes on a patients electrocardiogram can signal Wolff-Parkinson-White Syndrome, in which electricity travels an alternate route—or a shortcut—through tissue and arrives at the ventricles too soon.

Ventricular tachycardia is most often the result of scar tissue from a previous or acute heart attack; this tissue is irritable and prone to arrhythmias. Rarely, ventricular tachycardia can be due to electrolyte abnormalities (usually potassium or magnesium) or birth defects in the heart's electrical system. Due to the danger for compromised blood flow, most patients who have an episode of ventricular tachycardia will get an ICD, in case they have any recurrent episodes.

Ventricular Fibrillation

Ventricular fibrillation is also characterized by a quivering of the ventricles. This leads to a drop in blood flow and is a medical emergency, requiring immediate defibrillation by shocking. Similar to ventricular tachycardia, ventricular fibrillation is commonly the result of a previous or ongoing heart attack, where a part of the ventricles either has or is developing a scar that is susceptible to electrical irritability. Ventricular fibrillation, combined with ventricular tachycardia, is the most common cause of death in patients who die suddenly from a heart attack. Less commonly, patients with other very severe medical illnesses or electrolyte abnormalities can experience ventricular fibrillation.

Wolff-Parkinson-White Syndrome

Congenital malformations of the heart are relatively rare causes of arrhythmias in general. However, one of the most common anomalies of the heart's electrical system is the existence of an accessory pathway—that is, alternative tissue conducting beats to the ventricles, aside from the His-Purkinje system (see page 107). This tissue can cause beats to reach the ventricles even faster than usual, activating them early (called *pre-excitation*). Normally, patients do not have symptoms.

The existence of an accessory pathway makes it much easier for the heart to experience circu-

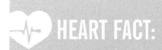

itous arrhythmias; the electrical current can just go around and around and around! This is experienced as palpitations, lightheadedness, flushing, or dizziness. Rarely, these episodes can represent life-threatening ventricular tachycardia. For this reason, patients with such symptoms are recommended for treatment. They can be treated with medications or they may undergo catheter-based or surgical ablation of the accessory pathway, a curative procedure.

Bradyarrhythmias

Although it is less common than hearts that beat too quickly, hearts can beat too slowly, a condition called bradyarrhythmia. This condition is usually not the result of extra circuits or abnormal tissue within the heart; therefore, ablation and defibrillation do not work. Occasionally, low heart rates can be from an ongoing heart attack. More commonly, they are caused by abnormal AV nodes or His-Purkinje systems. Patients with dangerous bradyarrhythmias receive permanent pacemakers to ensure that their hearts beat regularly at an appropriate rate.

Q. & A. with Dr. Cannon

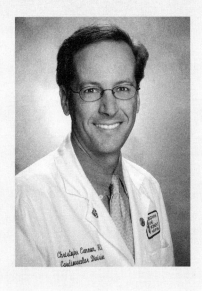

Christopher Cannon, MD
Cardiovascular Division

Q. I am taking warfarin for my atrial fibrillation and will be having knee surgery next month. What should I do about the warfarin?

A. It is usually necessary to stop your warfarin briefly to undergo surgery (and other major procedures). Typically, warfarin is stopped three days prior to surgery to allow the effects to wear off, but your doctor will need to determine how long (or if at all) it should be stopped prior to surgery or a procedure.

Q. We always hear about the risk of heart attack with cholesterol and high blood pressure. What risks exist with atrial fibrillation?

A. The biggest risk is a stroke. A blood clot can form inside the top chamber of the heart (atrium) and then break off and go to the brain, leading to a stroke. This is a greater risk in patients who have certain risk factors (see the CHADS2 score on page 96). It is important to strongly consider taking blood-thinning medications to prevent a stroke.

Q. Is installing a pacemaker a dangerous procedure?

A. No. Having a pacemaker implanted is a relatively minor procedure with very rare complications. Sometimes patients will get some swelling or bleeding where the pacemaker is placed, but it will usually resolve.

Q. My doctor said my heart is weak and I should have an implantable cadioverter defibrillator (ICD). Is that worth it?

A. Yes. ICDs are one of the great advances in preventing sudden cardiac death, which impacts more than 300,000 patients each year in the United States. Former vice president Dick Cheney had one put in to prevent sudden death.

chapter 6:

STRUCTURAL HEART DISEASE

STRUCTURAL HEART DISEASE

℞ THE PRESCRIPTION

This diagnosis may lead your doctor to prescribe a wide range of medicines. If your disease is caused by a disorder unrelated to the heart—an infection, for example, or even a rheumatologic disorder such as lupus—the first task will be to treat that condition. This may involve antibiotics, steroids, or other medications. Your doctor may not prescribe medicine if the defect is discovered as the result of routine tests, your heart is functioning well, and you have no symptoms.

Many of the therapies for structural heart disease are familiar to patients with heart failure or high blood pressure. The therapeutic goals for all three conditions are the same: to relieve stress on the heart, optimize heart function to prevent progression to heart failure, and relieve symptoms. However, it is important to note that none of these medicines can fix a structural problem with the heart; for many defects, catheter-based procedures or open heart surgery is the only treatment.

STRUCTURAL DEFECTS AND DISEASES

Mitral stenosis, atrial septal defect (ASD), and patent ductus arteriosus (PDA)—these are just some of the major structural defects that occur in the complex architecture of the heart. They range from heart defects that occur at birth, called congenital defects, to diseases of the heart valves that occur over a lifetime. Because many of the therapies and diagnostic procedures that treat them are the same, we have grouped them together in this chapter. They are as follows:

Valvular Heart Disease

Mitral Stenosis

Mitral Regurgitation

Aortic Stenosis

Aortic Regurgitation

Tricuspid Stenosis

Tricuspid Regurgitation

Pulmonary Valve Disease

Endocarditis

Congenital Heart Disease

Atrial Septal Defect

Ventricular Septal Defect

Patent Ductus Arteriosus

Transposition of the Great Arteries

Tetralogy of Fallot

A quick glance at the heart's structure will help you understand how and where these defects and diseases occur and how they affect the heart's functioning (see chapter 8 for a tour of the heart).

Heart Primer

The heart is divided into two sides, left and right, with two chambers on each side. The chambers are called atria and ventricles; each of us has a left atrium and ventricle and a right atrium and ventricle. The atria receive blood, and the ventricles pump blood out. The left side of the heart receives oxygenated blood from the lungs and pumps it out to the rest of the body; the right side of the heart takes blood back from the body after the oxygen has been depleted and pumps it into the lungs, where the cycle begins again. In a healthy heart, blood flowing through the left and right sides doesn't mix.

Four heart valves ensure that blood moves in the correct direction when the ventricles contract: one valve between each atrium and ventricle, and one at the outflow of each ventricle.

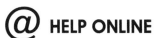 **HELP ONLINE**

For general information from the National Institutes of Health Information on Congenital Heart Defects: www.nhlbi.nih.gov/health/dci/Diseases/chd/chd_what.html

For information on valvular disease: www.nhlbi.nih.gov/health/dci/Diseases/hvd/hvd_whatis.html

TREATING STRUCTURAL HEART DISEASES WITH MEDICINE

Diuretics Help Remove Fluid

Many of the symptoms patients experience from structural heart diseases are related to having too much fluid, which can accumulate in the legs, abdomen, or lungs. This is generally a result of poor blood flow to the kidneys, where urine is produced. Diuretics increase the amount of urine produced by the kidneys, even when the flow to them is reduced, so you urinate more and retain less fluid. Diuretics can also be used to decrease blood pressure by lessening the amount of circulating fluid. Here are some examples of typical diuretics:

- Furosemide (Lasix)
- Bumetanide (Bumex)
- Torsemide (Demadex)
- Chlorothiazide (Diuril)
- Hydrochlorothiazide (HydroDiuril, Microzide)
- Metolazone (Zaroxolyn)

Every diuretic has pros and cons, and not all patients respond the same way to the same drug. The preceding list includes diuretics that mainly act on the kidney to increase urine output. However, other types of diuretics act differently—they can influence not only urine output, but also other hormonal effects in the body, and thereby improve heart function. These include the following:

- Spironolactone (Aldactone)
- Eplerenone (Inspra)

WHAT'S NEW:

Fewer Side Effects with Eplerenone

What's eplerenone? This new medication is an aldosterone blocker, similar to spironolactone. It works by blocking a chemical (aldosterone) in your body, which in turn lowers the amount of sodium and water the body retains. Both eplerenone and spironolactone are important therapies for heart failure and some structural heart diseases. However, through some of its hormonal actions, spironolactone can result in unpleasant side effects such as excessive breast development in men. Eplerenone provides the hormonal benefits to the heart with lower frequency of such side effects. It is also used to lower high blood pressure.

Are there any risks? Before taking eplerenone, tell your doctor if you have kidney or liver disease, high cholesterol, or high triglycerides. To be sure this medication is helping your condition and is not causing harmful effects, your blood pressure and potassium levels will need to be checked on a regular basis. If you are taking this medication, don't miss any scheduled appointments! Keep using this medicine as directed, even if you feel well. Hypertension often has no symptoms, so you may not know when your blood pressure is high.

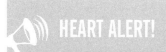

ADJUST THE BLOOD PRESSURE

Another way to manage structural defects of the heart is to adjust blood pressure. In many of these cases, patients experience symptoms and progression to heart failure because blood is not flowing well in the correct direction. This can occur in hearts with congenital defects and in hearts with valves that are diseased.

As the ventricles squeeze, blood moves out through the easiest path. In a healthy heart, valves prevent backflow of blood, and there are no structural defects or "holes" through which blood can escape. However, in hearts with such defects, the normal outflow to the body's blood vessels is decreased as blood escapes through a leaky valve or a hole in the heart. Think of a garden hose, with a leak between the open spigot and the sprinkler; turning off the sprinkler will worsen the leak in the hose, because that is the only escape route for the water. However, as the sprinkler is opened to allow more water out, the water flowing through the leak decreases. It has an alternate pathway of less resistance through the sprinkler. This is the key to treating defects of the heart—maintaining a pathway of less resistance through which blood can flow.

Thus, in hearts with various "leaks" or inappropriate blood flow, therapies that make it easier for blood to flow into the vessels of the body (where it is supposed to go) can help decrease stress on the heart. This is usually accomplished by dilating the body's blood vessels. Several medicines do this, which we describe in the following sections.

ACE Inhibitors and ARBs Dilate Blood Vessels

Angiotensin-converting enzyme (ACE) inhibitors and angiotensin-receptor blockers (ARBs) are two closely related, very popular medications commonly used for the treatment of high blood pressure. They are very good at dilating the body's blood vessels and are commonly used in patients with congenital or valvular heart disease. Common ACE inhibitors include the following:

- Benazepril (Lotensin)
- Captopril (Capoten)
- Enalapril (Vasotec)
- Fosinopril (Monopril)
- Lisinopril (Prinivil, Zestril)
- Quinapril (Accupril)
- Ramipril (Altace)
- Trandolapril (Mavik)

ARBs work similarly to ACE inhibitors and are sometimes better tolerated than ACE inhibitors. Examples of ARBs include the following:

- Candesartan (Atacand)
- Irbesartin (Avapro)
- Losartin (Cozaar)

- Telmisartin (Micardis)
- Valsartan (Diovan)

In addition to their ability to dilate blood vessels and help control blood flow in patients with structural heart disease, these medications may help the heart through a process called *remodeling*, in which they prevent a stressed-out heart from developing severe muscle dysfunction.

However, your doctor may not prescribe these medications if your blood pressure is already somewhat low. Additionally, one significant side effect of ACE inhibitors and ARBs can be a decline in kidney function, particularly when combined with diuretics (see earlier discussion). Therefore, your doctor will monitor your labs closely. Rarely, patients may also experience a cough or a rash from ACE inhibitors; these patients may better tolerate an ARB.

Hydralazine, a Reliable Dilator

Hydralazine is an older medication, less commonly used for the treatment of high blood pressure because it usually must be taken several times each day. However, it is very potent at dilating the body's blood vessels, can do so with more efficacy than ACE inhibitors or ARBs, and is less likely to affect the kidneys. Thus, it can be particularly useful in helping a heart with structural defects. However, it does not help the heart in productive remodeling, as ACE inhibitors and ARBs can.

Side effects of hydralazine include headache, nausea or vomiting, diarrhea, or sometimes high heart rates. Rarely, patients taking hydralazine can experience a rash or lupus-like syndrome; this is usually reversed once therapy is stopped.

Calcium-Channel Blockers

Another class of medications that are very effective at dilating the body's blood vessels is a certain type of calcium-channel blocker. These are different from the calcium-channel blockers described in chapter 5 that are used to treat diseases of the electrical system—verapamil and diltiazem. The class of calcium-channel blockers called *dihydropyridines* is much less likely to affect the calcium channels in the heart. Instead, they affect calcium channels in the blood vessels, causing them to relax or dilate. Common dihydropyridine calcium-channel blockers include the following:

- Amlodipine (Norvasc)
- Felodipine (Plendil)
- Nifedipine (Procardia)
- Nicardipine (Cardene)
- Nimodipine (Nimotop)

These medications are potent vessel dilators and are highly effective at treating high blood pressure. They can therefore be very effective in controlling blood flow in patients with structural heart disease. However, care must be taken that blood pressure does not drop too much.

Antibiotics Prevent Endocarditis

Patients with many types of structural heart disease, both congenital and valvular, are at increased risk of bacterial infections at the site of the defect. Bacteria in the bloodstream can "seed" these locations and grow into a dangerous and damaging infection known as endocarditis (described later in this chapter). Bacteria can transiently enter the bloodstream during many routine procedures, such as dental procedures or any surgeries. Thus, if you have a heart defect, your doctor may prescribe antibiotics for you to take prior to any medical or dental procedures.

Heart Defects and the Dentist

The following conditions usually require antibiotics to prevent endocarditis in the setting of surgical or dental procedures:

- Artificial prosthetic cardiac valve or prosthetic material used for valve repair
- Previous infective endocarditis
- Congenital heart disease (CHD):
  - Unrepaired cyanotic CHD or CHD with palliative shunts or implanted "tubes"
  - Completely repaired CHD with prosthetic material or device, whether placed by surgery or by catheter intervention, for six months after the procedure
  - Repaired CHD with residual defects at the site or adjacent to the site of a prosthetic patch or prosthetic device
- Cardiac transplantation recipients who develop valve disease

The following heart defects generally do not require antibiotic administration prior to dental or surgical procedures:*

- Congenital cardiac valve malformations, particularly those with bicuspid aortic valves, and patients with acquired valvular dysfunction (e.g., rheumatic heart disease)
- Patients with an isolated secundum ASD, or those who are six or more months past a successful surgical or catheter-based repair of an ASD, ventricular septal defect (VSD), or PDA
- Patients who have hypertrophic obstructive cardiomyopathy
- Patients who have undergone valve repair
- Most patients with mitral valve prolapse in the absence of mitral regurgitation
- Patients with physiological, functional, or innocent heart murmurs
- Patients with evidence of physiologic mitral or tricuspid regurgitation on an echocardiogram, in the absence of a murmur and with structurally normal valves

*Note: These guidelines have recently changed. Some doctors may still recommend antibiotics for certain conditions.

Source: American Heart Association (AHA) 2007 and 2008 guidelines

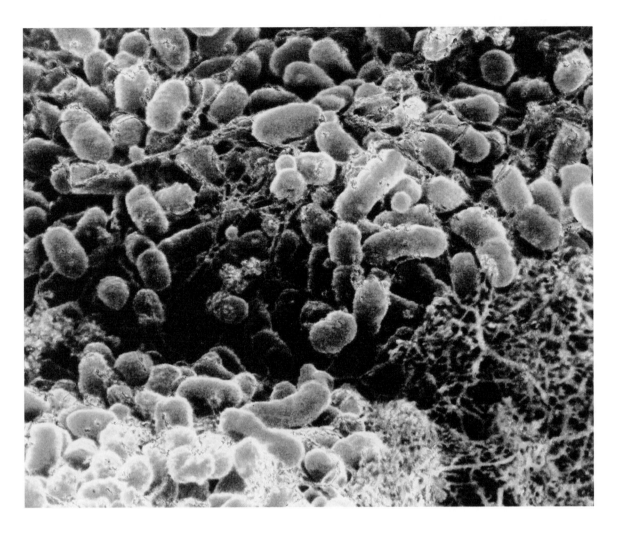

Actinobacillus actinomycetemecomitan. Close-up of the bacteria, actinobacillus actinomycetemecomitans, which can cause endocarditis, inflammation of the internal lining of the heart.

These may include any of the following:

- Amoxicillin
- Amoxicillin/clavulanate (Augmentin)
- Clindamycin (Cleocin)
- Azithromycin (Zithromax)

Although these agents do not affect the structural defect in the heart, they may prevent dangerous infections from complicating already diseased hearts. They are relatively well-tolerated medications whose major side effect is often upset stomach.

SURGICAL REPAIR OF STRUCTURAL DEFECTS

For the majority of structural defects of the heart, both congenital and valvular, medicines alone do not correct the problem. Rarely, these defects may correct by themselves, and sometimes they simply do not pose a big enough problem to require further treatment. However, many do require surgical intervention. This typically involves an invasive surgical procedure using a heart-lung bypass machine so that the heart can be stopped to operate on it. But do not fear! In the many years in which surgeons

Heart Valve Replacements

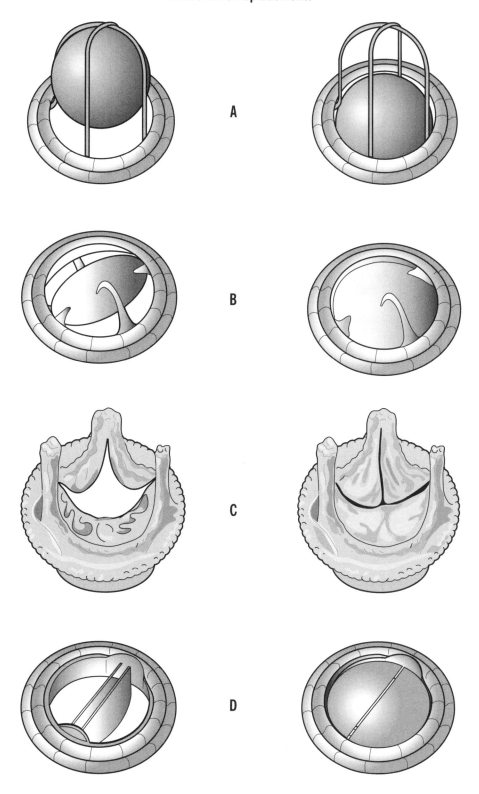

Examples of heart valves. Mechanical valves: **A, B, D**. Valve made from cow tissue: **C**.

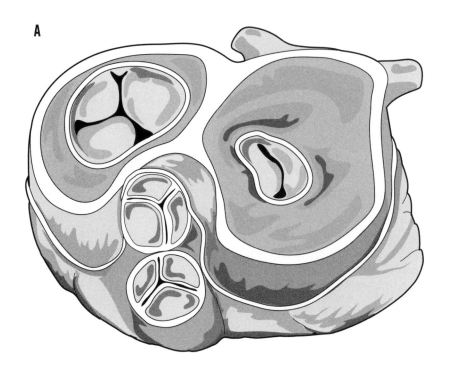

A

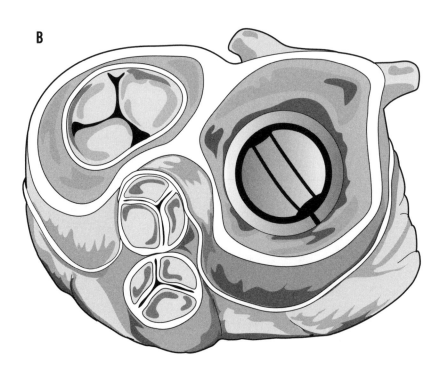

B

Before and after a heart valve replacement. Cross sections of the heart showing a dysfunctional mitral valve **(A)** and a mechanical replacement **(B)**.

have been perfecting this technique, it has become quite common—hundreds of thousands of such operations are performed each year.

Surgery on the Valves

Operations to replace dysfunctional heart valves are fairly straightforward. As with other structural heart diseases, valve dysfunction can be treated only temporarily with medicines. If the disease progresses, it invariably requires surgery. Occasionally, the surgery may simply involve a repair of the valve; however, this is less common, given that by the time surgery is required, the valve is usually long past repair. Typically, an entire valve is replaced with either an entire synthetically manufactured valve, composed of various composite plastics and metals or a valve sewn from other animal tissue, attached to a metal ring, and inserted in the place of the patient's native valve.

Of the two choices, the latter, so-called bioprosthetic valves are typically composed of either pig valves or the heart lining from cows. Of course, they are chemically treated to eliminate any risk of infection or reaction to the tissue. Their greatest advantage is that they do not require thinning the blood for more than six weeks; this is in contrast to entirely synthetic (metal) valves, which require long-term anticoagulation, or blood thinning, to prevent blood from clotting on the valve. Blood clots on such valves are dangerous for two reasons: They can degrade the competence of the valve, and they can travel to other parts of the body and clog arteries, most dangerously in the head, where they can cause strokes. However, the trade-off is that entirely synthetic valves can last much longer (more than twenty years) than bioprosthetic ones, which usually degrade over eight to fifteen years.

Congenital Defect Repair

Surgery for congenital heart disease is highly variable depending on the type of malformation. Occasionally, repairs can be done with minimally invasive techniques, using large catheters inserted in the groin during a cardiac catheterization. However, more commonly, congenital heart defects require more invasive open-heart surgery to repair. Typically, these operations involve using a heart-lung bypass machine to take over the functions of the heart and lungs while the heart is stopped so that surgeons can operate on it. The type of repair and operation varies widely with the type of defect, and we will discuss each one in detail.

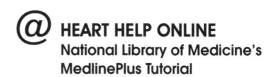

HEART HELP ONLINE
National Library of Medicine's MedlinePlus Tutorial

Heart Valve Replacement Tutorial: www. nlm.nih.gov/medlineplus/tutorials/ heartvalvereplacement/htm/index.htm

TESTS AND DIAGNOSIS OF STRUCTURAL HEART DISEASE

Initial evaluation of patients for structural heart disease is typically the result of symptoms that have developed or the detection of a murmur by a primary care physician. In children, the diagnosis of congenital heart disease may derive simply from a baby that is not growing as quickly as expected, or who is much less active than his peers of similar age. No matter the symptoms, your doctor will first listen to what is going on and examine you. There may be other causes for your symptoms besides your heart, and your doctor may investigate these as well. The exams may include an electrocardiogram (an ECG or EKG), detailed in chapter 5. However, the most helpful study of your heart structure is currently the echocardiogram.

Echocardiogram

An echocardiogram (or echo) is a sonogram for the heart—the same technology used to look at a fetus inside the uterus is used to look at the heart. It is incredibly useful. An echocardiogram can first assess how well the heart is functioning, how well different parts are beating and contracting, and whether any parts are lagging behind. It can also assess for normal anatomy—that is, are all the parts hooked up correctly? Are there any holes where there shouldn't be? It can even give a limited assessment of pressures in various parts of the heart. Lastly, the echocardiogram can provide an excellent assessment of the function of each of the four valves in the heart—how well each of them is allowing blood through and how well they are preventing backflow of blood. It can also identify any infections or other potential obstructions of the valves.

Transesophageal Echo

Typically, an echo is performed by placing the probe over your chest to look at the heart. However, if this does not give a good enough view, your doctor may order a transesophageal echocardiogram. This means a smaller probe is used to look at the heart from the esophagus (throat). Don't worry; patients are usually sedated during the test , and it remains a very low-risk study.

Invasive Cardiac Catheterization

Less commonly, an echocardiogram is not sufficient to characterize structural defects of the heart—this can be particularly true for congenital defects. Furthermore, an echo cannot definitively assess all of the different pressures in every part of the heart; its evaluation is limited. For those reasons, your doctor may recommend a cardiac catheterization. This is a procedure very similar to that performed for coronary artery disease or heart attacks—large catheters are inserted in the groin, or less commonly in the neck, and are threaded to the heart where they take measurements of pressures in various parts of the heart. A cinematic X-ray, or fluoroscopy, can also be performed during this procedure, to get a better look at the structures of the heart.

STRUCTURAL DEFECTS EXAMINED

Valvular Heart Disease

The most common form of structural disease of the heart involves the valves and their dysfunction. The four valves of the heart control blood flow at two points in the contraction cycle on both the left and right sides. The mitral valve controls flow from the left atrium to the left ventricle, and the tricuspid valve controls flow from the right atrium to the right ventricle. The aortic valve is the gateway from the left ventricle to the aorta and the rest of the body, whereas the pulmonary valve maintains forward flow from the right ventricle to the lungs through the pulmonary artery.

The general purpose of each valve is to ensure that blood flows in one direction; that when the ventricles contract, there's only one way for the blood to go, and it cannot reflux back toward the ventricles after it is ejected. The mitral and tricuspid valves are composed of flaps—the mitral has two, and the tricuspid has three—that swing open in one direction, from atria to ventricles. These "doors" are tethered like swinging kitchen doors that have a rope tied to one side, allowing them to swing in only one direction. This prevents them from swinging back into the atria, thereby preventing blood from flowing back into the atria.

By contrast, the aortic and pulmonary valves are flaps built into the walls of the major vessels exiting the ventricles. These flaps remain compressed against the vessel wall as blood is ejected out from the ventricles, and then fall out to prevent blood from refluxing or "regurgitating" back into the ventricles.

Dysfunction of the heart valves can be broadly categorized into two mechanisms: either the valve is obstructed or stenotic (stiff) and does not open to accommodate blood flow in any direction, or the valve is incompetent and does not prevent blood from flowing backward, causing a backup of blood. The former is called stenosis of the valve; the latter is referred to as either valvular regurgitation or insufficiency. Each valve can experience either type of mechanical malfunction for a variety of reasons, which will be discussed here.

Mitral Stenosis

Mitral stenosis is relatively common among valvular heart diseases. It is characterized by poor movement of the flaps of the mitral valve, not allowing blood to flow from the left atrium to the left ventricle. Imagine swinging trapdoors that are rusted shut. Naturally, the flaps are not totally shut; we could not survive if there was *no* flow. However, the stenosis of these valves makes it increasingly difficult for blood to move from the left atrium to the left ventricle.

Over long periods of time, mitral stenosis leads to multiple changes in the heart. First, the backup of blood in the left atrium stretches it out, weakening it and making it more susceptible to arrhythmias, or disturbances of the electrical signals that coordinate heart movement. More importantly, when the mitral valve obstructs flow, blood has no where to escape but to back up in the lungs. Depending on the severity of this backup, patients may be asymptomatic, may experience mild shortness of breath, or may be severely symptomatic with fatigue, shortness of breath, and limited exercise tolerance. With such blockage of the mitral valve, less blood gets to the ventricle, and thus less blood is available to be propelled to the rest of the body.

Causes of Mitral Stenosis

Mitral stenosis is usually caused by two potential factors. Historically, patients who had rheumatic fever (also called group A streptococcus infections) as children were at risk for progression of the infection to affect the mitral valve. It is not the actual infection but the body's abnormal response to it that affects the mitral valve. That is, in certain patients the streptococcus infection confuses the body's immune system, which attacks the valve thinking it is the infection. However, this complication is relatively

A Healthy Heart

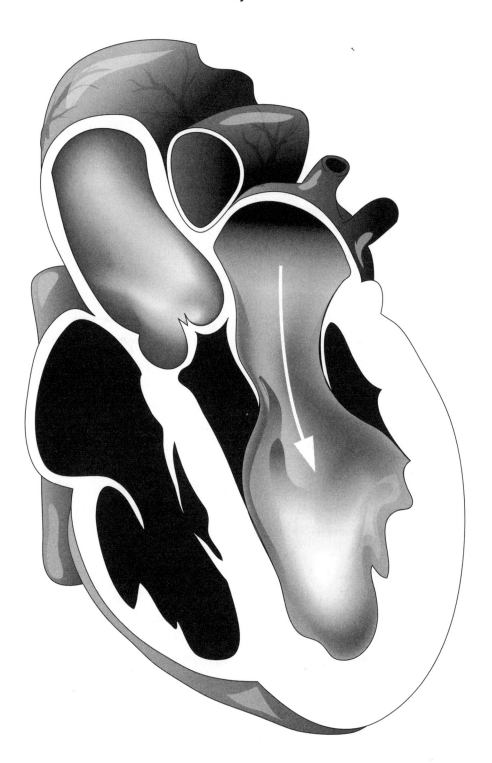

An internal view of a healthy heart showing a functioning mitral valve.

Mitral Valve Stenosis

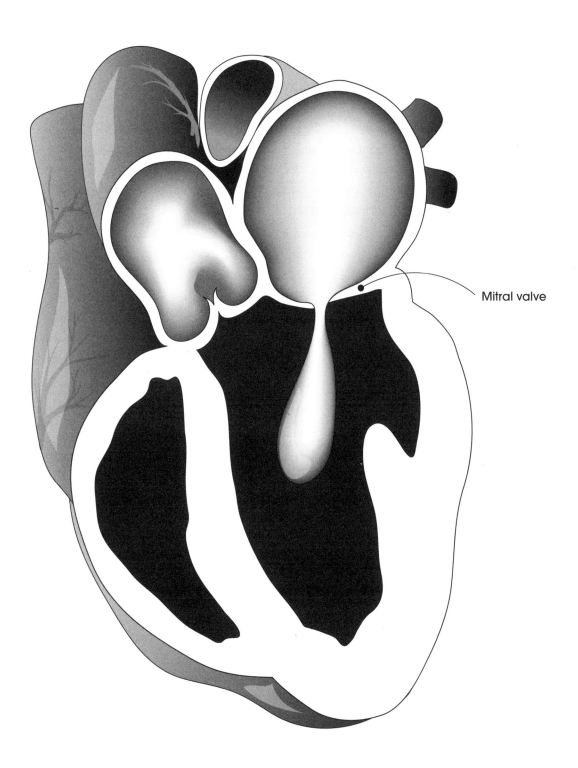

Mitral valve

An internal view of a heart with mitral valve stenosis showing decreased flow through the valve.

rare, and with the advent in the early twentieth century of antibiotics that are highly active against streptococcus, the incidence of rheumatic heart valve disease has dropped dramatically.

More commonly, mitral stenosis is the result of atherosclerotic disease on the mitral valve. Atherosclerosis is the process by which blood vessels and heart valves become laden with hard, calcium-containing plaques. Multiple factors contribute to atherosclerosis (as described in chapter 1). In brief, atherosclerosis is partly the result of high blood pressure and elevated cholesterol and likely is affected by our genes as well. This complicated process results in calcium deposits in the walls of blood vessels and on the flaps of the heart valves. This leads the vessels and valves to become hard and noncompliant, making the vessels more susceptible to rupture and the heart valves stiffer and less likely to open.

Mitral Stenosis Symptoms

Mitral stenosis may remain benign for several years. For severe, symptomatic mitral stenosis, many medications may be prescribed to help prevent its progression to heart failure. However, the ultimate therapy is surgical valve replacement. Surgery is currently recommended for patients who are not candidates for a catheter-based approach and who experience profound symptoms with mild or no exertion. These patients can barely perform functions of daily life because they are short of breath and tired. Surgery may also be performed in patients who have significant mitral stenosis *and* mitral regurgitation.

Mitral Regurgitation

Mitral regurgitation is the opposite problem of mitral stenosis; blood moves through the valve with ease—both ways. A trapdoor meant to open in one direction is instead swinging both ways without

preventing flow in either direction. Thus, as the left ventricle contracts, blood is ejected not just out the aortic valve to the aorta but also back through the mitral valve and into the left atrium.

The causes of mitral regurgitation are many. Rheumatic heart disease can cause mitral regurgitation. Infections on the valve, (endocarditis, described later in this chapter), and atherosclerosis can cause mitral regurgitation. As we discussed, the flaps of the mitral valve have tethers or tendons that keep them from refluxing back into the atrium. When one of these tethers ruptures or breaks, mitral regurgitation can result. This can occur during heart attacks—if blood flow to these structures is compromised, tendon rupture can occur. Mitral valve prolapse syndrome, a common condition, can also lead to mitral regurgitation. This usually benign syndrome describes a significant proportion of the population whose mitral valves not only close during left ventricular contraction, but also get pushed back into the left atrium slightly.

Effects of Mitral Stenosis

Mitral regurgitation presents several problems. Most obviously, it allows blood that was just pumped from the left atrium into the left ventricle back into the left atrium. This is not very productive and is essentially wasted work performed by the heart. What's worse, similar to mitral stenosis, this reflux into the left atrium causes the atrium to become overloaded, to dilate (expand), and in severe cases to back up blood into the lungs. Additionally, when the left ventricle squeezes a certain amount of blood during each contraction, less of that blood is going out to the aorta and more is going back into the left atrium. This process decreases flow to the rest of the body and compromises the function of other organs.

Mitral Regurgitration

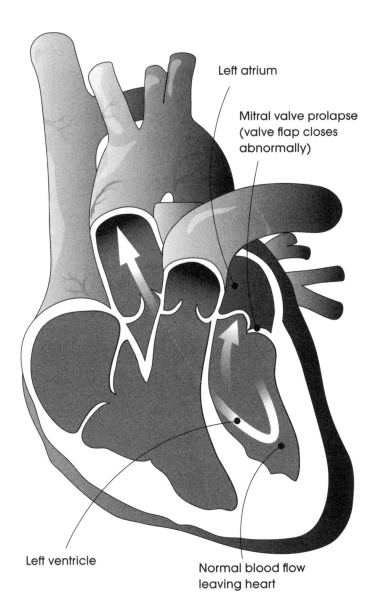

Left atrium

Mitral valve prolapse
(valve flap closes
abnormally)

Left ventricle

Normal blood flow
leaving heart

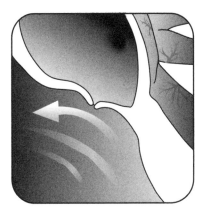

Normal closed mitral valve

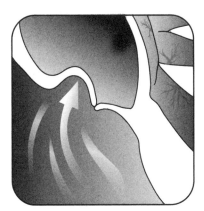

Blood pushes on valve

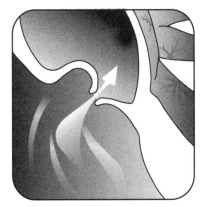

Blood regurgitated back into
atrium

An internal view of a heart and close-ups showing mitral valve regurgitation.

However, many patients with mild mitral regurgitation may have few to no symptoms at all. For patients with severe disease, medications can do only so much. They cannot prevent progression to ventricular dysfunction, at which point surgical replacement of the valve is favored. Patients who benefit from surgery include those with severe symptoms during mild or minimal exertion and those with signs of other consequences from mitral regurgitation—they may have significantly depressed ventricular function, elevated pressures in the lungs, or arrhythmias. Often, surgical repair of the mitral valve is preferred to complete replacement.

Aortic Stenosis

Similar to mitral stenosis, aortic stenosis is characterized by the stiffening and lack of movement of the flaps of the aortic valve. They no longer compress against the wall of the aorta and remain out of the way, but instead stand in the way of outgoing blood flow from the left ventricle. Thus, the aortic valve is an obstruction that greatly decreases flow from the left ventricle to the rest of the body.

Aortic stenosis is evaluated by measuring the size of the valve opening. Patients with a healthy aortic valve may have 3–4 cm^2 of area through which to push blood, whereas those with severe aortic stenosis might have less than one-quarter of that, or is less than 1 cm^2. Similarly, your doctor may measure the pressure drop or gradient across the valve. That is, as the valve increasingly obstructs outflow, the difference between pressure in front of it and behind it increases. These are just a few of the things your doctor will look at when evaluating aortic stenosis.

Causes of Aortic Stenosis

The causes of aortic stenosis are similar to those of mitral stenosis. Rheumatic fever was a significant cause of aortic stenosis in patients sickened with group A streptococcus infections as children. This condition leads to aortic stenosis in which the leaflets of the valve fuse together, decreasing their ability to move out of the way when the aorta contracts. The more common cause is atherosclerosis, which deposits calcium plaques on the leaflets, hardening and stiffening them to the point of inflexibility. Patients at risk for atherosclerosis and therefore aortic stenosis include those with hypertension and/or high cholesterol, smokers, and those with atherosclerosis in other parts of the body (i.e., the aorta, the coronary vessels, the mitral valve, or vessels to the kidney).

Lastly, aortic stenosis can be the result of a birth defect in which patients are born with only two leaflets to the aortic valve. Although this condition can be a benign malformation and does not cause aortic stenosis in the majority of patients, it can also indicate that there are underlying structural malformations in the walls of the major blood vessels and valves in the body. Patients with such a defect in their aortic valve are also at risk for defects in the wall of the aorta, such as aneurysms (bulging) or dissections (splitting) of the wall.

Aortic Stenosis Symptoms

Similar to other valve disorders, patients with mild aortic stenosis may not experience many symptoms, if any. However, the heart knows when the aortic valve is obstructed—the left ventricle must work harder to pump blood to the body to overcome this blockage. Think of the hose that is kinked (without opening the spigot any more); flow out the end is markedly decreased. Furthermore, to generate pressure on the other side of the kink or obstruction, greater pressure must be generated in front of it. Thus, the heart must work much harder to pump

Aortic Stenosis

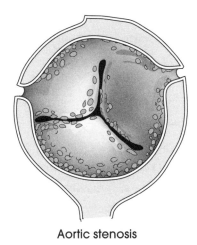

Aortic stenosis

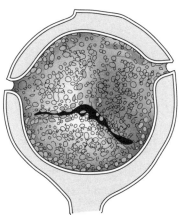

Bicuspid aortic stenosis

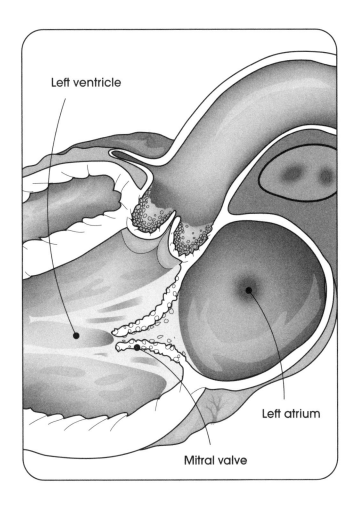

Left ventricle

Left atrium

Mitral valve

A depiction of aortic stenosis, characterized by the stiffening and lack of movement of the leaflets of the aortic valve.

blood through the body at the same pressure than it would without such an obstruction. This presents several problems for the heart.

Primarily, over long periods of time, the heart starts to thicken, or hypertrophy. Just like any other muscle in the body, when the heart works out more than normal it bulks up like a bodybuilder's biceps. Unfortunately, this is not advantageous for the heart.

As described in chapter 4, thickening of the heart muscle means less space in the heart for blood to fill and less ability for the heart to stretch to accommodate blood filled from the left atrium (which leads to diastolic heart failure). Although this is more commonly the result of high blood pressure from the rest of the body, aortic stenosis represents a similar process for the heart, only worse.

As the aortic valve becomes more stenotic, it opens less and there is less space for blood to squeeze through—the leaflets are stuck closer and closer to each other without budging. Not only does the heart become increasingly thick and less accommodating of blood filling it, but the blood it does squeeze has no choice but to escape back into the left atrium. Though this is similar to worsening mitral valve stenosis or regurgitation, the overall problem is worse. In the mitral valve disorders we have some medications that can help to alleviate the burden on the heart and lungs. Unfortunately, because the aortic valve is at the exit of the left ventricle and is so important to blood flow, treatment of this disorder with medications is limited. For patients with severe aortic stenosis and life-changing symptoms, surgery to replace the defective valve is the best and only remedy.

Surgery is typically recommended for patients who experience symptoms from their aortic stenosis (either at rest or with exertion), those who have dysfunction of the heart muscle due to aortic stenosis, or those who have severe aortic stenosis and are having another cardiac surgical procedure (and the valve replacement can be performed at the same time).

WHAT'S NEW:

Minimally Invasive Surgery to Replace Aortic Valves

How have valve replacements traditionally been done? Since the introduction of the first man-made heart valve in the 1960s, doctors have improved the quality—and even saved the lives—of hundreds of thousands of patients. Aortic valve replacement is one of the most common forms of open-heart surgery and is performed throughout the world. Typically, this procedure involves cutting open the chest, stopping the heart, and using a heart-lung machine to maintain circulation.

What's the problem? Patients with aortic stenosis often don't have symptoms for several years. When they do become symptomatic, their prognosis is limited if the valve is not replaced. However, elderly people with additional health problems are high-risk candidates for open-heart surgery with a heart-lung machine.

Is a solution on the horizon? The latest research in this area indicates that using a stent to replace a diseased valve may be the way to go. Stents would be placed in the heart through a catheter as in other balloon procedures. Scientists are currently developing stents that are the appropriate size to replace heart valves.

In addition, several companies are working on ways to replace heart valves percutaneously, which describes a procedure in which doctors gain access to the inner body through a needle puncture, rather than opening the body with a scalpel.

Aortic Valve Replacement

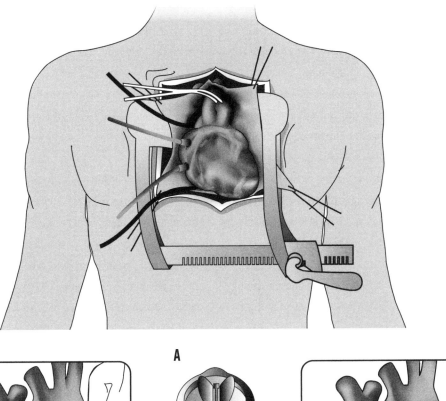

A

B

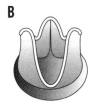

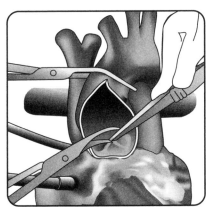

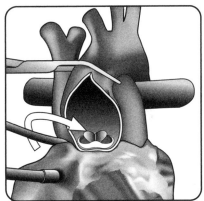

A depiction of an aortic valve replacement. Mechanical **(A)** and tissue **(B)** replacement valves are shown.

Aortic Regurgitation (Aortic Insufficiency)

The last disorder of left-sided valves is aortic regurgitation, also called aortic insufficiency. This disorder describes the inability of the aortic valve to properly prevent the backflow of blood from the aorta into the left ventricle; in other words, the valve is incompetent. As you'll recall, the aortic valve is composed of three flaps or leaflets that line the inside of the aorta, just outside the left ventricle. Aortic regurgitation may be the result of a defect in one or more of these flaps. They may get stuck against the wall, they may be torn, or they may no longer be strong enough to catch the blood as it backflows.

Aortic regurgitation can be the result of several distinct problems. In some respects, it is a disease primarily of the valve itself. Conditions such as rheumatic fever and patients born with only two aortic valve leaflets can both develop aortic regurgitation, in addition to the possibility of aortic stenosis. Furthermore, aortic regurgitation may be the result of processes extrinsic from the valve itself. It is common for defects in the wall of the aorta, specifically dilation of the aorta, to lead to aortic regurgitation by stretching so much that the leaflets no longer cover the entire opening. Additionally, systemic infections in the bloodstream can progress to involve the valve and eat away at leaflets. Less commonly, disorders such as lupus, certain types of arthritis, or vasculitis (inflammation of blood vessels) can lead to aortic regurgitation.

Effects of Aortic Regurgitation

Regardless of the cause of aortic regurgitation, the effect on the ventricle is the same: too much blood. When the aortic valve is incompetent, a fraction of all blood the ventricle ejects is washed right back at it. As the amount of backflow increases, the scenario becomes a Sisyphean state: akin to the legendary Greek hero doomed to repeatedly push the same boulder up the hill, only to see it come crashing down time after time. The severity can progress to the point where the left ventricle is pushing the same blood out, only to see it fall back again. Of course, there is always some forward movement of blood; if not, patients with aortic regurgitation could not survive. However, the constant backflow can take its toll.

In many patients, this backflow of blood represents a small fraction of the entire amount the heart pumps, and many patients' hearts can compensate for the extra work. However, in a subset of patients, the left ventricle can become stretched out from all the blood, weaken, and develop what we described in chapter 4 as systolic heart failure. Although several medications can help prevent these changes, heart failure is an unfortunate consequence of aortic regurgitation. Initially, these patients may remain asymptomatic. However, dysfunction of the heart muscle is the first sign that surgery may be needed to replace the valve. Once this dysfunction becomes symptomatic—that is, the patient experiences fatigue, shortness of breath, or chest pain—surgery becomes increasingly important for those who are appropriate candidates.

Tricuspid Stenosis

Stenosis of the tricuspid valve, located between the right atrium and right ventricle, is most commonly caused by rheumatic fever. Less commonly, the tricuspid valve may be poorly formed at birth and therefore obstructed. With such an obstruction, blood cannot get from the body through the valve to the right ventricle. Thus, there is a backup, and patients may experience symptoms such as swelling in their legs or abdomen. They may also experience a sense of fullness in the neck, as blood cannot escape from the upper body and head into the heart. As this

Aortic Valve Operating Normally

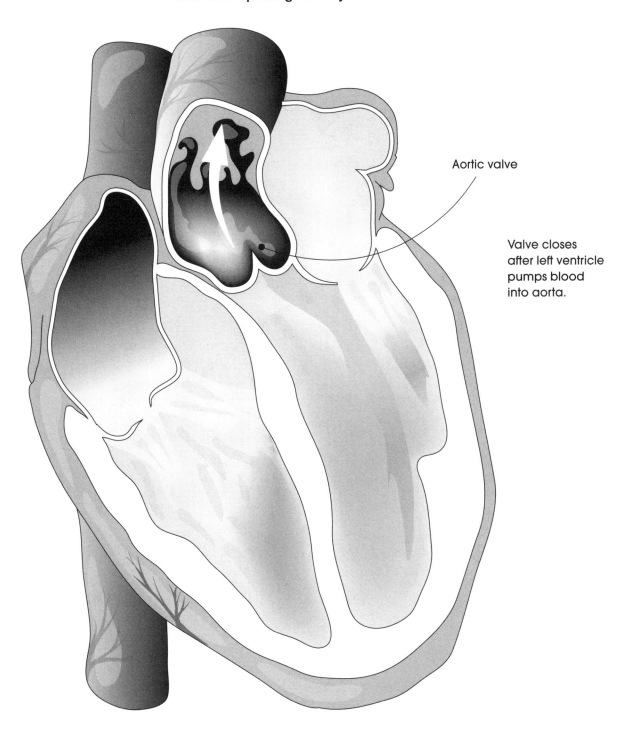

Aortic valve

Valve closes
after left ventricle
pumps blood
into aorta.

A cross section of a heart showing a healthy aortic valve and the normal flow of blood.

Aortic Regurgitation

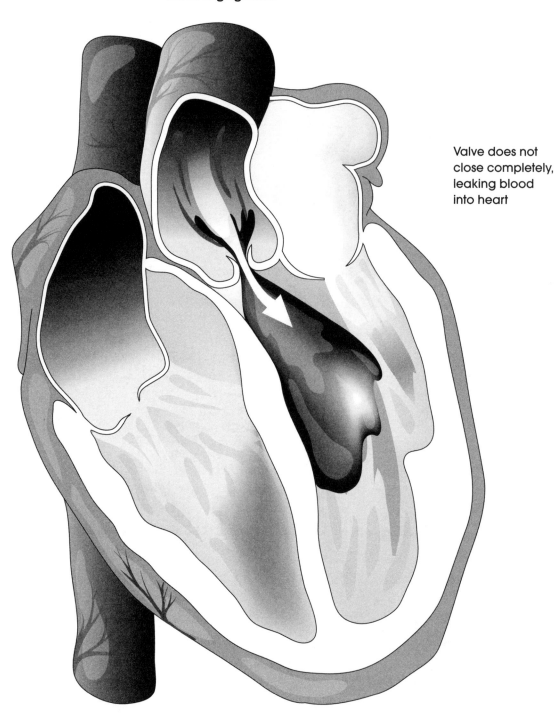

Valve does not close completely, leaking blood into heart

A cross section of a heart showing an unhealthy aortic valve and leakage of blood.

Tricuspid Stenosis

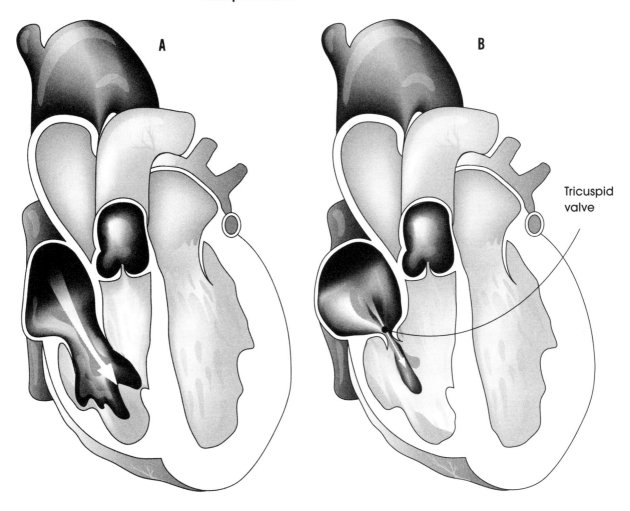

Tricuspid
valve

A heart with a healthy tricuspid valve showing the normal flow of blood into the right ventricle **(A)**, and a heart with tricuspid valve stenosis, in which blood cannot get through the valve to the right ventricle **(B)**.

condition progresses, the right atrium enlarges, similar to the left atrium in mitral stenosis.

Although medicines may help alleviate symptoms and possibly delay surgery for tricuspid stenosis, they are not definitive forms of therapy. Surgery is ultimately required to repair—or more likely replace—the valve. However, in patients with tricuspid stenosis, the vast majority have disease of other heart valves as well, such as mitral stenosis. It is therefore important to repair both defects at once.

Tricuspid Regurgitation

Abnormal backflow through the tricuspid valve, or tricuspid regurgitation, is most commonly unrelated to any specific disease of the tricuspid valve. Instead, enlargement of the right ventricle, which occurs in heart failure as well as diseases of the blood vessels to the lungs, causes the leaflets of the pulmonary valve to stretch. Thus, even when the leaflets open and close normally, they no longer come together to block the opening between the right atrium and the right ventricle. The result is blood leaking back

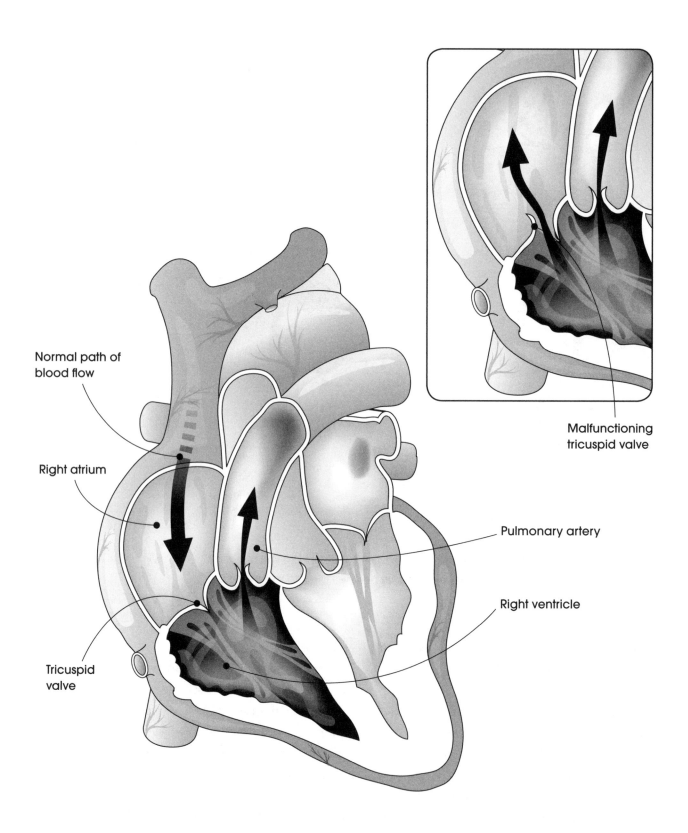

Normal path of
blood flow

Right atrium

Tricuspid
valve

Malfunctioning
tricuspid valve

Pulmonary artery

Right ventricle

A heart with a healthy tricuspid valve showing the normal flow of blood, and a close up of a malfunctioning tricuspid valve allowing blood to flow back into the right atrium (inset).

through the residual opening. Therefore, treatment of tricuspid regurgitation is specifically geared toward resolving the underlying disease—treating the heart failure or lowering the pressures in the pulmonary vessels so that there is less stress on the right ventricle.

Pulmonary Valve Disease

Diseases of the pulmonary valve are relatively rare. Pulmonary stenosis is most commonly associated with congenital defects (as in tetralogy of Fallot) or rheumatic disease, and pulmonary regurgitation is most commonly seen in disorders where the valve is stretched (similar to tricuspid regurgitation) or in cases of endocarditis. The diseases are rarely severe enough to require surgical repair. In instances where the effect on the right ventricle is substantial enough to warrant surgery, replacement of the pulmonary (and tricuspid) valves is almost always with bioprosthetic valves (i.e. valves made from biologic sources, such pig tissue). This is related to the fact that pressures in the right atrium and right ventricle are significantly lower than those on the left side. Thus, bioprosthetic valves last longer in these positions, as the wear and tear on them is less severe than it would be on the left (see the discussion of surgery on valves on pages 118–121). Furthermore, the lower pressure and lower flow characteristics of the right side make synthetic valves a higher risk for clot formation than they are on the left.

Endocarditis

Endocarditis refers to an infection of the valves of the heart. The valves can be particularly susceptible to infection because they are inert tissue—there is no direct blood supply to the valve itself and thus no way to carry infection-fighting cells to it. Furthermore, any defect in the valves can create a nidus or

⟋⟋⌐ WHAT'S NEW:

Catheter-Based Repairs for Pulmonary Valves

The research pouring into catheter-based repairs for the aortic valve was first applied to the pulmonary valve because this valve is more easily reached and tolerates less-than-perfect results better than the aortic valve. The procedure to repair pulmonary valves—most easily, pulmonary stenosis—can be accomplished by inflating a balloon within the valve to dilate it, allowing more blood to flow through.

How does it work? The Cribier-Edwards valve, which has been successfully placed within the aortic valve as well as the pulmonary valve, integrates a balloon-expandable, wire-mesh, stainless-steel stent that serves to anchor it in place, with tissue leaflets that ensure one-way blood flow.

The balloon-mounted valve is compressed to the diameter of a pencil and then inserted at the tip of a long, thin, plastic catheter through a small incision in the groin and delivered through the veins to the heart. The catheter is passed through the right atrium to the right ventricle, which pumps blood to the lung, through the pulmonary valve.

Endocarditis

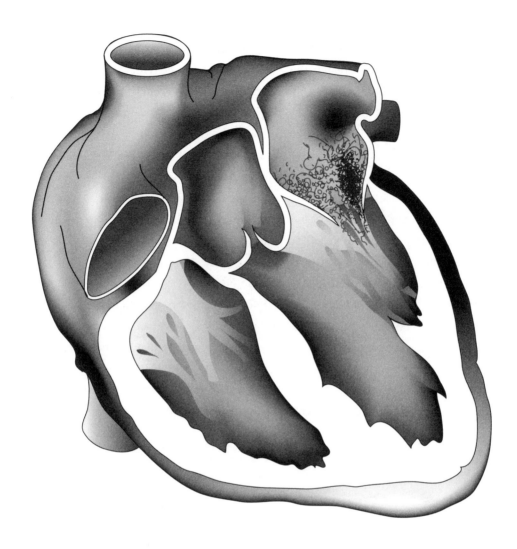

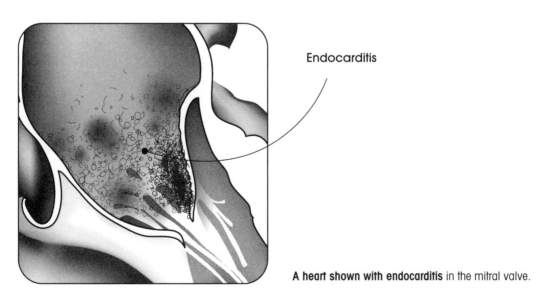

Endocarditis

A heart shown with endocarditis in the mitral valve.

"sticky spot" on which bacteria can land and grow. Therefore, certain groups of patients are particularly at risk for developing endocarditis. They include patients with the following conditions:

- Artificial prosthetic cardiac valve or prosthetic material used for valve repair
- Previous infective endocarditis
- Congenital Heart Disease:
  — Unrepaired cyanotic CHD or CHD with palliative shunts or implanted tubes
  — Completely repaired CHD with prosthetic material or device, whether placed by surgery or by catheter intervention, for six months after the procedure
  — Repaired CHD with residual defects at the site or adjacent to the site of a prosthetic patch or prosthetic device
- Cardiac transplantation recipients who develop valve disease

Development of endocarditis is frequently spontaneous. We are all exposed to bacteria in our blood on a daily basis, and these routine exposures provide the most risk for endocarditis. Occasionally, endocarditis is related to a procedure or event during which bacteria transiently entered the bloodstream: surgery, dental procedures, nonsterile intravenous injections, or injuries. Therefore, many patients with structural heart disease are advised to take antibiotics prior to most surgeries or procedures.

Endocarditis Symptoms

Patients with endocarditis typically feel profoundly ill. They develop fatigue, malaise, diffuse pain, and often, high fevers. As infections grow on the valves, they may appear as "vegetations" or large "burdens" of bacteria. Pieces of theses vegetations can break off and travel through the blood stream, similar to a clot; only instead of obstructing the artery they travel through, they cause small infections everywhere they land. This diffuse infection, combined with the lack of direct blood supply to the valves, makes endocarditis particularly difficult to treat.

Typical therapy for endocarditis involves six weeks of intravenous antibiotics to help kill the infection. In many patients, surgery is required to replace the infected valve because either the infection is not clearing with antibiotics or the infection is spreading into other tissues in the heart. Furthermore, in patients who have infections of a replacement valve, the odds of clearing the infection with antibiotics alone are low. Surgery is almost always required for a repeat valve replacement.

CONGENITAL HEART DISEASE (CHD)

Congenital heart disease refers to those diseases of the heart which occur during the development of the heart in the fetus and are then present at birth. Structural heart defects are some of the most common birth defects to occur in babies today, and believe it or not, many are relatively benign and do not need much intervention. However, some defects do require extensive surgery to correct. Fortunately, these techniques and the outcomes from surgery have improved dramatically over the past fifty years.

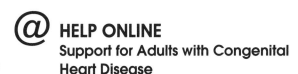

HELP ONLINE
Support for Adults with Congenital Heart Disease

The Adult Congenital Heart Association: www.achaheart.org

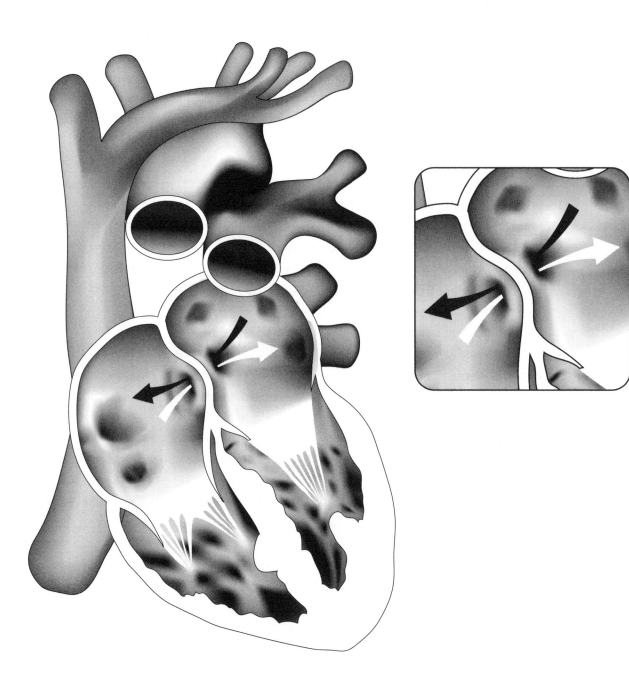

A depiction of atrial septal defect, in which blood can flow across the septum in either direction.

Atrial Septal Defect

An atrial septal defect, or ASD, is a defect in which the two atria, left and right, are not properly separated. The septum, or piece of tissue between them, does not fully develop. In fact, it's not supposed to be completely formed in the fetus, which has special circulation that necessitates this connection remain open until birth, when it closes in the vast majority of healthy babies. However, this connection can remain open through childhood. In many cases, it is a relatively small hole in the septum and is known as a *patent foramen ovale (PFO)*. This is often a benign condition that can last into adulthood without causing problems of blood flow. However, if you have PFO and you develop a blood clot in your legs (such as after a long plane ride), which breaks off, it could cross over to the left side of your heart, travel to your brain, and cause a stroke.

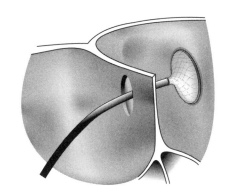

Effects of ASD

In patients who have a significant ASD, blood from the left and right atria mixes. The result is that blood high in oxygen in the left atrium can be contaminated with blood low in oxygen from the right atrium and blood from the left atrium can spill into the right atrium. What determines which way the blood goes? It's all about the pressures; most commonly, the pressure in the left atrium is higher than that in the right atrium, and thus blood spills out of the left atrium into the right. This might not seem so bad, since highly oxygenated blood is still moving from the left atrium to the left ventricle and out to the rest of the body. Unfortunately, it also means excess blood is spilling into the right atrium, in addition to all of the blood returning from the body.

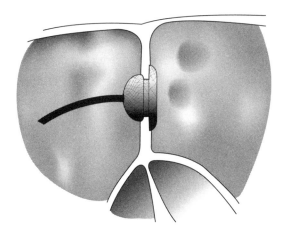

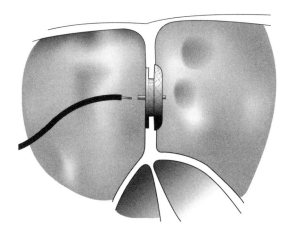

Three possibilities for repairing an atrial septal defect using catheter-based techniques.

The right side of the heart was not designed to handle all of this blood flow. It can cause it tremendous stress, resulting from trying to force all the excess blood into the lungs, where it can back up. Over time, the muscle of the right side of the heart tires out, weakens, and gives out under the burden of all this extra blood.

Surgical Treatments for ASD

Thus, in patients with an ASD and significant flow across it, definitive repair is often recommended. Fortunately, minimally invasive catheter-based technologies can sometimes close these types of defects. During such a cardiac catheterization, a closure device is placed across the ASD. The closure device consists of two discs on each side of the hole, fastened together to form a kind of sandwich across the defect. This closes such a defect, and over time the heart's own tissue will grow over it to form a smooth layer. However, when such a minimally invasive approach cannot be taken, surgical intervention is required. This typically involves either placing a synthetic patch over the hole, or simply sewing it closed. Such an operation can often be performed without stopping the heart or using the heart-lung bypass machine.

Ventricular Septal Defect

One of the most common congenital heart defects, ventricular septal defect (VSD), is characterized by the incomplete formation of the ventricular septum—the muscle that separates the left and right ventricles. However, unlike the atrial septum, the ventricular septum is supposed to develop in the fetus fully formed, without any holes. Unfortunately, in some babies it does not completely close. This presents a similar problem to that of an ASD; the higher pressure in the left ventricle causes blood to leak into the right ventricle. However, pressures in the left ventricle are typically significantly higher than in any other part of the heart. Therefore, this shunt

of blood is more likely to be problematic, causing overloading of the right ventricle.

If a significant amount of blood is leaking across the VSD, it is important to have such defects repaired before the right ventricle begins to weaken and give out. Compared to an ASD, a VSD is less amenable to a minimally invasive, catheter-based approach. However, surgical techniques for these repairs have been refined over more than fifty years. Complications are now uncommon. As with an ASD, surgical options include closing the hole by simply sewing it shut or by placing a synthetic patch over it. Over time, the heart's tissue will grow over the patch.

Patent Ductus Arteriosus

One of the less common structural anomalies, a patent ductus arteriosus (PDA), represents another possible transmission between blood that is high in oxygen and blood that is low in oxygen. Like an ASD, a PDA is the result of the circulation of the fetus persisting after birth. In the healthy fetus, blood going to the lungs from the right ventricle is not actually getting oxygen—the fetus is not breathing inside the womb; he or she is provided oxygen from mom via the umbilical cord. But blood is still pumped from the right ventricle to the lungs, in preparation for birth. However, without being full of air, the lungs cannot accommodate this much blood flow, and the pressure increases. Therefore, blood is diverted from the pulmonary artery to the aorta through a conduit known as the ductus arteriosus. Once the baby is born, this conduit is supposed to close on its own within days of birth, without complication. However, in some children, it remains open, resulting in the patent ductus arteriosus. The PDA allows blood to move across it just like before the child was born—except that now the pressures are reversed and blood flows from the aorta to the pulmonary artery. Similar to an ASD and a VSD, this excess flow to the lungs can overwhelm them and cause them to accumulate fluid.

Fortunately, many of the children born with PDAs are asymptomatic, and the PDA closes (later than usual) on its own. In those children who are symptomatic or in whom the PDA does not close spontaneously, medications called indomethacin or ibuprofen (Advil) can actually expedite closing of the defect. This is one of the rare cases in which a medicine can actually cure a structural heart defect. In cases where medication fails, intervention is required to close the PDA. Once again, catheter-based approaches are available and widely used to close PDAs. They are successful in up to 85 percent of cases. This is the preferred method of closure since it is lower risk than open heart surgery. However, in cases where the PDA is too large for catheter-based closure or in which catheter-based closure has failed, surgery to tie the conduit closed is recommended.

Transposition of the Great Arteries

One of the most severe congenital cardiac anomalies, transposition of the great arteries (TGA), is characterized by the reversal of the major vessels leaving each ventricle. In a healthy heart, the left ventricle pumps into the aorta, a massive artery supplying blood to the entire body. The right ventricle usually pumps into the pulmonary artery that leads to the lungs, allowing blood from the body to saturate again with oxygen. However, in patients with TGA, these two massive vessels have formed in reverse. The left ventricle, which still receives blood from the lungs, then pumps out to the pulmonary artery, back into the lungs. Analogously, the right ventricle, which still receives the body's blood from the right

atrium, pumps the same blood low in oxygen out to the aorta and back to the body. This results in two totally independent circuits.

In this scenario, there is no way for the blood going to the body from the right atrium to get oxygen from the lungs. Therefore, babies born with this condition must have another abnormality—some other connection between the left and right systems—to survive. This is typically an ASD, VSD, PDA, or other remnant of fetal circulation that allows them to survive through birth. However, without surgical correction, babies born with such abnormal circulation cannot live more than a year, with nearly one-third dying in the first week of life.

Immediately following birth, medicines may be used to keep children with TGA alive. However, major cardiac surgery is the only definitive treatment option for TGA. The main goal is to reverse the two major arteries: the aorta is connected to the left ventricle, and the pulmonary artery is attached to the right ventricle. This is a major operation, and frequently is complicated by other factors. TGA is often accompanied by other defects that are highly variable among patients, and it must be verified that each ventricle can accommodate the new anatomy and the pressures it will generate.

Tetralogy of Fallot

Perhaps one of the most well-known congenital heart defects, tetralogy of Fallot is characterized by a confluence of four defects, as the name suggests. They include the following:

1) Pulmonary valve stenosis: The valve that controls blood flow from the right ventricle to the pulmonary artery and the lungs is obstructed.

Normal Heart

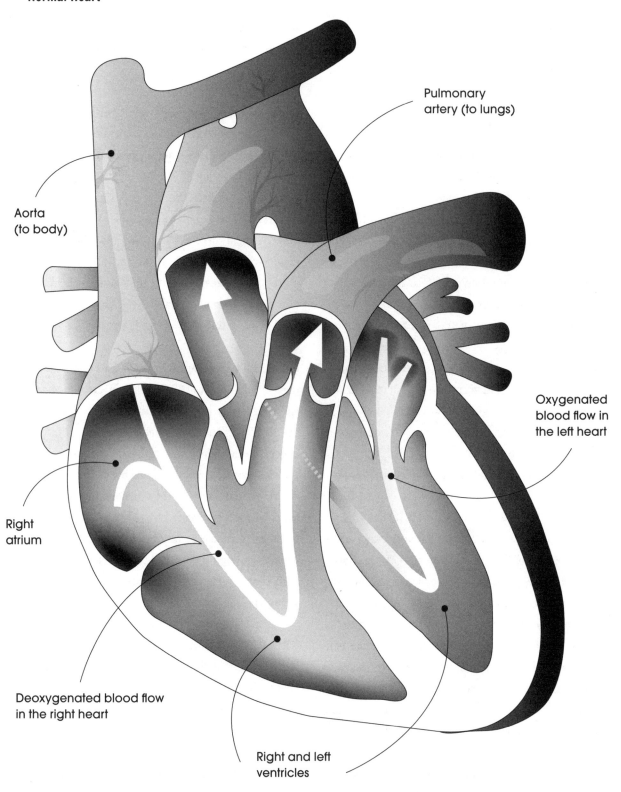

Pulmonary
artery (to lungs)

Aorta
(to body)

Oxygenated
blood flow in
the left heart

Right
atrium

Deoxygenated blood flow
in the right heart

Right and left
ventricles

Cross section of a normal heart for comparison to the Tetralogy of Fallot, opposite.

Heart with Tetrology of Fallot

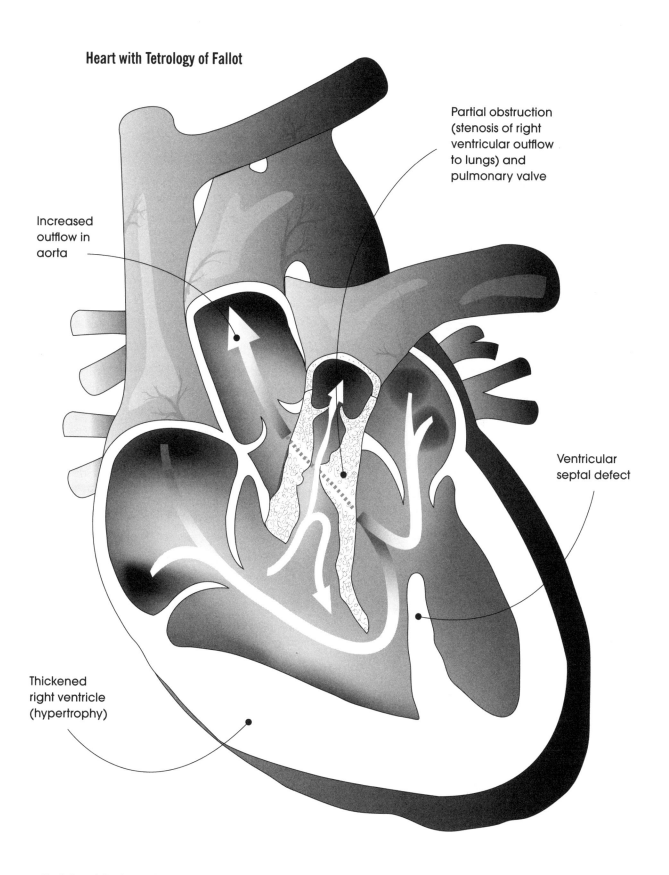

Partial obstruction (stenosis of right ventricular outflow to lungs) and pulmonary valve

Increased outflow in aorta

Ventricular septal defect

Thickened right ventricle (hypertrophy)

Depiction of the four defects of Tetralogy of Fallot: pulmonary valve stenosis, ventricular septal defect, overriding aorta, and an enlarged right ventricle.

Tetralogy of Fallot and the History of Pediatric Cardiology

Historically, tetralogy of Fallot was characterized by *tet spells,* during which children with the disorder would become cyanotic, or blue. This occurred when the flow across the VSD changed so that more blood that was low in oxygen in the right ventricle shifted over to the left side and out the aorta to the rest of the body, causing the child to look blue. Children quickly learned that one way to reverse this process was to squat down, which increased the pressure in the aorta and the left ventricle, thus preventing blood from shifting from the right side.

The first surgical procedures to correct tetralogy of Fallot were part of incredible advances in invasive cardiac surgical techniques performed at The Johns Hopkins Hospital in the 1950s. The success of these initial surgical procedures was due to an unlikely trio, including the first pediatric cardiologist and first female president of the American Heart Association, Helen Taussig; a famous Hopkins surgeon, Alfred Blalock; and his African American lab assistant, Vivien Thomas, who performed the first such operations on animals in Dr. Blalock's lab. Their story was portrayed in the 2004 HBO movie, *Something the Lord Made.*

2) VSD: As described earlier, a VSD allows inappropriate communication between the left and right ventricles.

3) Overriding aorta: The main artery exiting the left ventricle, partly due to the VSD, appears at the opening of both the left and right ventricles.

4) Enlarged right ventricle: Due in part to the force that is required to squeeze blood through the obstructed pulmonary valve, the right ventricular muscle becomes thickened (also called right ventricular hypertrophy).

These four abnormalities are characteristic of tetralogy of Fallot. The majority of children born with the disorder have highly variable anatomy. The degree of each defect varies with each child, and often there are other accompanying structural anomalies. Accordingly, outcomes for children with tetralogy of Fallot vary based on the severity of their disease. The vast majority require some form of surgical correction, the complexity and extent of which vary with the degree of disease.

Q. & A. with Dr. Cannon

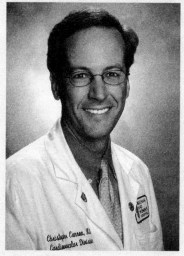

Christopher Cannon, M.
Cardiovascular Division

Q. My daughter has congenital heart disease and is just "graduating" from her pediatric cardiologist. Can she choose any adult cardiologist, or should she look for a specialist in congenital heart disease?

A. Although any cardiologist is trained to treat adults with congenital heart disease, because it is a relatively rare condition—at least compared to, say, diabetes or heart attack—I would generally recommend seeing a cardiologist who specializes in patients with congenital heart disease. Sometimes, if there is no such doctor nearby, you might have *both* a regular cardiologist that you see more often and a specialized congenital heart disease cardiologist that you consult periodically.

Q. I have mitral valve prolapse and have always taken antibiotics before going to the dentist. My cardiologist says I no longer need to take them. Why the change?

A. New national guidelines from the American Heart Association were released in 2007 that no longer recommend use of antibiotics for patients with mild heart valve problems. It was noted that the risk of developing an infection on a mildly abnormal heart valve is exceedingly low, and that antibiotics have not actually been shown to reduce that risk. Thus, it was felt unnecessary to treat many such patients with antibiotics. Also, people sometimes develop allergic reactions to the antibiotics. However, if you have more serious valvular or structural heart problems, such as having had a valve replacement, antibiotics are still recommended.

Q. I have aortic stenosis, but my doctor says it is only "mild to moderate" at present. I get an echo each year. Will I eventually need to have a valve replacement?

A. It is not certain that you would need to have one, but it is hard to predict. That is why we monitor the valve function each year with an echo—to see whether it is getting worse. Also, we monitor any symptoms you have; do you get short of breath when exerting yourself, or get lightheaded, or feel chest pressure? If the symptoms become significant, and the valve looks to be more severely narrowed, valve surgery would generally be recommended.

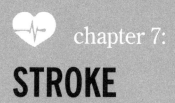 chapter 7:

STROKE

STROKE

℞ THE PRESCRIPTION

Your treatment plan depends on the type and underlying cause of the stroke.

Ischemic Stroke

When there is a blockage (also known as a clot) in the vessels carrying blood to the brain, treatment is aimed at restoring blood supply. The blood clot might form in the carotid artery (the main artery to the brain) at the site of a cholesterol plaque (as in heart attacks) or could come from elsewhere in the body—such as the heart, via the blood vessels—in which case it is called an embolic stroke. If this clot is short-lived and resolves on its own by natural mechanisms, stroke symptoms would be temporary and you would experience a transient ischemic attack (TIA).

Hemorrhagic Stroke

A hemorrhagic stroke is a bleeding stroke, due to a leak or rupture in a blood vessel in the brain. Treatment in this case is aimed at preventing further bleeding and reducing pressure on brain cells due to the excess blood. The bleeding can be in the brain tissue itself; in the arachnoid space, or the dura surrounding the brain. Treatment differs depending on where the bleeding occurs.

In any case, therapy consists of four essential components:

➡ Emergency treatment with medication

➡ Surgery and other interventional procedures

➡ Control of risk factors

➡ Rehabilitation and recovery

STROKE: A MEDICAL EMERGENCY

During a stroke—also known as a "brain attack" or a cerebrovascular accident—you may experience one or more of the following typical symptoms:

- Sudden numbness, weakness, or paralysis of a leg, arm, or one side of the face
- Sudden blurry vision, double vision, or visual loss in one or both eyes
- Sudden confusion, slurred or garbled speech, or trouble understanding others
- Sudden trouble walking due to dizziness or loss of balance or coordination
- Sudden severe headache without any apparent cause

Less commonly, you may develop sudden nausea, vomiting, or brief loss or change in consciousness (fainting, seizures, or coma).

Beware the Mini Stroke

A transient ischemic attack (TIA), or "mini stroke," can also cause these symptoms, but by definition, a TIA generally does not last more than twenty-four hours and does not cause permanent brain damage. Typically, symptoms disappear within an hour. TIAs are often a precursor or warning sign of a stroke, just as chest pain (angina) is a precursor to a heart attack. One-third of the people who have had one or more TIAs will go on to have a stroke. In about half the cases, the stroke occurs within one year of the TIA. However, most strokes are not preceded by a TIA.

The most important point to remember is that *a stroke is a medical emergency*. In fact, one reason why a stroke is now often called a brain attack is to underline its similarity to a heart attack—both need immediate recognition of symptoms and urgent medical attention.

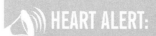

HEART ALERT:

"Time Is Brain!"
The sooner you call 9-1-1, the lesser the brain damage. Also, note the time when you first observe symptoms, as this information will be crucial in deciding optimal therapy.

EMERGENCY TREATMENT WITH MEDICATION—ISCHEMIC STROKE

Two types of medications are most commonly used to help resume normal flow of blood to the brain. These include blood-clot-dissolving medications called thrombolytics and anticlotting medications that are either antiplatelet or anticoagulant agents. Of course, your doctor will always rule out a hemorrhagic stroke before using these drugs, as their use can be life-threatening in the presence of bleeding in the brain.

Thrombolytics

Commonly known as clot busters, thrombolytics are highly effective in the treatment of ischemic strokes and can improve recovery and decrease the chance of disability. Thrombolytics work by dissolving any clots that might be obstructing blood flow to the brain. The thrombolytic alteplase (Activase) is a recombinant, or genetically engineered, form of the enzyme tissue plasminogen activator (t-PA). T-PA is naturally found in our body where it helps to dissolve blood clots; recombinant (genetically engineered) forms are referred to as rt-PA. These medications are usually given in your vein (i.e., intravenously), but they can also be given through catheters put directly into the brain arteries.

The most important side effect of these drugs is bleeding in the brain. As a result, patients are carefully selected using some standard criteria. The key condition is the "three-hour window"—thrombolytics can be used only within three hours of the onset of symptoms. After that time, any further benefit is unlikely, while the risk of complications remains.

Thrombolytic drugs cannot be used if your blood pressure is too high. Antihypertensive drugs such as labetalol (a beta blocker) may be used to lower your blood pressure to an acceptable level before using thrombolytics. Typically, labetolol is used for a systolic pressure greater than 220 mm Hg or diastolic pressure greater than 120 mm Hg. Medication may also be used to control fever and blood glucose levels.

Antiplatelet/Anticoagulant Agents

Aspirin acts on platelets by decreasing their ability to clump together and form a clot. Early aspirin use in ischemic stroke reduces long-term death and dependency and also reduces the risk of having another stroke. Aspirin is used within forty-eight hours after symptoms are first observed, but it should not be used within twenty-four hours of therapy with t-PA. Sometimes aspirin is used in combination with other antiplatelet drugs such as clopidogrel (Plavix) or ticlopidine (Ticlid). Even after a TIA, aspirin is used to decrease the likelihood of another stroke.

Blood thinners (anticoagulants) such as warfarin (Coumadin) and heparin are less commonly used for emergency treatment of an ischemic stroke, but are usually given if the stroke was embolic and/or in patients with atrial fibrillation.

WHAT'S NEW:

A Longer Window of Opportunity for Thrombolytics

How soon should patients receive rt-PA? One-third to one-half of stroke patients do not receive rt-PA treatment within the recommended three-hour window after their first symptoms appear because they delay seeking treatment. The three-hour limit is a matter of safety; patients should be treated as soon as possible.

Fortunately, recent studies suggest that rt-PA may be beneficial for some patients outside the three-hour window. Although not yet approved by the U.S. Food and Drug Administration (FDA), these drugs show potential for benefit up to four and a half hours after the onset of symptoms.

Patients with basilar artery occlusion (BAO), a severe type of stroke, have a longer window of opportunity.

Because BAO has a fluctuating course, these patients may be considered for thrombolytic treatment twenty-four to forty-eight hours after symptoms begin.

Where should I seek treatment? If you live near a stroke center that should be your first choice. The need to expedite evaluation of stroke patients with laboratory, radiology, and clinical neurological testing has been a driving force behind the establishment of stroke centers. Some stroke centers do emergency angiograms of the brain blood vessels and can safely give thrombolytic drugs directly into the blockage within six hours of the onset of symptoms.

EMERGENCY TREATMENT WITH MEDICATION—HEMORRHAGIC STROKE

Medical treatment alone is typically used in most mild and moderate cases, and is aimed at removing the underlying cause. High blood pressure may cause bleeding in the brain. When systolic pressure is greater than 170 mm Hg, antihypertensive drugs such as labetalol are used. Excessive anticoagulation may also cause bleeding. If this is the suspected cause, all anticoagulant medications are discontinued immediately and additional drugs may be given to reverse their effects.

Along with prescribing medication, your physician will carefully monitor you for signs of increased pressure on the brain, such as restlessness, headache, confusion, and difficulty following commands. Bleeding may cause edema (swelling) of adjacent brain tissue, and drugs called hyperosmotic agents (Mannitol, glycerol, and hypertonic saline solutions) may be administered to reduce this pressure. Pain relievers (analgesics), sedatives, and antianxiety medications may also be needed.

Other medication may be used to prevent or treat seizures, as well as to control fever and blood glucose levels.

For subarachnoid hemorrhage (a type of hemorrhagic stroke), a calcium-channel blocker (see chapter 1) called nimodipine (Nimotop) is used. It has been shown to reduce brain cell loss by preventing a complication called vasospasm.

SURGERY AND OTHER INTERVENTIONS—ISCHEMIC STROKE

Two types of procedures—carotid endarterectomy and angioplasty with stenting—are commonly used after an ischemic stroke to remove clots and blockages in the internal carotid artery (the main artery to the brain which runs up along the sides of the neck).

Carotid Endarterectomy

In carotid endarterectomy, the blocked area of the carotid artery is opened, the obstruction is removed, and the artery is then widened or repaired and closed. It is usually performed in patients with symptoms of stroke or TIA that can be attributed to a 70 percent to 99 percent narrowing of the internal carotid artery.

Angioplasty with Stenting

Angioplasty with stenting is a less-invasive procedure that is done as an alternative, especially if surgical risk for endarterectomy is too high. It involves

HEART ALERT:

Caution Before Starting Aspirin!

Unlike a heart attack where sometimes your doctor might recommend taking an aspirin while waiting for emergency services to arrive, this is *not* a good idea in the case of a stroke. This is because some strokes are caused by bleeding (hemorrhagic), and aspirin could worsen those cases. In fact, you should let your emergency team and doctors know whether you have already taken your daily aspirin. After evaluation and imaging tests, aspirin will likely be given to ischemic stroke patients.

inserting a catheter into a blood vessel in your leg or arm, gently threading it through to the carotid artery, opening the artery using a balloon (angioplasty), and finally placing a stent in the artery to keep it open (similar to coronary stenting).

SURGERY AND OTHER INTERVENTIONS— HEMORRHAGIC STROKE

Surgery is rarely performed for hemorrhagic strokes due to risk of rebleeding and brain damage from the surgery itself. It may be considered for large *subdural hematomas* (a collection of clotted blood outside the blood vessels) in the back of the brain or for superficial hematomas. In that case, the hematoma is opened through the skull and drained. For subarachnoid hemorrhage, surgical procedures vary with the underlying cause.

Clip Ligation and Coil Embolization for Aneurysms

An aneurysm is a localized blood-filled bulge in a blood vessel which may rupture and cause bleeding. It is usually present at birth, weakens over time, and usually does not cause symptoms until it ruptures. Clip ligation involves clamping off the aneurysm from the rest of the vessel using a metal clip to prevent further bleeding. Coil embolization is a less-invasive procedure which uses a catheter, inserted through a leg or arm artery and guided to the aneurysm, to deposit a coil that clots and seals the aneurysm.

Surgery, Stereotactic Radiosurgery, and Coil Embolization for AVMs

An arteriovenous malformation (AVM) is a congenital abnormal connection between an artery and a vein, which may burst and cause bleeding. A small AVM in an accessible area of the brain may be removed surgically. For less-accessible areas, stereotactic radiosurgery is preferred, where a focused beam of radiation is used to "clot off" the AVM. Coil embolization can also be used for AVMs.

CONTROL OF RISK FACTORS

After a stroke, it is essential to control your stroke risk factors, such as high blood pressure, high cholesterol, diabetes, or atrial fibrillation. For an ischemic stroke or TIA, you might have to take aspirin or other antiplatelet medicines. If you have chronic atrial fibrillation or certain other heart, blood-clotting, or blood vessel abnormalities, you may need to take anticoagulants to prevent another stroke. You may also need to take medicines to lower your cholesterol or your blood pressure (see chapter 11).

You can also improve your lifestyle by stopping smoking, reducing alcohol intake, exercising regularly, and eating a balanced diet.

REHABILITATION AND RECOVERY

Stroke rehabilitation (which is often shortened to "rehab") is an important and effective way of recovering after a stroke. Stroke rehab aims to make you as independent as possible and help you adjust to the effects of the stroke on your brain and body. In stable patients, rehab can begin in the hospital within two days after the stroke and can be continued after discharge in an inpatient, outpatient, or home-based setting.

In rehab, a team of doctors and nurses along with physical, occupational, and speech therapists will help you regain basic skills such as walking, eating, dressing, bathing, writing, and speaking. Other health profes-

Devices to Treat Stroke

Penumbra System

This is a clot-retrieval device that uses suction to remove blood clots in larger vessels of the brain to treat acute ischemic stroke. This system is effective if used within eight hours of the first symptoms, an option for those diagnosed beyond the three-hour window for receiving clot-busting therapy with recombinant tissue-type plasminogen activator (rt-PA). The Penumbra System became available for use in the beginning of 2008.

Penumbra is delivered into the brain using a catheter inserted through a small puncture in the groin. Using X-ray guidance, the device is maneuvered through the blood vessels of the body to the site of the clot in the brain. A separator is advanced and retracted through the catheter to dislodge the clot, and a suction device removes it.

MERCI Retriever

Cleared by the FDA in 2004, this tiny, cork-screw-shaped device works by wrapping around the clot and trapping it. It is threaded to the location of the clot via a catheter (as in coil embolization), and the clot is then retrieved and removed from the body. Most importantly, this system can be used for patients who are beyond the three-hour window for t-PA (only 3 percent to 5 percent of stroke patients arrive at hospitals within that window) and also in those who are ineligible for t-PA or fail to respond to t-PA. It has been proven to restore blood flow in the larger vessels of the brain.

PFO Closure Devices

A patent foramen ovale (PFO) is an opening between the right and left atria, detected in 10 percent to 15 percent of the adult population. A remnant of a baby's circulation while in the womb, a PFO is usually not a problem and is not associated with right-to-left shunting of blood. However, it can cause a condition called paradoxical embolus, in which a blood clot or foreign matter circulating in the veins moves into the arteries through a PFO, resulting in a stroke or TIA.

PFO and atrial septal aneurysm have been identified as potential causes for recurrent cerebrovascular problems. This is especially true in younger patients with no identifiable cause of a stroke (cryptogenic stroke). In case-control studies involving patients younger than fifty-five years of age, the prevalence of PFO was about three times greater in those with unexplained cerebral ischemic events than in the general population.

Therefore, there has been interest in surgical closure of PFOs in patients with a history of embolic stroke of unknown cause. Investigational closure devices are now available that can close PFOs.

The Penumbra System

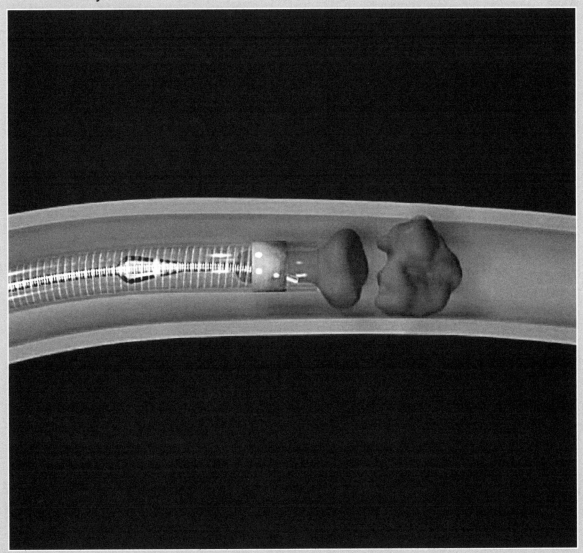

Enlarged photograph of the Penumbra system, a clot retrieval device.

sionals including psychologists, social workers, and vocational counselors can help deal with sadness and depression (which are very common after a stroke) and get you back into the community and to work.

More than half of the people who have a stroke regain the ability to take care of themselves. Many people relearn most of the lost skills, but some may have permanent deficits.

Stroke rehab should ideally begin as soon as the patient is stabilized and can last for several months to years, depending on the severity of symptoms after the stroke.

TESTS AND DIAGNOSIS OF STROKE

Initial exams and tests will aim to confirm the diagnosis of stroke and distinguish between an ischemic stroke or a hemorrhagic stroke (as drugs used for ischemic stroke can be life-threatening in the presence of a brain bleed). Other tests will help to determine the cause for the stroke. Most of these tests would also be performed within twenty-four hours of a TIA.

Your doctor will first gather information about your symptoms by getting a focused medical history and asking about any risk factors for stroke or heart disease that you might have. Your doctor will then perform a quick physical and neurological exam and listen to your heart and to the arteries in your neck with a stethoscope to assess for any abnormality.

Computed Tomography (CT) Scan

A CT scan is is usually the first test done for suspected stroke as it can quickly distinguish between an ischemic or hemorrhagic stroke. A CT scan involves a series of X-ray images to visualize the brain.

Magnetic Resonance Imaging (MRI)

MRI uses a magnetic field to generate a three-dimensional view of the brain. This test helps to accurately determine the extent of brain tissue damaged by an ischemic stroke, within minutes.

Blood Tests

Blood may be drawn to test for blood sugar, electrolytes, cholesterol, and liver and kidney function, as well as to assess blood clotting. These results help your doctor choose the correct treatment options and help rule out conditions that may cause symptoms similar to a stroke.

Electrocardiogram

An electrocardiogram is done to check for a cardiac cause of symptoms, including atrial fibrillation (see chapter 5) and other abnormalities in heart rhythms.

Carotid Ultrasonography/Doppler Scan

Ultrasonography uses sound waves that travel through tissues, are reflected back, and create images that can be deciphered for any abnormalities. A carotid ultrasonography/Doppler scan test shows narrowing or clotting in the carotid arteries and also the flow of blood through them.

Echocardiogram (Echo)

An echo is an ultrasound of the heart which is done if your doctor suspects a cardiac cause: blood clots, pumping or structural abnormalities, and valve disorders. A contrast echocardiogram (sometimes called a bubble study) can determine whether there is an opening (a PFO) between the left and right sides of the heart that could have allowed a blood clot in the legs to cross over to the left side of the heart and go to the brain.

Holter or Telemetry Tests

Holter and telemetry tests further assess heart rhythms by continuous EKG monitoring and may be used if your doctor suspects an underlying irregular heart rhythm.

Arteriography and Computed Tomographic/ Magnetic Resonance Angiography (CTA/MRA)

CTA/MRA tests use a dye and X-rays (for arteriography and CTA) or a magnetic field (for MRA) to look for narrowing, blockage, or malformations (such as aneurysms or AVMs). Arteriography is more invasive, as the dye is injected through a catheter threaded to the neck arteries; however, it gives more detailed information.

STROKE EXPLAINED

A stroke occurs when blood flow to the brain is impaired, either by blockage or by a rupture of an artery to the brain, leading to sudden death of brain cells due to lack of oxygen. When cells in an area of the brain die, the functions controlled by that part of the brain are lost. Symptoms depend on the location of the stroke as well as the extent of the brain damage (see below). However, one or more of the typical stroke symptoms (as discussed earlier in this chapter) are usually present.

Ischemic Strokes

Ischemic strokes account for more than 80 percent of all strokes (see Figure 4). There are two distinct types of ischemic strokes: embolic and thrombotic.

Embolic Stroke

An embolic stroke occurs when a blood clot forms at another location (usually the heart) and travels through the vessels (either whole or in fragments)

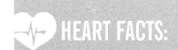

HEART FACTS:

Stroke

- Stroke is the third largest cause of death in the United States, behind diseases of the heart and cancer.

- Strokes kill more than 150,000 people every year. That's around one of every sixteen deaths.

- Each year, about 795,000 Americans suffer a new or recurrent stroke.

- Almost every forty seconds in the United States, a person experiences a stroke, and every three to four minutes, someone dies of it.

- Of every five deaths from stroke, two occur in men and three in women.

- More than four million adults in the United States live with the effects of a stroke. It is the number one cause of adult disability.

The American Stroke Association, a division of the American Heart Association, estimates that strokes cost the U.S. economy $68.9 billion in 2009. This projection includes costs paid by the government, insurance companies, and individual patients.

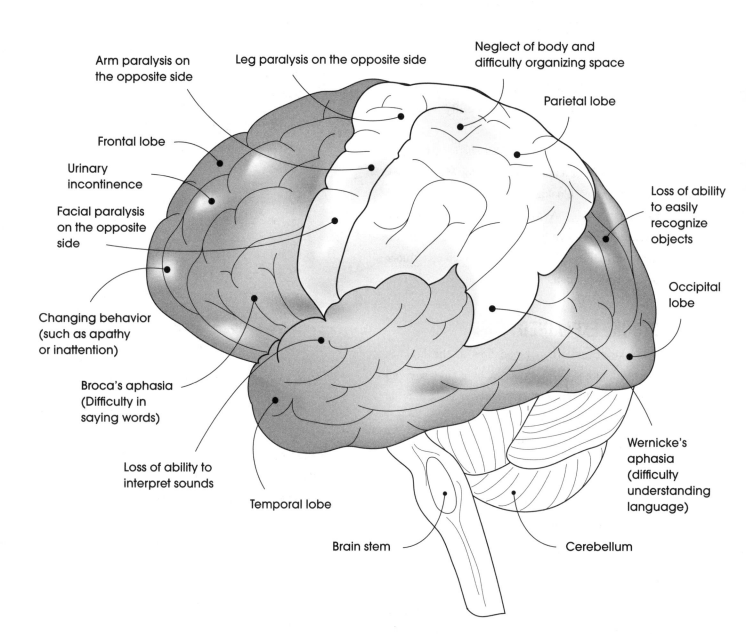

Arm paralysis on the opposite side

Leg paralysis on the opposite side

Neglect of body and difficulty organizing space

Parietal lobe

Frontal lobe

Urinary incontinence

Facial paralysis on the opposite side

Loss of ability to easily recognize objects

Occipital lobe

Changing behavior (such as apathy or inattention)

Broca's aphasia (Difficulty in saying words)

Wernicke's aphasia (difficulty understanding language)

Loss of ability to interpret sounds

Temporal lobe

Brain stem

Cerebellum

Areas of the brain that may be damaged by strokes and the dysfunctions that may occur as a result of loss of blood flow.

to your brain. Such a blood clot is called an embolus. Once in your brain, the clot eventually gets stuck in a vessel too small to let it pass and obstructs blood flow through the vessel, causing a stroke. Atrial fibrillation is an important cause, as it creates favorable conditions in the heart for a clot to form, break off, and go to the brain. Sometimes the heart will have a hole (a PFO) between the two atria. This opening would allow a blood clot in the leg veins to cross over to the left side of the heart and into the brain to cause a stroke.

Thrombotic Stroke

Atherosclerotic plaques are fatty deposits that form over time within the inner walls of your arteries, including those that supply the heart and the brain. In thrombotic stroke, a clot usually forms

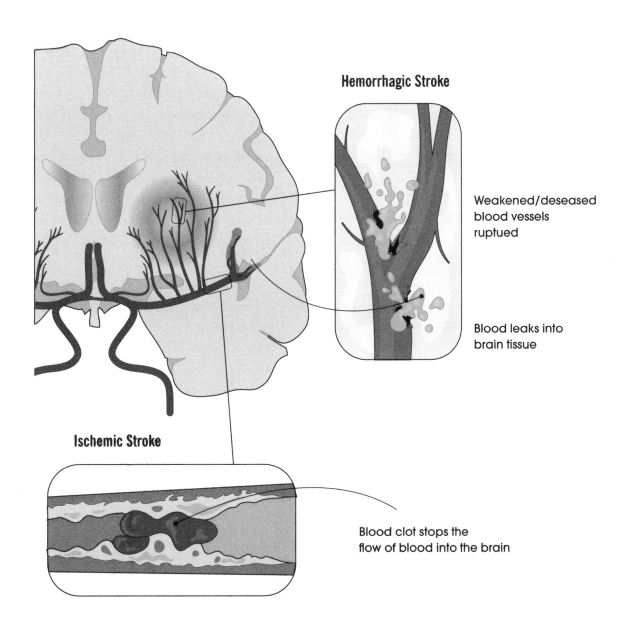

Hemorrhagic Stroke

Weakened/deseased blood vessels ruptued

Blood leaks into brain tissue

Ischemic Stroke

Blood clot stops the flow of blood into the brain

Depictions of an ischemic stroke and a hemorrhagic stroke and their affect on the brain.

around areas of the vessel wall damaged by atherosclerotic plaques leading to blockage of blood flow. Thrombotic stroke can be divided into two types: large-vessel thrombosis and small-vessel disease.

Large-vessel thrombosis is the most common type of thrombotic stroke. It is caused by sudden clot formation on a preexisting atherosclerotic plaque in a larger brain vessel. Patients who have large-vessel thrombosis are also likely to have risk factors and symptoms of coronary artery disease.

Small-vessel disease (lacunar infarction) occurs when blood flow is blocked to a very small arterial vessel in the brain. This type is closely related to high blood pressure.

Hemorrhagic Stroke

Hemorrhagic strokes account for less than 20 percent of all strokes (see Figure 5). They occur when a weakened blood vessel ruptures and bleeds into the adjacent brain tissue. Two types of weakened blood vessels that usually cause hemorrhagic strokes are aneurysms and AVMs.

There are two types of hemorrhagic stroke: subarachnoid and intracerebral hemorrhages. A third type of bleeding in the brain is a subdural hematoma.

A subarachnoid hemorrhage is bleeding into the area between the membranes surrounding the brain. It usually occurs spontaneously from a burst large-artery aneurysm but may also result from head trauma. It commonly strikes with a rapidly developing severe headache ("thunderclap headache"), vomiting, and an altered level of consciousness.

An intracerebral hemorrhage occurs due to bleeding from vessels within the brain into the surrounding tissue. High blood pressure is the most important cause of this type of hemorrhage. It is more likely to be fatal when compared to ischemic strokes or subarachnoid hemorrhage.

A subdural hematoma is bleeding outside the brain just under the skull. It occurs usually after trauma to the head (such as after a fall). This puts pressure on the brain and can make it function in an abnormal manner.

Some conditions which look like a stroke due to similar symptoms and must be ruled out by further testing include a tumor in the brain; an abscess (a collection of pus usually due to bacteria); viral infection of the brain (viral encephalitis); dehydration abnormalities in electrolytes (sodium, calcium, or glucose); and overdose of certain medications.

Q. & A. with Dr. Cannon

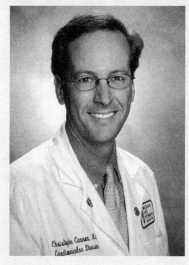

Q. Is it as important to get to the hospital for a stroke as it is for a heart attack?

A. Yes—in fact, it may be even more important! Current treatment for thrombotic stroke includes use of clot-busting medicines called thrombolytic drugs. These need to be given within the first three hours from the start of stroke symptoms to be of benefit. Thus, it is critical that you get to the hospital as quickly as possible.

Q. Are there new treatments that can be given to patients who have had a stroke but who don't seek medical attention until after three hours from the start of stroke symptoms?

A. Yes, new studies have suggested that benefit of the clot-busting medications might also occur if given between three and four and one-half hours after the onset of symptoms. This use is not yet approved by the FDA or in national guidelines, but new studies have just been completed. In addition, if patients go to a major stroke center, where angiograms of the brain arteries can be performed, clot-busting medications can be given through catheters directly into the blocked brain artery up to six hours after the start of symptoms.

Q. Is it necessary to take cholesterol-lowering medications after a stroke?

A. Yes. Multiple clinical trials suggest reductions in second strokes, heart attacks, and death if you take a statin after a stroke.

PART II:

THE MOST EFFECTIVE WAYS TO MAINTAIN YOUR HEART'S HEALTH

chapter 8:

YOUR HEART: A GUIDED TOUR

WHAT DOES THE HEART DO?

For many people, the heart represents the soul and the source of our feelings. But what about the heart as an organ in the body? What does it do, and how does it work?

The heart is the pump that drives blood through our bodies. All organs and tissues in our bodies require blood to function, and the heart gets it to them. Let's take a tour.

See figure 8.6 on pages 174–175.

HEART STRUCTURE

The heart is composed almost entirely of muscle and is very similar to other muscles in our bodies, such as those in our arms or legs. However, heart muscle is specifically designed for its purpose—to rhythmically contract, or squeeze, over and over, without our "remembering" to tell it to. Of course, many factors can alter the rate and strength of heartbeats. Intrinsic to the muscle of the heart is a desire to "beat"—even heart muscle in a glass dish will "beat" on its own, for seconds, minutes, or even indefinitely in ideal lab conditions. It's designed that way. The heart has specialized fibers that act as an electrical system—a natural pacemaker in the top of the heart and "wires" that go to the various parts of the heart to make it beat in a coordinated fashion.

The structure of the heart is uniquely designed to handle its job: delivering blood that is high in oxygen from the lungs to the body and returning blood low in oxygen from the body back to the lungs for a refill. And this has to be accomplished without mixing blood that is low in oxygen with newly oxygenated blood from the lungs.

Thus, the heart is divided into four chambers: two on the left and two on the right. Each side has an atrium, where blood is received, and a ventricle, from which blood is pumped out. In the healthy heart, the left and right sides are separated entirely, allowing for the separation of blood that is low in oxygen (returning from the body) from blood that is high in oxygen (coming from the lungs).

See figure 8.1 on page 169.

The heart makes sure blood flows in the correct direction through the use of four one-way valves. Let's follow the path of blood as it makes its tour through the heart.

THE CIRCUIT OF LIFE

As we breathe, our lungs saturate blood with oxygen and return that blood to the left atrium of the heart. As the left atrium contracts, it pushes blood through the mitral valve, which separates the left atrium from the left ventricle. The left ventricle is the major muscle of the heart; when it contracts, it expels blood out of the heart through the aortic valve to the entire body via the major artery leaving the heart—the aorta. This massive vessel runs out of the heart and down the body, with various arteries branching off to deliver oxygenated blood to the various parts of the body: the head, arms, abdomen and all of its internal organs, and finally, the legs. Arteries branch into smaller and smaller vessels as the blood gets farther from the heart.

See figure 8.4 on page 172.

The body and its organs then extract oxygen and other nutrients from the blood while it is in tiny vessels called capillaries. Capillaries have special channels that allow for such transport. Capillaries then switch to become small veins, called venules. In turn, the venules empty into larger veins that eventually pour into the two main veins of the body: the inferior vena cava (collecting blood from the lower half of the body) and the superior vena cava (collecting blood from the upper half of the body).

DIRECTIONAL FLOW

The inferior and superior vena cavae meet at the heart to return the body's blood to the heart's right atrium. When the right atrium contracts it pushes blood through the tricuspid valve and into the right ventricle. This valve keeps blood flowing only from the right atrium into the right ventricle. The right ventricle is similar to the left ventricle, but not as strong. As it contracts, the tricuspid valve closes, preventing blood from back-flowing to the right atrium, and blood flows out through the pulmonary valve to the lungs to receive oxygen once again. And the cycle continues.

See figure 8.3 on page 171.

A CLOSER LOOK AT THE HEART'S CHAMBERS

Atria Receive Blood to Load into the Ventricles

The two atria, the left and the right, act as receiving chambers in the heart—hence the name *atria*. They are a bit like a waiting room before seeing the doctor. Blood waits in the atria to enter the pumping chambers of the heart—the ventricles. The right

Nomenclature of the Heart

The chambers of the heart are separated into left and right *atria* and left and right *ventricles*. The atria accept blood into the heart; the ventricles eject blood to its destination. The heart tissue that separates the left and right sides is called a *septum*; there is an atrial septum and a ventricular septum. The contraction sequence of the heart is termed *systole*—the act of squeezing to push blood out. The time during which the heart muscle is relaxing is called *diastole*—while it fills with blood. The left ventricle pumps blood into the major artery that supplies the entire body: the *aorta*. The aorta branches into smaller and smaller arteries, called *arterioles*, then *capillaries*. Capillaries fill small veins, called *venules*, which fill into bigger and bigger veins. The major veins that return blood to the heart are the *superior vena cava* (from the upper body) and the *inferior vena cava* (from the lower body). Arteries that serve the heart muscle directly are the *coronary* arteries; arteries that serve the lungs are the *pulmonary* arteries. The major vein draining the heart's own supply of blood is the *coronary sinus*, whereas blood returning from the lungs comes via the *pulmonary veins*.

What's an Artery? What's a Vein?

An artery carries blood that has lots of oxygen from the heart to all the organs in the body. A vein carries blood that's low in oxygen from the body back to the heart. Because of the different jobs of arteries and veins, they are structured differently; arteries tend to have thicker walls to contain the higher pressures that come from the left ventricle, whereas veins tend to have thinner walls and lower pressures.

There are two exceptions to the preceding statements: The *pulmonary* arteries carry blood *low* in oxygen away from the heart to the lungs, and the *pulmonary* veins carry blood high in oxygen back to the heart from the lungs. Both the pulmonary arteries and the pulmonary veins have relatively low pressures.

atrium receives blood from the superior and inferior vena cavae. It also receives blood from the coronary sinus, a special vein that drains blood from the heart muscle itself. The left atrium receives blood from the lungs, via the pulmonary veins.

Both atria contract and push blood into their respective ventricles, which eject blood to either the body (on the left side) or the lungs (on the right side). Because blood from the atria is not going far, the atria do not have to contract strongly—and can't; they have relatively thin walls with much less muscle than the ventricles.

The contractions of the atria are helpful to keep blood moving; however, they are not essential to life. In certain diseases of the heart (e.g., atrial fibrillation, see chapter 5), the atria do not contract well, yet most patients may not feel much different than they would otherwise. This is because as the ventricles relax and enlarge, they can "suck" blood in from the atria, whether the atria contract or not. Ventricular function is essential to life.

Ventricles Flush Blood from the Heart

The ventricles are the workhorses of the heart—they are all muscle, and they work all the time. The right ventricle is responsible for moving blood into the lungs, and the left ventricle delivers blood to the body. The two ventricles are divided by a piece of muscle called the septum; this barrier keeps blood in each chamber totally separate. Because the left ventricle has to push blood to a much larger distribution, it generates much higher pressure and requires much more muscle.

(continued on page 177)

THE FOUR CHAMBERS OF THE HEART

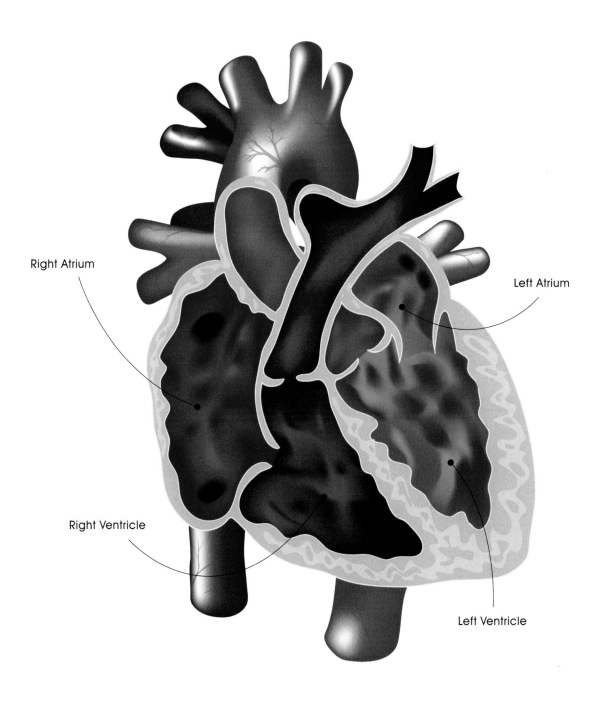

Right Atrium

Left Atrium

Right Ventricle

Left Ventricle

Figure 8.1

The heart is divided into four chambers, two on the left and two on the right. Each side has an atrium, where blood is received, and a ventricle, from which blood is pumped out. In the healthy heart, the left and right sides are divided, preventing blood returning from the body, which is low in oxygen, from mixing with blood high in oxygen coming from the lungs. The right ventricle pumps blood to the lungs, where it gets oxygen, and the left ventricle pumps blood out to the body. Four one-way valves ensure that blood flows in the correct direction through the chambers.

THE ELECTRICAL SYSTEM OF THE HEART

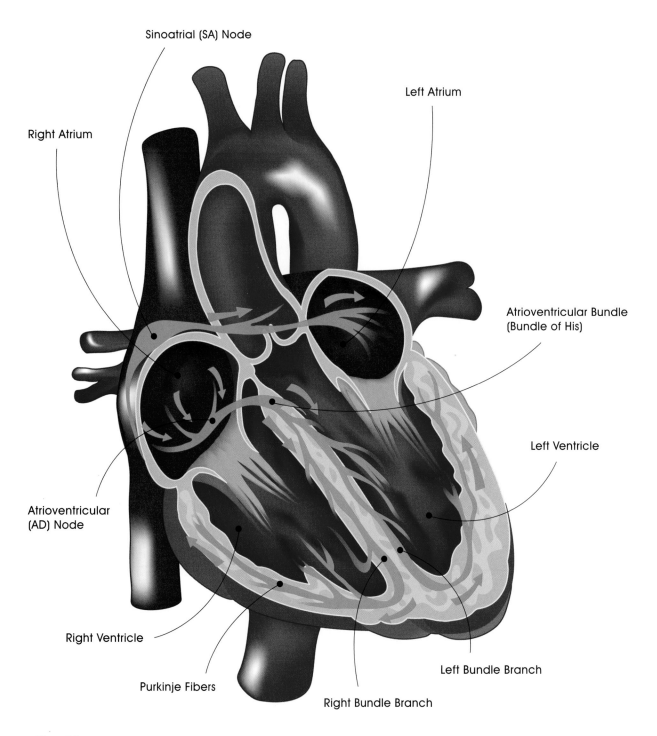

Sinoatrial (SA) Node

Left Atrium

Right Atrium

Atrioventricular Bundle
(Bundle of His)

Atrioventricular
(AD) Node

Left Ventricle

Right Ventricle

Purkinje Fibers

Left Bundle Branch

Right Bundle Branch

Figure 8.2

The heart's electrical activity begins in the right atrium where the sinoatrial (SA) node—the heart's pacemaker—initiates each beat. The impulses from the SA node spread through the muscle of the right and left atria, which contract in response to these signals. The AV node is connected to electrical fibers embedded in the muscle of the ventricles, called the His-Purkinje system. The fibers of the His-Purkinje system are specifically designed to conduct electrical impulses quickly. The His-Purkinje system is divided into two sections—a right bundle branch and a left bundle branch, each supplying their respective ventricles.

THE AORTIC, MITRAL, AND TRICUSPID VALVES OF THE HEART

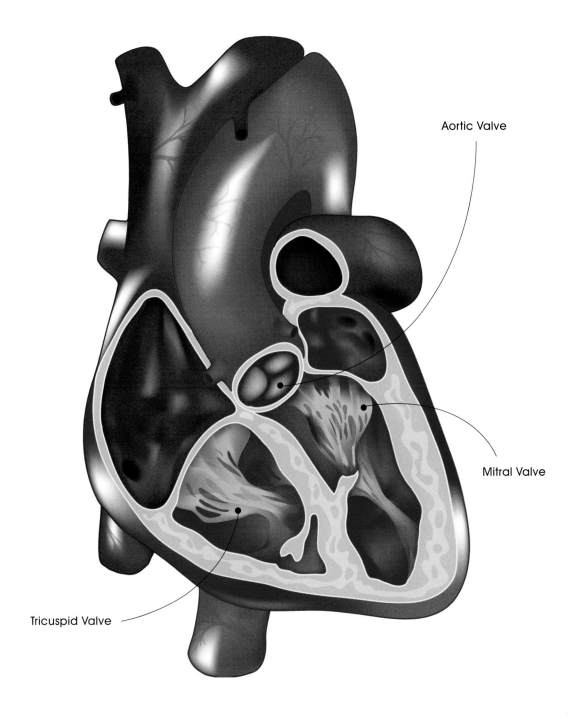

Aortic Valve

Mitral Valve

Tricuspid Valve

Figure 8.3

Blood is pumped through the heart's chambers with the help of four heart valves. The valves open and close to let blood flow in one direction from one chamber to another. Three valves are shown here: the aortic valve which is between the left ventricle and the aorta, the mitral valve, which is between the left atrium and the left ventricle, and the tricuspid valve, which is between the right atrium and right ventricle. The pulmonary valve—hidden under the aorta—is the valve between the right ventricle and the pulmonary artery going to the lungs.

DIRECTIONAL FLOW OF BLOOD THROUGH THE HEART

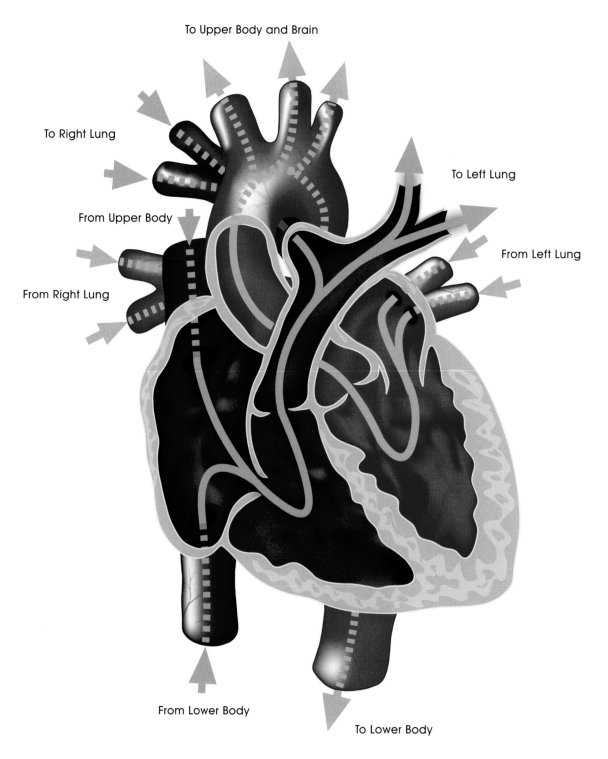

Figure 8.4

This diagram shows the directions that blood flows through the heart. De-oxygenated blood (in blue) is returned to the heart from the body at the right atrium. When the right atrium contracts, it pushes the blood through the tricuspid valve and into the right ventricle. The right ventricle is similar to the left ventricle but not as strong. As it contracts, the tricuspid valve closes, preventing blood from back-flowing to the right atrium, and blood flows out through the pulmonary valve to the lungs to receive oxygen.

VIEWS OF ALL FOUR VALVES IN NORMAL STATES

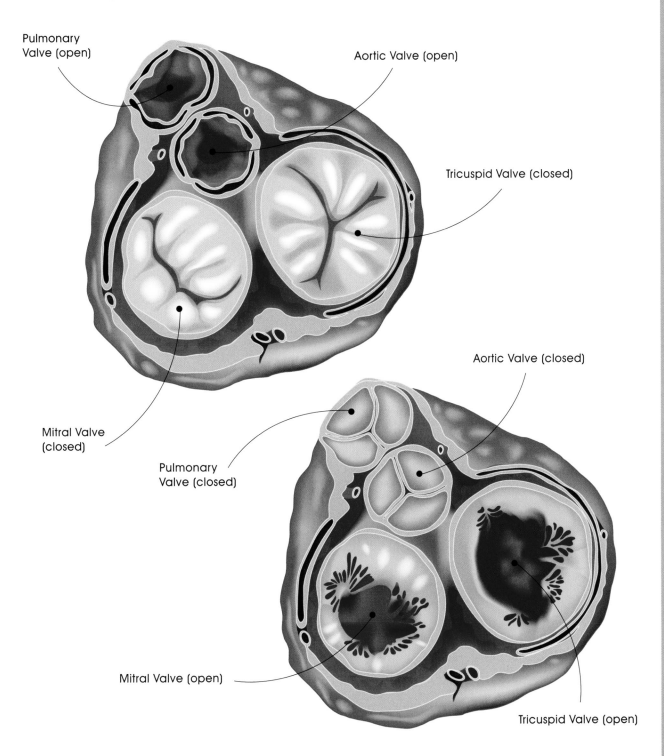

Pulmonary Valve (open)

Aortic Valve (open)

Tricuspid Valve (closed)

Mitral Valve (closed)

Aortic Valve (closed)

Pulmonary Valve (closed)

Mitral Valve (open)

Tricuspid Valve (open)

Figure 8.5

Figure 8.5 portrays the four valves of the heart in their open and closed positions. The valves control flow at two points in the contraction cycle of the heart. The mitral valve controls flow between the left atrium and the left ventricle, while the tricuspid valve controls flow from the right atrium to the right ventricle. The aortic valve is the gateway from the left ventricle out to the aorta and the rest of the body, while the pulmonary valve maintains forward flow from the right ventricle to the lungs through the pulmonary artery.

THE CIRCULATORY SYSTEM

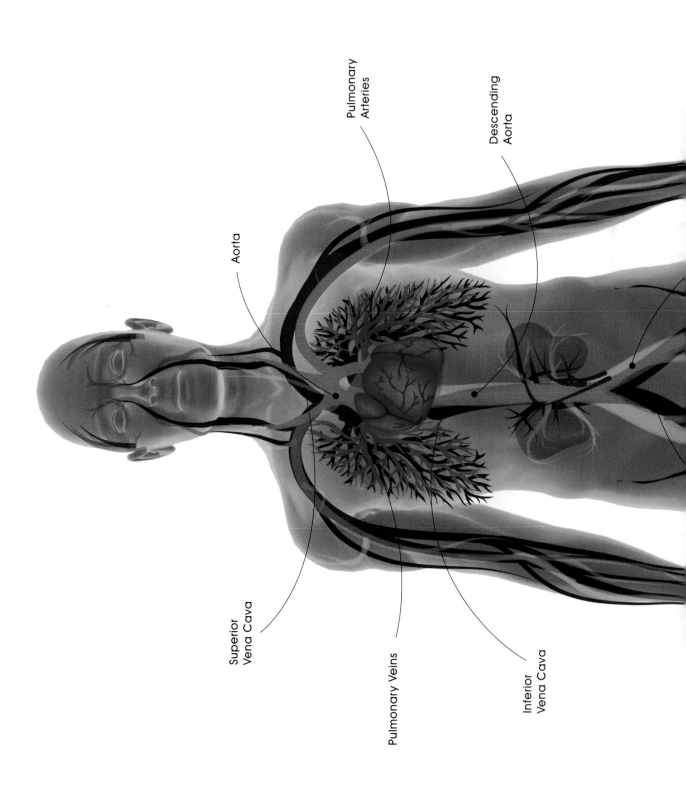

Pulmonary Arteries

Descending Aorta

Aorta

Superior Vena Cava

Pulmonary Veins

Inferior Vena Cava

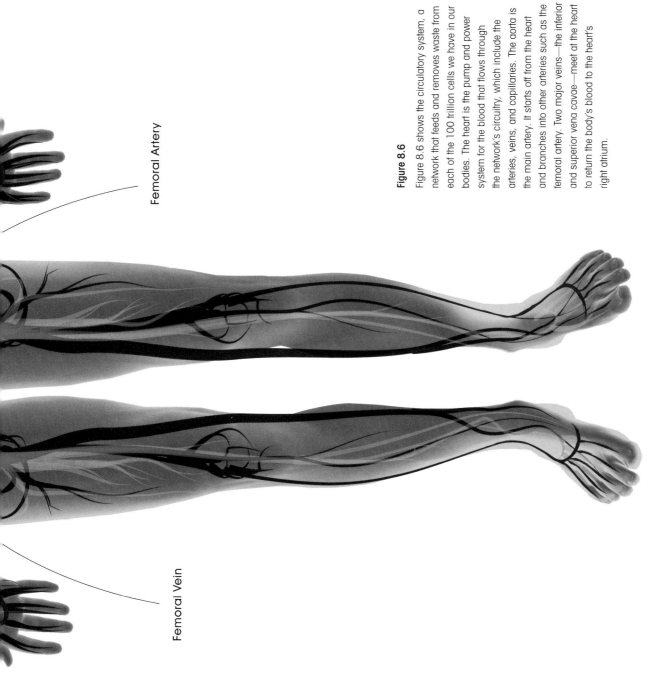

Femoral Artery

Femoral Vein

Figure 8.6

Figure 8.6 shows the circulatory system, a network that feeds and removes waste from each of the 100 trillion cells we have in our bodies. The heart is the pump and power system for the blood that flows through the network's circuitry, which include the arteries, veins, and capillaries. The aorta is the main artery. It starts off from the heart and branches into other arteries such as the femoral artery. Two major veins—the inferior and superior vena cavae—meet at the heart to return the body's blood to the heart's right atrium.

THE HEART: A VIEW FROM THE OUTSIDE

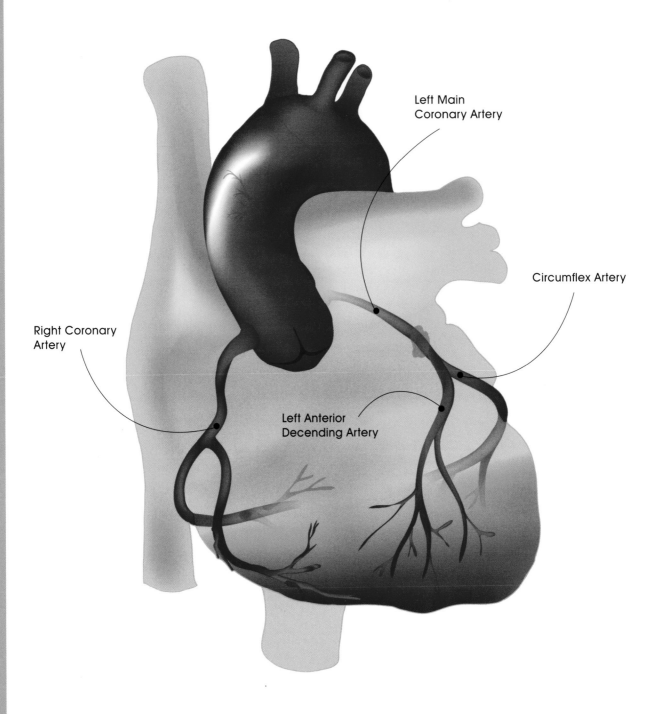

Left Main
Coronary Artery

Circumflex Artery

Right Coronary
Artery

Left Anterior
Decending Artery

Figure 8.7

Figure 8.7 shows the outside of the heart. The coronary arteries feed the heart muscle with the oxygen-rich blood it needs to perform its demanding job. The coronary arteries consist of two main arteries: the right main coronary artery and the left main coronary artery. The right coronary artery supplies the right atrium and right ventricle. It branches into the posterior descending artery, which nourishes the bottom of the left ventricle and back of the septum. The left main coronary artery branches into the circumflex artery, which supplies blood to the left atrium, and side and back of the left ventricle, and the left anterior descending artery, which supplies the front and bottom of the left ventricle and the front of the septum.

Unlike the atria, the ventricles go through an elaborate cycle of contraction and relaxation; the size of the ventricles varies widely throughout this cycle. Following each contraction, the ventricles relax and enlarge to accommodate another load of blood from the atria, thereby sucking blood from the atria into the ventricles. As the ventricles expel blood, the aortic and pulmonary valves prevent it from falling back into the ventricles from the body or lungs, respectively. Following this relaxation, the atria start the next contraction cycle, pushing another load of blood into the ventricles. When fully loaded, the ventricles squeeze, their size decreasing from the largest they can get to the smallest to force blood out.

As you can imagine, such coordinated motion of all of the heart's chambers requires an intimate communication network. This is accomplished through an elaborate system of electrical impulses that tell each part of the heart when to contract.

THE HEART'S ELECTRICAL SYSTEM

The heart's electrical system involves several features with two main goals: to keep the heart beating at regular intervals at an appropriate rate and to coordinate the beating of all parts of the heart at the appropriate times.

The heart's electrical activity begins in the right atrium with a special piece of tissue that acts as the heart's pacemaker, initiating each beat. This is called the sinoatrial (SA) node. The heart cells here are special; they beat spontaneously and provide the initiating spark of electricity for the rest of the heart to follow. The timing of these sparks—or how fast the heart is supposed to beat—is controlled by many factors: Nerve signals from the brain, responding to emotions, can speed up or slow the heart rate; different hormones in the blood, such as adrenaline, serve to increase heart rate; low oxygen levels in the blood drive the heart to beat faster; and changes in the body's electrolytes, low blood pressure, or high temperature can also cause the SA node to increase its rate.

See figure 8.2 on page 170.

The impulses from the SA node spread through the muscle of the right and left atria, and they contract in response to these impulses. Because the electricity is simply traveling through the thin muscle of the atria, this is a relatively slow conduction. However, the impulses then reach another piece of special tissue called the atrioventricular (AV) node. As labeled, this special electrical tissue sits at the junction of the atria and ventricles. It is here at the AV node that the speed of conduction picks up, and that is a good thing!

Once the impulses hit the AV node, they are on an electrical superhighway. The AV node is connected to electrical fibers embedded in the muscle of the ventricles, called the His-Purkinje system. The fibers of the His-Purkinje system are specifically designed to conduct electrical impulses and to conduct them fast.

The His-Purkinje system divides into two sections—a right bundle branch and a left bundle branch, each supplying their respective ventricles. The left bundle branch further divides into an anterior fascicle and a posterior fascicle—delivering impulses to the front and back of the left ventricle, respectively. This is how the ventricles can coordinate the elaborate contraction cycle we discussed earlier; electrical impulses coming down the His-Purkinje system reach all parts of the ventricles nearly simultaneously, thus creating a highly coordinated contraction of both the left and right ventricles. And *voilà*! Blood is pumped out of the heart.

A CLOSER LOOK AT HEART VALVES

Mitral Valve: Separating Left Atrium and Left Ventricle

The mitral valve controls the flow between the left atrium and the left ventricle. It is composed of two leaflets, analogous to a trapdoor between the two chambers. As blood moves into the left ventricle, the trapdoor falls open. When the left ventricle contracts to move blood out to the body, the doors swing shut to prevent backflow into the left atrium. The leaflets or doors are tethered by strings of muscle to prevent them from swinging all the way back into the left atrium. Thus, blood in the left ventricle cannot flow back into the left atrium and must escape out to the aorta.

See figures 8.3 and 8.5 on pages 171 and 173.

Aortic Valve: Controlling Flow from the Left Ventricle to the Body

After the left ventricle contracts to move blood out to the body, it must relax and fill with more blood from the left atrium. What prevents it from filling with blood it has already pushed out to the body? This critical task belongs to the aortic valve. It is positioned just outside the left ventricle at the beginning of the aorta, the major artery that connects the heart to the body.

The aortic valve is composed of three leaflets attached to the wall of the aorta. As blood flows out of the heart, the leaflets are compressed against the wall of the aorta, out of the way of blood flowing to the rest of the body. Between ventricular contractions, blood sinks back toward the left ventricle and is caught by the three leaflets. This process is also important for the heart's own blood supply.

See figures 8.3 and 8.5 on pages 171 and 173.

Tricuspid Valve: Separating the Right Atrium and the Right Ventricle

As blood returns to the right atrium of the heart from the rest of the body, forward flow from the right atrium to the right ventricle is controlled by the tricuspid valve. This valve functions very similarly to the mitral valve, with the exception that it has three leaflets or doors that swing open when the right atrium contracts to pump blood into the right ventricle. Similar to the mitral valve, these three trapdoors swing shut when the right ventricle contracts, tethered by muscle to hold them in place, and blood slams against them. Thus, blood is ejected out to the lungs.

See figures 8.3 and 8.5 on pages 171 and 173.

Pulmonary Valve: Controlling Flow from the Right Ventricle to the Lungs

The pulmonary valve controls blood flow from the right ventricle to the lungs. Similar to the aortic valve on the left side, the pulmonary valve is the mechanism that prevents blood ejected into the lungs from falling back into the right ventricle as it relaxes. Like the aortic valve, these three enveloping cusps are compressed out of the way to allow blood to flow toward the lungs and catch any backflow to the right ventricle. Notably, the blood going to the lungs does not have far to go, so the right ventricle does not generate nearly the same amount of pressure as the left ventricle. Thus, the structures on the right are generally weaker and thinner than those on the left, as they do not experience the wear and tear from higher pressures.

See figures 8.3 and 8.5 on pages 171 and 173.

HOW DOES THE HEART MUSCLE GET BLOOD?

Just like every other part of the body, the heart requires blood to function. In fact, pound for pound, the heart and brain require the most oxygen of any of the body's organs! And although it is constantly bathed in oxygen-rich blood from the lungs, not all of the heart's muscle can absorb these nutrients simply through the heart chambers; they have to be delivered deep into the heart tissue by other blood vessels. Thus, the heart has its own arteries, the coronary (or crown) arteries, which feed blood to different parts of the heart.

There are three major coronary arteries that begin as two arteries from the aorta. Initially, the left coronary artery is one artery, called the left main coronary artery. It then separates into two segments—the left anterior descending (LAD) artery and the left circumflex artery (LCA). The LAD usually runs *down* the *front* of the *left* ventricle, carrying blood to a major portion of left ventricle muscle (hence the name left *anterior descending*). The LCA wraps around the left side of the heart, feeding the left side of the left ventricle, the back of the left ventricle, and the left atrium.

The right coronary artery comes off the aorta and feeds most of the right side of the heart, including the atrium and ventricle, and then goes on to feed the back part of the left ventricle. It is also mainly responsible for supplying blood to the major electrical tissues of the heart. Interestingly, there is some overlap in the territories supplied by the left coronary and right coronary arteries—which is a good thing. The overlap means a decrease in flow to one side can occasionally be supported by redundant flow from the other. However, a major obstruction in any of these arteries often leads to a significant heart attack.

See figure 8.7 on page 176.

The coronary arteries are attached to the aorta right next to the aortic valve; in fact, they are positioned between the leaflets of the valve. Yet, as blood is ejected out and the leaflets are compressed against the side walls of the aorta, the coronary arteries do not fill. As the left ventricle relaxes, the ejected blood begins to fall back toward the aortic valve. As the valve's leaflets catch the backflow of blood, blood fills the coronary arteries. Thus, while the rest of the body gets blood when the heart contracts, the heart's arteries, the coronary arteries, fill while the heart is relaxing. This is important; it is much easier for blood to get to the muscle of the heart when it is relaxed than when it is tight and contracted.

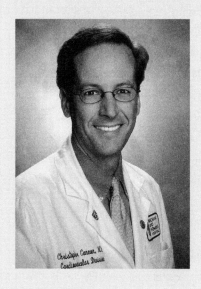

Christopher Cannon, M.D.
Cardiovascular Division

Q. What is the "lub-dub" of the heartbeat?

A. The two sounds of the heartbeat are the sounds of the valves closing. The "lub" is when the mitral and tricuspid valves close when the heart ventricles *start* a heartbeat. The "dub" is when the aortic and pulmonary valves close at the *end* of a heartbeat.

Q. Can I live if my electrical system fails?

A. Yes, but you might need an artificial pacemaker. The normal heartbeat starts in the SA node, but it can age and malfunction. It may simply beat too slowly. The other electrical tissues can beat at forty to seventy beats per minute to keep you alive, but you'll feel weak and thus may need a pacemaker implanted.

Normal heart function usually provides a resting heart rate of fifty-five to seventy beats per minute, but it can vary among individuals. We usually use a simple calculation to determine one's maximum possible heart rate: 220 minus your age. Thus, a twenty-year-old can usually achieve a heart rate of 200, whereas a sixty-year-old may be able to achieve a maximum heart rate of only 160. But again, this varies.

Q. I have been told I have a murmur. What is it exactly?

A. A murmur is simply an abnormal sound of blood moving in the heart. Most often, this is due to a problem with one of the heart valves, which is leaky (or not closing properly) or calcified (not opening enough). When blood moves through the valve, it makes extra noise that can be heard with a stethoscope. A murmur is not necessarily dangerous. Many people have murmurs that will not affect them; however, in some circumstances a murmur can represent abnormalities in the heart's structure or function that will require medical attention. It is important to discuss this with your doctor if you do have a murmur.

chapter 9:

HOW TO DETERMINE YOUR RISK

RISK FACTORS FOR HEART DISEASE

More people die every year from heart disease than from any other cause. Cancer, the second largest killer, accounts for a little more than half as many deaths.

The good news is that coronary heart disease (CHD)—the most common form of heart disease—is largely preventable. Yet many people are not aware of the factors that increase the odds of developing heart disease and the things they can (and shouldn't) do to reduce those odds.

The first, simple—but significant—step toward prevention is to understand these factors. The next step is to assess your level of risk and figure out areas in which you can make positive changes, with the support of your health care team.

KNOW YOUR RISK FACTORS

Any condition or disease that increases your odds of developing heart disease is called a *risk factor*. Major risk factors have been proven to significantly increase the risk of heart disease. We know by how much they add to cardiovascular risk; how they cause heart attacks and heart disease; and how many heart attacks we can prevent by controlling them.

Major risk factors are classified into two categories:

- *Modifiable risk factors* (such as smoking) can be controlled or treated by adopting heart-healthy habits and taking medications that your doctor might prescribe. You and your health care team will primarily focus on changing these risk factors for the better to lower your level of cardiovascular risk.

- *Nonmodifiable risk factors* (such as advanced age) are beyond your or your doctor's control. These factors will persist throughout your life. Your only option is to make extra effort to tackle your modifiable risks with added urgency and intensity.

MODIFIABLE RISK FACTORS

Cholesterol and Other Fats (Lipids)

Cholesterol is a waxy, fatlike substance produced in the liver, ideally in quantities that are just enough to take care of your body's requirements. An excess of cholesterol is usually caused by diet. This extra cholesterol accumulates in our arteries (a process called atherosclerosis), leading to blockages and eventually heart disease. As we describe in chapter 11, cholesterol exists in our blood in two important forms: low-density lipoprotein (LDL) and high-density lipoprotein (HDL) cholesterol. The relationship between your total, LDL, and HDL cholesterol levels determines your cardiovascular risk.

LDL is the "bad cholesterol" that carries cholesterol to your vessel walls and deposits it there. HDL is the "good cholesterol" that does the reverse—it removes fatty buildup from your arteries. Total and

LDL cholesterol levels have a continuous and graded relationship with heart disease risk, so higher numbers will always mean a higher risk. Low HDL adds to this risk to some extent.

Smoking

The rate of heart attacks is increased sixfold in women and threefold in men who smoke at least twenty cigarettes per day, compared to people who never smoked. Smoking accounts for about one in five heart disease deaths. Smokers are two to four times more likely to develop heart disease compared to nonsmokers, and this risk increases with the number of cigarettes smoked daily.

Notably, marijuana use is not an established risk factor for heart disease, but it does act as a rare trigger for a heart attack. It increases the heart rate and blood pressure within the first hour and thus increases the risk of heart attack by about five times. (For cocaine, this number is about twenty-four times).

Exposure to second-hand smoke (passive smoking) also increases cardiovascular risk. When cigarette smoking acts in the presence of other existing risk factors, it enhances your risk from those factors as well. Smoking lowers HDL, increases blood pressure, increases fibrinogen (a protein that promotes blood clotting), and injures the vessel walls, making them more susceptible to fatty buildup. To know more about smoking and keys for quitting, see chapter 14.

High Blood Pressure (Hypertension)

Hypertension is more prevalent than any of the other major risk factors. It increases your risk of developing heart disease and stroke, and this risk becomes greater as your blood pressure climbs. When high blood pressure exists with few or none of the other

HEART HELP:

Cholesterol Screening

In all adults twenty years of age or older, a blood test called a *fasting lipoprotein profile* should be obtained once every five years. This test measures levels of total cholesterol, LDL cholesterol, HDL cholesterol, and triglycerides. The results are accurate only if the test is done after a nine- to twelve-hour fast. If the test is done nonfasting, only the values for total cholesterol and HDL cholesterol are usable. In this case, if your total cholesterol is equal to or greater than 200 mg/dL or if your HDL is equal to or greater than 40 mg/dL, your doctor will order a repeat lipoprotein profile, which must be done in a fasting state.

Cholesterol screening may begin at an early age if your doctor feels you may be at risk, usually due to presence of heart disease or some genetic abnormalities in the way your body processes cholesterol.

Triglycerides are a distinct group of fats found in the bloodstream that also raise your cardiovascular risk. Elevated triglycerides are usually seen in people with diabetes or those who are obese. Increased triglycerides are linked to high LDL and low HDL levels. Lp(a) is a genetic variant of LDL cholesterol that may separately contribute to heart disease risk by promoting fatty plaque formation. To learn more about lipids, see chapter 11.

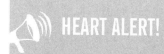

Metabolic Syndrome

Metabolic syndrome is a constellation of risk factors that tend to cluster together and increase the risk of heart disease. It is characterized by central obesity (fat in and around the belly), abnormal lipid levels favoring plaque formation, insulin resistance (utilization of insulin and glucose is inadequate), high blood pressure, and a situation that favors inflammation and clot formation in the blood vessels. Metabolic syndrome is diagnosed if three out of the following five criteria are present:

- Central obesity, defined by waist circumference equal to or greater than 40 inches (102 cm) in men and equal to or greater than 35 inches (89 cm) in women

- Fasting triglycerides equal to or greater than 150 mg/dL

- HDL cholesterol equal to or greater than 40 mg/dL in men and equal to or greater than 50 mg/dL in women

- Blood pressure equal to or greater than 130/equal to or greater than 85 mm Hg

- Fasting glucose equal to or greater than 100 mg/dL

Metabolic syndrome is becoming increasingly prevalent and promotes the development of diabetes and heart disease. In fact, having this syndrome can increase your risk for developing heart disease by one and a half to three times.

risk factors, the overall risk is relatively less. But if many other risk factors are present, cardiovascular risk increases several times. It has been estimated that if diastolic blood pressure is reduced by 5 to 6 mm Hg, one-quarter of the deaths from heart disease can be prevented. To learn more about hypertension, see chapter 12.

Physical Inactivity

If you lead a sedentary life, you're almost twice as likely to suffer a heart attack as someone who exercises regularly. Exercise can raise HDL levels and reduce blood pressure, insulin resistance, and obesity. Regular exercise has been shown to actually prolong life. Even moderate exercise can lower your risk. To learn more about exercise, see chapter 14.

Obesity

Obesity is defined in terms of body mass index (BMI). BMI is calculated by dividing your weight (in kilograms) by your height (in meters) squared (i.e., height × height) (BMI = W [kg]/H [m^2]). A person with a BMI higher than 25 is considered overweight, whereas a person with a BMI higher than 30 is considered obese (see page 249 for a handy table of BMI ratings arranged by height and weight). Overweight or obese people have a higher rate of heart disease and are more likely to develop diabetes. Obesity is linked to high blood pressure, elevated triglycerides, decreased HDL, and an increased risk of death from all causes. Excess weight is more dangerous if it is around the waist, compared to weight around the hips. To read more about weight control, see chapter 14.

Diabetes Mellitus

In people with type 2 diabetes, the risk of a heart attack or stroke is increased two- to fourfold, while the risk of death from any cause is doubled. About three-quarters of people with diabetes die of some form of cardiovascular disease. The cardiovascular risk of having diabetes is similar to that associated with having a prior heart attack. In other words, if you have diabetes, your level of risk is the same as somebody who has already had a heart attack and has CHD. Also, people with type 2 diabetes have higher rates of death during and after a heart attack. Thus, diabetes is categorized as a *CHD risk equivalent*. Diabetics have higher rates of hypertension and obesity, elevated fibrinogen, elevated triglycerides, and abnormal blood lipids. In fact, higher levels of blood glucose may be associated with increased cardiovascular risk, even in people without diabetes. To learn more about diabetes, including type 1, see chapter 13.

NONMODIFIABLE RISK FACTORS

Increasing Age

Approximately four out of every five people who die from heart disease are sixty-five years of age or older. The amount of fatty deposits (plaques) in the arteries increases over time. These plaques are ultimately responsible for most heart attacks. So as we age, our risk for heart disease increases. Younger men (younger than forty-five) and women (younger than fifty-five) are less likely to be affected by this condition.

Gender

In general, men have a higher risk of heart attack than women at any given age, although this difference considerably narrows as women pass menopause. Men have heart attacks at earlier ages compared to women. The level of risk in women lags about ten to fifteen years behind that of men. However, CHD is the leading cause of death even among women.

Women are relatively protected from heart disease due to the effect of estrogen and other sex hormones. However, after menopause, this protective effect is somewhat lost. In fact, women who have heart attacks at an old age are more likely than men to die from them.

Heredity

Sometimes it's just in your genes. Heart disease tends to cluster in families. If either of your parents had heart disease (especially "prematurely"), you are more likely to develop it and your risk may be higher if both parents were affected. Similarly, presence of heart disease in siblings also increases cardiovascular risk. If your father, brother, or grandfather developed heart disease before the age of fifty-five or your mother, sister, or grandmother developed it before age sixty-five, you have a family history of premature heart disease, which increases your cardiovascular risk.

Race

Certain groups have higher rates of heart disease than others. For example, African Americans have high rates of heart attacks, stroke, high blood pressure, and heart failure. More than one-quarter of Mexican Americans have some form of heart disease. American Indians and native Hawaiians also have increased rates. People of South Asian descent are at very high risk, but people of Japanese descent are a low-risk group.

OTHER RISK FACTORS

Stress and Psychosocial Factors

How successfully you deal with stress may affect your risk of heart disease. Different people respond differently to stressful situations. Hence, the effects of stress are not completely understood. Stress may act on the body directly by increasing your heart rate and blood pressure, by exposing your body to stress hormones (such as adrenaline and cortisol) that further increase blood pressure, and by increasing clotting factors in the blood and promoting clot formation. Stress may also act indirectly; people tend to smoke, drink alcohol, and eat in greater amounts when they are "stressed out." They also exercise less and may become overweight. Other psychosocial conditions such as depression and anger may also add to cardiovascular risk.

Alcohol

Recent research suggests that moderate alcohol consumption has a protective effect on heart disease. Alcohol raises your HDL cholesterol and decreases the formation of blood clots by preventing platelets from clumping together.

However, drinking too much alcohol can increase your triglyceride level, your blood pressure, and your calorie intake. It can cause high blood pressure, cardiomyopathy (an enlarged and weakened heart), stroke, and heart failure. There are also several adverse effects of alcohol consumption outside of the heart (cancers, motor vehicle accidents, social effects, etc.). Many of the beneficial effects of drinking alcohol can also come from safer alternatives such as a healthy diet, exercise, and taking niacin and aspirin.

Chronic Kidney Disease (CKD)

In this condition, there is a gradual decline in your kidneys' ability to remove waste and toxins from the blood. The result is that these harmful substances accumulate in the body. Heart disease kills a majority of people with this condition. CKD may worsen heart disease even before it has caused any major damage to the kidneys themselves.

Inflammation (Assessed by C-Reactive Protein)

Heart disease involves some amount of inflammation of the blood vessels. C-reactive protein (CRP), which can be determined through blood tests, is a marker of inflammation that is linked to development of heart disease, stroke, and death. For more information on C-Reactive Protein see the box on the right.

CALCULATE YOUR RISK

Now that you know your risk factors, you can start assessing your level of risk. The best way to do this is by using a validated risk factor score. All risk factors are not equal; some increase your risk to a greater extent than others. Further, risk is also affected by the magnitude of individual risk factors; for example,

HEART ALERT!

Drink Alcohol in Moderation

If you drink, do so in moderation. The upper limit is one to two drinks per day for men and one drink per day for women. If you are a non-drinker, do *not* start drinking just to decrease your risk for heart disease.

if two people have cholesterol levels elevated above normal, the person with the higher level would be at greater risk. Thus, using a score is more accurate as it accounts for the effect and magnitude of each risk factor.

Most doctors use the Framingham risk score to evaluate heart disease risk in patients. This score is based on data from the Framingham Heart Study, which began in Framingham, Massachusetts, in 1948 with more than 5,000 people. Since then, researchers have followed three generations of this population to identify cardiovascular risk factors and determine their effects on heart disease.

Calculating your risk is beneficial in many ways:

- An accurate understanding of your risk helps your doctor adjust the intensity of treatment. For example, if you are high risk, you will need to be treated aggressively. However, you may not need such intensive treatment if your risk is low.
- Using a risk-assessment tool ensures that all potentially modifiable risk factors are identified and treated.
- Knowing your risk will motivate you to make that extra effort and closely follow your doctor's instructions.

CRP Test

Research suggests that injury and subsequent inflammation of the arteries plays an important role in the process of atherosclerosis. The body produces CRP during any inflammatory condition. High-sensitivity CRP (hs-CRP) testing is a simple blood test that can detect a heightened level of inflammation in your body by measuring CRP.

Initial studies have suggested that elevated CRP levels are at least as good, if not better, in predicting heart disease risk as cholesterol levels. It has also been suggested that this test can identify high-risk patients who may otherwise go undetected by usual cholesterol-based screening.

Elevated CRP can increase the risk of having a heart attack (by two to three times) and dying from heart disease. It also adds to the risk of having a second heart attack or a second stroke. One recent large-scale study has shown that when apparently healthy individuals with raised CRP but normal LDL levels are treated with a statin drug, the risk of heart attacks and stroke is reduced by about one-half.

The decision to perform this test is usually based on your ten-year Framingham risk score:

- If your risk score is less than 10 percent, this test may not be required.

- If your ten-year risk score is between 10 percent and 20 percent, currently this test is warranted. This is because if CRP levels are elevated in people with "intermediate" ten-year risk, they are treated as aggressively as people who are in the "high" risk group (with risk scores greater than 20 percent).

- If you already have CHD or any of the CHD risk equivalents (including a greater than 20 percent risk score), you will be treated intensively regardless of hs-CRP levels. This test will add very little to the way your risk factors are managed, although some doctors will check to see if the level went down after medical treatment.

FIVE STEPS TO CALCULATING RISK

There are five steps that you and your doctor should take to determine and lower your risk for heart disease.

Step 1: Fasting Lipid Profile

First, your doctor will order a test called a complete fasting lipoprotein profile. Based on the results, you will know whether your LDL, HDL, triglycerides, and total cholesterol numbers are within the normal range.

Increased LDL cholesterol is linked to increasing heart-disease risk. In addition, many research studies have shown that LDL-lowering therapy reduces risk for heart disease. So, lowering LDL cholesterol will be the main target for you and your doctor. Your other risk factors will determine how aggressively your LDL should be lowered.

Step 2: Medical History

Next, your doctor will ask whether you have any of the following:

- Clinical CHD: a prior heart attack, current or prior stable/unstable angina, or any prior procedures such as bypass surgery or angioplasty
- Symptomatic carotid artery disease: a transient ischemic attack (a mini stroke) of carotid origin or if your doctor discovers a greater than 50 percent narrowing on angiography or ultrasound of the carotid artery
- Peripheral artery disease (PAD): painful cramping in your hip, thigh, or calf muscles after walking or climbing stairs (intermittent claudication); numbness, weakness, or coldness in your lower leg or foot; nonhealing sores, change in the color of your legs, hair loss, or nail changes in your foot or leg
- Abdominal aortic aneurysm: a weakened and bulging area in the aorta, the main artery that supplies blood to the body

The last three conditions are caused by the buildup of fatty plaque in the arteries of the leg, the carotid artery, and the abdominal part of the aorta, respectively. This buildup is due to atherosclerosis, which also affects the coronary arteries (vessels of the heart). In fact, coronary atherosclerosis and noncoronary atherosclerosis share the same risk factors, and the presence of one often predicts the presence of the other. So, these conditions are treated as CHD risk equivalents, as cardiovascular risk is approximately equal to that in established CHD. As mentioned previously, diabetes is another CHD risk equivalent.

Step 3: Count Risk Factors

Your doctor will count the number of major risk factors (other than LDL) that you have. The major risk factors are as follows:

- Cigarette smoking
- Hypertension (blood pressure greater than 140/90 mm Hg or on blood-pressure-lowering medication)
- Low HDL cholesterol (lower than 40 mg/dL)
- Family history of premature CHD (see the "Heredity" section earlier in this chapter)
- Age (men forty-five years or older; women fifty-five years or older)

Good news: High HDL (greater than 60 mg/dL) is considered a negative risk factor due to its protective effect. If you have high HDL, one risk factor will be subtracted from your total count.

Step 4: Find the Framingham Score

Your doctor will then use the Framingham risk score to calculate your CHD risk. You can also calculate your risk online using an online tool called the Risk Assessment Tool for Estimating Your 10-Year Risk of Having a Heart Attack, which can be found on the official website of the National Heart, Lung, and Blood Institute. (Go to http://hp2010.nhlbihin.net/atpiii/calculator.asp). In this scoring system, all major risk factors (age, total cholesterol, smoking, HDL, and blood pressure) are divided into categories according to increasing severity. Each category is assigned points, with the more severe categories receiving higher points. These points are then added to calculate point totals, which in turn correspond to the ten-year CHD risk percent.

As an example, if your ten-year CHD risk is 20 percent, it means there is a one in five chance that you will have a major coronary event (heart attack or death from heart disease) within the next ten years.

Three levels of ten-year risk are identified: Less than 10 percent means low risk, 10 percent to 20 percent is intermediate risk, and higher than 20 percent is high risk. A person with a ten-year risk of greater than 20 percent is considered to have a CHD risk equivalent and will be treated as aggressively as someone who already has heart disease. In fact, most people with other CHD risk equivalents (such as diabetes, carotid artery disease or PAD, or an abdominal aortic aneurysm) will also have a ten-year risk of greater than 20 percent. If you have any of these conditions, you are presumed to be at high risk for heart disease, and calculation of the Framingham risk score is not needed. Similarly, if you have one or none of the major risk factors mentioned earlier, it is most likely that your ten-year risk score will be less than zero. Thus, you are presumed to be at low risk and a ten-year risk assessment is not necessary.

Step 5: Determine LDL Goal

Once your risk has been calculated, your doctor will use this risk estimate to determine your LDL goal. If you are above the goal, your doctor can use your ten-year risk to decide whether to treat you with lifestyle changes alone or to add drug therapy.

For more information on treatment of abnormal cholesterol levels, see chapter 12.

Q. & A. with Dr. Cannon

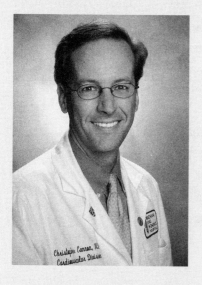

Q. Should I have screening tests such as a carotid ultrasound test or ankle brachial index to see whether I have a blockage in my neck or leg arteries?

A. Screening tests are not currently recommended for all people. The issues are that it would cost lots of money to screen all patients with these tests, and sometimes tests can lead to complications and additional tests. However, in selected patients, testing may be appropriate.

Q. I have heard of a blood test called CRP. Should I get that when I have my cholesterol checked?

A. Yes. CRP stands for C-reactive protein. It is a relatively new test that indicates inflammation in your body. Generally (if you do not have lupus, rheumatoid arthritis, any infection, or any other major illness), it is an indicator of irritation in the blood vessels, and it correlates with a higher risk of having a heart attack or stroke—over and above cholesterol levels.

Q. I am forty years old and my father had a heart attack at age forty. What should I do to assess my risk?

A. You should have a physical with your doctor to measure your blood pressure and your BMI, and to have a cholesterol panel and CRP performed. Then, calculate your Framingham risk score. If that is elevated or if your CRP is greater than 2 mg/L, check with your doctor about beginning lifestyle modification and an exercise program to improve your risk profile, and possibly taking a statin medication.

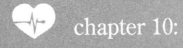 chapter 10:

LIVING WITH HEART DISEASE

LIVING WITH HEART DISEASE

Thanks to tremendous advances in medical science and quality of care, more people are now living with heart disease, rather than dying of it.

Having a heart attack or being diagnosed with heart disease can be traumatic and life-changing for you and your family. Without the right information and support, this change is often for the worse—patients may resign themselves to a dependent, depressed, and sedentary life, leading to further worsening of their heart condition. However, with some commitment from you and support from your family and medical team, it is possible to use this event as a driving force for the better.

Surviving a heart attack (or heart surgery) is just the beginning of a long journey. Recovery from heart disease, in fact, can be a difficult physical and emotional roller-coaster ride. There is good news, however: Most people lead full and active lives despite having heart disease. Over time, people often emerge feeling better and healthier after a heart attack (or heart surgery) than before it.

Remember, heart disease is a permanent, chronic condition. *Once you have heart disease, you can control it but you cannot make it go away.* So, it is vital that you treat this event as a wake-up call and as an opportunity to take immediate, persistent, and positive action to manage and enhance your heart health.

CARDIAC REHABILITATION

Cardiac rehabilitation, or cardiac rehab, is a medically supervised exercise, education, and counseling program designed to improve your physical, psychological, and social functioning. Cardiac rehab forms part of the comprehensive recovery process for patients with heart attack, heart disease, or heart surgery.

In cardiac rehab, you will work with a specialized team consisting of cardiologists, nurses, and other health care professionals such as dietitians, occupational therapists, physical therapists, exercise physiologists, psychologists, psychiatrists, social workers, and vocational counselors.

Cardiac rehab will help you recover from a heart attack or heart surgery, identify your risk factors and suggest lifestyle changes you can bring about to control them, get you back to work and to the community as safely and quickly as possible, and improve your overall health and quality of life.

Who Needs Cardiac Rehab?

Cardiac rehab benefits a wide variety of heart disease patients. You should be in rehab if you have or have had any of the following:

- A heart attack
- Coronary bypass surgery
- Percutaneous coronary intervention
- Stable angina
- Heart valve repair or replacement
- Heart or heart-lung transplant
- Heart failure

Everyone—men, women, the young, and the elderly—can benefit significantly from rehabilitation.

WHAT WILL HAPPEN DURING REHAB?

Typically, cardiac rehab is divided into three phases.

Phase I: Baby Steps

Phase I is the inpatient phase, which ideally should begin as soon as your condition has stabilized. This phase will prepare you for the day-to-day activities you will need to perform after discharge from the hospital. While you are in intensive care, a nurse will help you exercise your arms, legs, hands, and feet (called range-of-motion exercises). You may then start with simple things such as sitting up or moving around in bed, sitting in a chair, and washing and dressing, either in intensive care or in the regular ward. You will eventually be able to walk up and down the hallways, climb stairs, and independently perform simple household tasks. Members of the rehab team may visit you in the hospital and give you some preliminary information about the recovery process and about improving your risk factors by changing your lifestyle.

Phase II: Outpatient Rehab

Phase II is the outpatient rehab process that typically begins two to six weeks after discharge from the hospital and continues on a regular basis (around three times per week) for about two to three months. This phase will help you gradually increase your exercise regimen under supervision and reduce your risk factors. Overall, you may spend two to six months in this stage of your recovery. Here are some details on outpatient rehab:

- Your doctor will need to provide a referral for a cardiac rehab facility where a specialized team will work with you. Home-based rehab is an option if you do not have any rehab centers nearby or it is too difficult to get to one. Talk with your doctor about your preferences and ask for a suitable referral.
- The process will begin with a medical assessment by your doctor (see the upcoming "Initial Medical Assessment" section).
- Your team will then determine the level of exercise you can safely tolerate (using a cardiac stress test) and design a structured exercise program. You will slowly build up your exercise levels into a stable regimen at the

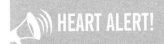

HEART ALERT!

The First Few Days

The first few days after discharge from the hospital are best spent getting enough rest and taking it easy. The key is to continue with the activities you were doing just before leaving the hospital and *not to try to do anything additional.* This could include light household activities, but you should avoid doing anything strenuous that would require additional energy. These activities would include lifting, pulling and pushing heavy objects, heavy yard work, shoveling snow, and so forth. Take a breather whenever you feel tired. Avoid working after a large meal, when it is very hot or cold, or at high altitudes.

Although it is recommended to gradually intensify your exercise regimen, this should only be done in a safe manner—that is, after an initial medical assessment and under medical supervision.

It is also important to take all your medications exactly in the amount and manner prescribed by your doctor. Remember to keep your follow-up appointment with your doctor and also contact him or her immediately if you have any symptoms you feel might be related to your heart condition or to side effects of your medications.

end of this phase. Your exercise will be under constant medical supervision. You will be educated about heart-healthy nutrition, quitting smoking, and other changes you can make in your lifestyle to prevent your heart condition from worsening. Counseling and support for emotional issues (stress, anxiety, depression, etc.) will also be available.

Phase III: Maintaining Recovery

This is the ongoing—or maintenance—phase of the recovery process, where you continue with the exercise regimen established in the preceding phase while maintaining a healthy lifestyle aimed at reducing your heart disease risk factors. Constant medical supervision and EKG monitoring is no longer necessary; most people develop a home-based or a gym-based exercise program, although you may continue at the cardiac rehab facility as well. Exercise is usually scheduled three times per week, although it will be customized to suit your needs and preferences.

ESSENTIAL PARTS OF A REHAB PROGRAM

Initial Medical Assessment

Your medical team will review your medical history, with a focus on any heart disease diagnoses and procedures you may have had, along with current and prior heart disease symptoms, medications, and risk factors. A physical exam and some tests (EKG, blood cholesterol, blood sugar, etc.) may also be done at this time. Based on this information, your doctor will create a treatment plan with short-term and long-term goals for controlling your risk factors, as well as strategies to achieve those goals.

Controlling Cholesterol Levels

The team will also review your medications and risk factors for abnormal cholesterol levels. Blood will be drawn to measure lipids (total cholesterol, high-density lipoprotein, low-density lipoprotein [LDL], and triglycerides) four to six weeks after hospitalization, and two months after starting or altering your lipid medication. For LDL, you will receive dietary counseling to help adopt a heart-healthy diet and will be started on a statin unless you have some conditions (such as liver or kidney disease) that might make you ineligible for taking statin drugs. Using these interventions, your doctor will aim to keep your LDL lower than 70 mg/dl (see chapter 12).

Tackling High Blood Pressure

Your doctor will measure your blood pressure in both arms during two or more visits as part of initial assessment for hypertension. Your blood pressure medications and lifestyle choices affecting blood pressure will also be reviewed (see chapter 13).

- If your systolic blood pressure is 120 to 139 mmHg or your diastolic blood pressure is 80 to 89 mm Hg, your doctor will suggest some changes in your lifestyle to lower your blood pressure.
- If your systolic blood pressure is equal to or higher than 140 or your diastolic blood pressure is equal to or higher than 90 mm Hg, you will be given medications to lower your blood pressure.
- If you have chronic kidney disease, heart failure, or diabetes, medication may be given—even for systolic blood pressure equal to or higher than 130 or diastolic blood pressure equal to or higher than 80 mm Hg.

Diabetes Care

If you have diabetes, your doctor will review your diabetes medications, diet, and blood sugar monitoring methods. You'll discuss symptoms related to diabetes complications along with any episodes of low (hypoglycemia) or excessively high (hyperglycemia) blood sugar levels. Your blood may be tested for levels of fasting blood sugar and glycosylated hemoglobin (HbA1c). You will be taught how to recognize hypoglycemia or hyperglycemia and what you can do to treat it. You will also be informed by a dietitian about the "diabetic diet."

Controlling Your Weight

Your weight, height, and waist circumference will be measured to calculate your body mass index (BMI). If you're overweight or have fat around your belly (BMI is greater than 25 kg/m² and/or waist is greater than 40 inches [102 cm] in men and 35 inches [89 cm] in women), your rehab team will help you set short- and long-term weight loss goals, which will help you lose weight in a safe and durable manner. For example, you may be asked to reduce body weight by 5 percent to 10 percent by shedding 1.5 lbs (0.7 kg) per week over six months. You can reach these goals by following the eating and exercise plans the team creates for you. A registered dietitian may help you decide on a diet geared toward weight loss (see chapter 14).

Quit Smoking

You will be asked about the amount and duration of smoking and as well as your willingness to quit. If you are not yet ready, your doctor will tell you about the risks associated with smoking and encourage you to kick this habit. If you are ready to quit, your doctor will help set a quit date and reinforce the risks of continued smoking. Your doctor will provide nicotine replacement with a nicotine patch or gum and

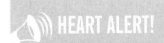

HEART ALERT!

Diabetes and Exercise

If you are on insulin or drugs that increase insulin secretion, your blood sugar levels can change rapidly with exercise. Therefore, you should monitor your blood sugar levels before and after every exercise session.

You will be advised not to inject insulin in your exercising limb and to avoid exercising for a certain time after taking your medication when insulin levels are highest in your blood. This is because exercise can lower blood sugar levels, and the effect is magnified if insulin levels are high, leading to hypoglycemia.

- You can safely exercise if your preexercise blood sugar levels are between 100 and 300 mg/dL.

- For levels lower than this, the recommendation is to delay your exercise by at least fifteen minutes. Your doctor might tell you to keep some candy or juice handy, to help you bump up your blood sugar immediately. If after fifteen minutes your blood sugar is higher than 100 mg/dL, you may start your exercise.

- For levels greater than 300 mg/dL, you should exercise only if you are not feeling sick or short of breath, you do not have ketones in your urine, and you keep yourself well hydrated.

For other diabetes medications, blood sugar checks are needed for only the initial six to ten sessions because the risk of hypoglycemia is low with these drugs.

may use drugs such as bupropion (Zyban) to help you quit. He or she may also refer you to a smoking cessation group program and may suggest supportive measures such as hypnosis, acupuncture, and self-help literature (see chapter 14).

Changing Your Diet

Nutritional counseling will be provided by a registered dietitian who will discuss your dietary habits, food choices, and intake of specific nutrients. You will be educated about specific areas of your diet where you can make changes, as well as some techniques to improve your eating behavior. Your customized dietary plan will aim to reduce calorie and fat intake. If required, dietary measures to reduce blood pressure and control diabetes may also be introduced (see chapter 14).

PRESCIPTION FOR EXERCISE

This is a structured, supervised exercise program that is custom-designed according to your needs and preferences by specialized professionals and then approved by your doctor. The main components of an exercise prescription are the mode, frequency, duration, intensity, and progression of exercise.

Mode: What Types of Exercise Are Good?

Aerobic training is the best form of exercise for cardiac rehab. It consists of low-impact activities such as walking, jogging, treadmill use, cycling, rowing, stair climbing, and similar exercises that require the use of the whole body or at least large muscle groups.

Resistance training uses cuff/hand weights, dumbbells, free weights, weight machines, calisthenics, elastic bands, or wall pulleys to increase muscle mass, strength, and stamina in an effort to improve performance of household chores and activities at work.

All rehab programs incorporate aerobic exercises; some also introduce components for strength training and increasing flexibility as your condition improves. Your rehab team will help you choose the exercises you like best and will adhere to most conveniently.

Frequency: How Often Should You Exercise?

For aerobic exercise, your target will be to exercise three to five times per week, while resistance exercises will be required two to three times per week to produce the desired benefits.

Duration: How Long Should You Exercise Each Time?

For aerobic exercise, each session should last for thirty to sixty minutes. For strength training, you will ultimately build up to one to three sets of eight to ten different upper- and lower-body exercises.

Actual intensive exercise lasts twenty to forty minutes in what is called the *conditioning phase*. Participants should warm up and cool down for five to ten minutes before and after the conditioning phase. The warm up/cool down phases include low-intensity activities such as stretching, which slowly increase or decrease the workload on your heart. Warming up also helps prevent muscle injury, while cooling down will reduce the chances of developing low blood pressure (hypotension) and irregular heart rhythm that may occur if exercise is stopped abruptly. Patients with heart failure and heart transplant will need longer warm-up and cool-down periods.

Intensity: How Hard Should You Go?

One of the first tests you will undergo before starting an exercise-based rehab program is a *symptom-limited exercise tolerance test* or a stress test (see appendix II). The results of the stress test will let your doctor know the *maximal* or *peak heart rate* you can reach before you start having symptoms (such as chest pain, shortness of breath, etc.). This peak heart rate will then determine the *target heart rate*—the range your pulse needs to be in for you to gain the most benefits without jeopardizing the safety of your heart.

Usually, the target heart rate range is 50 percent to 80 percent of the peak heart rate attained during the stress test. Patients with heart failure and heart transplant will exercise at lower intensity.

HEART ALERT!

Estimated Peak Heart Rate

When people start a fitness program at a gym or a health club, the trainer often uses a simple formula to estimate their peak heart rate:

Estimated peak heart rate = 220 – age (in years)

Although this estimation may work reasonably well for people without heart disease, it is not appropriate for people with heart disease. This is because people with heart disease are often on drugs which can slow down their heart (most commonly beta blockers) by varying amounts. You may develop symptoms at heart rates much lower than your target heart rate range, if it has been estimated using this formula. A stress test is much more accurate.

Exercise Progression

All exercise programs start at the lower end of your target rate, frequency, and duration. The heart rate may gradually increase by 5 percent to 10 percent until you reach the upper limit of your target range. In general, the duration and frequency are increased before increasing the intensity. Thereafter, you reach the maintenance stage, where no more changes are made to your exercise regimen.

Supervision

If your doctor thinks you are at moderate or high risk of cardiac complications from exercise (either you have had multiple heart attacks, you have severe heart failure, or very low ability to exercise), your exercise will be medically supervised with heart rate, blood pressure, and electrocardiogram monitoring for eight to twelve weeks until your regimen is declared safe.

Low-risk patients (with stable heart disease) may be initially monitored for six to twelve sessions. Once you are reassured about the safety of exercise and understand how to monitor exercise intensity, you may exercise without supervision. You will need to take your pulse or use a heart-rate monitor before, during, and after exercise. You may need to report these readings to your rehab team.

Physical Activity Counseling

Clinical studies have shown that moderate-intensity exercise has beneficial effects on heart disease. Physical activity counseling will help you incorporate activities and habits in your day-to-day routine that will provide adequate exercise and will be as effective as a structured exercise program. You will be encouraged to accumulate thirty to sixty minutes per day of moderate-intensity physical activity on at least five (preferably most) days of the week. Some changes that may be suggested include active yard work, actively playing with kids, parking farther away from entrances, walking two or more flights of stairs, walking during your lunch break, and walking at a brisk pace.

PSYCHOSOCIAL MANAGEMENT

After a heart attack, heart surgery, or other serious cardiac event, you may feel depressed, anxious, angry, or isolated or be in denial. It is important to get help for these conditions immediately. Depression can make your recovery longer and harder. It can cause physical problems such as an irregular heart rhythm, chest pain, reduced exercise capacity, less energy, and more fatigue, and it may even increase your risk of death. It can also affect your relationships, your family, or your marriage, and can keep you from returning to work.

Your rehab team will identify these and other potential problems such as sexual dysfunction and addiction to drugs and alcohol. Psychotherapy, counseling, and stress-management classes will be provided on a one-on-one basis or in small groups to help you cope with these emotions. Your doctor may also prescribe medications for these conditions. Trained personnel including psychologists, psychiatrists, and social workers will be available as part of your rehab program to educate and support you throughout this tough phase. Include family members or significant others in these discussions for maximum benefit.

Benefits of Cardiac Rehab

Cardiac rehab can help you live longer and reduce your chances of future heart problems. It can re-duce your risk of dying from a heart attack, keep you out of the hospital, decrease chest pain,

WHAT'S NEW:

"Wii-hab"

How does the Wii work? Nintendo's Wii is a popular gaming system that features a unique, motion-sensitive game controller used for games such as tennis, baseball, golf, bowling, and boxing. This new controller captures the player's movements so that the animated character on-screen can display a similar action. Instead of just pressing buttons on a traditional controller, the Wii requires players to actually swing their arm to hit a baseball or throw a punch when boxing.

How is it used? Some cardiac rehab centers have now started using the Wii alongside traditional rehab methods in individual or group sessions once or twice per week. The idea is that gaming movements will help increase strength, endurance, and coordination, while making the otherwise repetitive and boring exercise sessions more entertaining. Patients may then be more motivated to stick to their rehab regimen. Some may end up getting their own consoles so that they can continue their Wii-hab even when at home. Actual results from research studies about the benefits of Wii-hab are still limited, but some clinical trials are underway to evaluate this new therapy.

lower your need for medication, and possibly reduce the progression of atherosclerosis. Over the long term, you will improve your strength and stamina, adopt heart-healthy habits, and learn to manage stress and enhance your emotional health. Eventually, you will improve your quality of life and will be able to function independently in society and in the workplace.

RETURNING TO NORMAL ACTIVITY

Housework

You may perform light housework, such as dusting, cleaning, and cooking, within the first few days of returning from the hospital. You should attempt heavier work such as yard work, gardening, and work involving heavy loads weeks to months after returning home—depending on your exercise capacity at that point in time.

Work

The amount of time you remain away from work depends on the type of heart condition you have, the treatment you received, and the type of work (whether it involves heavy exertion or lots of stress) that you do. For example, after angioplasty for stable angina, you may return to work in days, but if you had a heart attack or surgery, it may be several weeks before you can get back to work. Consult with your doctor on this issue. Although most people can return to their original jobs, some people may need to change to a less tiring or less stressful vocation. It is also a good idea to let your employer know about your condition.

Driving

If you do not have chest pain or complications, you can generally start driving within a week. If you still have symptoms, they must be stable for a few weeks before you can drive again. As with getting back to work, the wait time is much longer if you have had a heart attack or heart surgery compared to someone who just has stable angina. Of course, each state has different laws regulating driving after serious illness—be sure to comply with state law.

Sexual Activity

Sex is also a form of exercise as it can increase your heart rate and blood pressure, thus adding to the workload on your heart. Many of the rules for exercise apply to sex as well. You may need to take it easy initially and gradually resume normal activity. Your doctor may decide to do another stress test before giving the all-clear signal. In general, most people can resume sexual activity within three to six weeks. Some positions (such as side by side or with your partner on top) are less stressful for your heart than others. Some of your medications may interfere with sexual functions. It is a good idea to keep your doctor posted if you have any sexual problems or develop any new heart-related symptoms.

Travel

Your doctor will tell you when you can start traveling. Most people who do not have symptoms can begin flying. While traveling, always pack light (so that you do not have to lift heavy bags), build plenty of time into your schedule (to avoid the stress related to a rushed schedule), keep your medications handy (you might need them), and avoid going to places that are very hot or cold or at high altitudes.

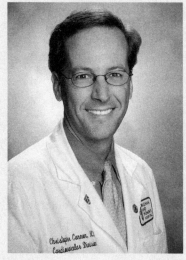

Q. I had a heart attack four months ago, and I didn't participate in a cardiac rehab program. Is it too late to join one now?

A. No, it is not too late. It is certainly reasonable to rest after a major heart attack, and it is a good idea to join a cardiac rehab program to help build up your exercise level and endurance. It also helps get many other aspects of life in order, with tips on and compliance with medications and a general understanding of the issues with heart disease and how to prevent any further heart problems.

Q. When exercising, do I need to target a specific heart rate, or should I just exercise as tolerated?

A. No, you do not need to target a specific heart rate. Some exercise programs will have you pay close attention to slower versus faster heart rates during exercise. Generally, doing moderate exercise is the key. If you find your heart rate goes very high (greater than 100 percent of your age-predicted heart rate), it might be a sign that you are pushing too hard too fast. I believe moderation is key.

Q. How often do you recommend exercising each week?

A. Our guidelines recommend exercising for thirty minutes each day of the week, but they allow for some days where you can't because of your schedule. Thus, five times per week is an "A" for exercise.

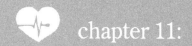 chapter 11:

ALL ABOUT CHOLESTEROL

HIGH CHOLESTEROL

Your doctor has told you that you have an excess of harmful cholesterol in your blood, often called simply "high cholesterol." Her diagnosis means there's a good chance you are developing *or already have* heart disease. Your doctor may have expressed her concerns to you in a number of ways: She may have revealed that you have *high* blood levels of low-density lipoprotein (LDL), the culprits that cause clogging in coronary arteries. Or she may have said you have *low* levels of high-density lipoprotein (HDL), which is the good cholesterol that helps eliminate harmful cholesterol from your blood. Perhaps she said you have high levels of triglyceride, a type of fat. (We'll explain these terms later in this chapter.) The all-important bottom line is that if you have high cholesterol, you need to get it under control to halt the development of heart disease.

THE PRESCRIPTION

When you have been told you have a cholesterol problem, the first step is to know your numbers. Knowing what your LDL and HDL cholesterol numbers are is key to getting them in a healthy range. Then, for extra credit, know your triglyceride level (the "other" bad cholesterol). Next we think about treatment, and this has two parts: lifestyle changes (including diet) and drug treatment.

The first treatment goal is to reduce the levels of LDL cholesterol in your blood. Important second and third goals are to increase HDL cholesterol levels and decrease triglyceride levels. The first measure for reaching all three goals is to clean up your lifestyle: Exercise regularly, keep a healthy weight, practice heart-friendly nutrition, and don't smoke (which helps increase your good cholesterol). For some people, making and sticking to lifestyle changes may be enough to lower their LDL levels. For example, if you eat a diet that is designed to help you lower your cholesterol and lose weight, and if you perform aerobic exercise for twenty to thirty minutes at least every other day, you can reduce your blood cholesterol levels by up to 15 percent.

Eat a Heart-Healthy Diet

It is trite but true: You are what you eat. After your body processes food, the bad things you eat show up in your bloodstream and artery walls. See the "Tips for Lowering Cholesterol" sidebar in this chapter for some practical guidelines to prevent this problem.

Exercise a Lot

A rule of thumb is to exercise aerobically (such as walking briskly) for twenty to thirty minutes *at least* five times per week. But this routine should be your baseline. In other words, think of this amount as an important minimum, and when possible, feel free to do much more, such as swimming, bicycling, gardening/yard work, or attending exercise classes. Remember, though, that you should consult a physician before starting any exercise program and slowly build up both the time and the frequency of exercise.

Don't Smoke

Smoking cuts levels of beneficial HDL in your blood, narrows blood vessels, and injures blood vessel walls, escalating the development of heart disease.

TREATING HIGH CHOLESTEROL WITH MEDICINE

For many people, lifestyle changes may not be enough to hit the targets that doctors have identified as protective against heart disease. This may be the situation for you if you have risk factors such as hypertension (see chapter 12), a family history of heart disease, if you are older than age forty-five (if you are male) or fifty-five (if you are female), if you carry excess weight in your midline, or if you are diabetic. In such cases, your doctor is likely to call on the heavy artillery of cholesterol control: lipid-reducing medications. A prescription for one of these is not a reason to back off on lifestyle changes but simply a reflection of the degree of cholesterol lowering needed.

Specifically, lipid therapy lowers your blood levels of LDL and triglycerides and boosts your levels of HDL. Lipid therapy includes five different types of drugs: statins, fibrates, bile acid sequestrants, cholesterol absorption factors, and niacin or nicotinic acid. The table below outlines common treatment approaches and goals based on LDL cholesterol levels. We discuss the specific measurements later in this chapter.

First, Lower LDL Levels

Because LDL cholesterol is the major culprit in heart disease, it is usually the first number that we tackle. We like to get those LDL numbers down—way down. Most people should aim for an LDL level lower than 130 mg/dL (3.4 mmol/L). If you have other risk factors for heart disease, your target LDL may be lower than 100 mg/dL (2.6 mmol/L). And if you already have had a heart attack, stroke, or blockages in your arteries anywhere (heart, brain, body) or if you have diabetes, you're at very high risk of developing a heart attack (or dying), so we recommend aiming for an LDL level lower than 70 mg/dL (lower than 1.8 mmol/L).

LDL Levels and Treatments

CONDITION	LIFESTYLE CHANGE INDICATED	DRUG THERAPY INDICATED	LDL TARGET (MUST GET TO)	IDEAL LDL TARGET (DR. CANNON RECOMMENDS)
One or no heart disease risk factors	LDL level exceeds 160 mg/dL	LDL level exceeds 190 mg/dL	Less than 160 mg/dL	Less than 130 mg/dL
Two or more heart disease risk factors	LDL level exceeds 130 mg/dL	LDL level exceeds 130 mg/dL or 100 mg/dL (optional)	Less than 130 mg/dL	Less than 100 mg/dL
Diagnosed heart disease	Always	LDL level exceeds 100 mg/dL	No more than 100 mg/dL	Less than 70 mg/dL

Source: Adapted from the National Cholesterol Education Program and the American College of Cardiology (www.cardiosmart.org)

HDL levels should be higher than or equal to 35 mg/dL and triglycerides should be lower than or equal to 150 mg/dL.

Statins

The most widely used and effective drugs to treat high cholesterol are called statins. These drugs block your liver from making cholesterol. They may also help your body remove cholesterol that has built up in artery walls. Statins can lower total cholesterol by 20 percent to 40 percent and LDL cholesterol by 40 percent to 50 percent or more. They also reduce the levels of triglycerides in the blood. Here are some commonly used statins and the percentage decrease in LDL a maximum dose provides:

- Atorvastin (Lipitor): 50 percent
- Fluvastatin (Lescol): 35 percent
- Lovastatin (Mevacor/generic): 40 percent
- Pravastatin (Pravachol/generic): 34 percent
- Rosuvastatin (Crestor): 55 percent
- Simvastatin (Zocor/generic): 47 percent

It is important to understand that if you can successfully take a statin drug, you will probably be a "lifer." In other words, you will need to keep taking the medication for the rest of your life to keep your cholesterol levels low and your cardiovascular system healthy. If you are considering stopping a statin, be sure to talk to your doctor first.

Cholesterol Levels in Children and Adolescents Two to Nineteen Years of Age

CATEGORY	TOTAL CHOLESTEROL (MG/DL)	LDL CHOLESTEROL (MG/DL)
Acceptable	Lower than 170	Lower than 110
Borderline	170–199	110–129
High	200 or higher	130 or higher

Although statins are well tolerated by most people, they do have some side effects, including:

- Muscle and joint aches
- Nausea
- Diarrhea
- Constipation

And there are two serious side effects of statins that your doctor will watch for:

Elevated liver enzymes: Your doctor will periodically draw your blood to test your liver function. He is checking for an increase in liver enzymes, which can indicate liver damage. If your enzymes have increased, your doctor will tell you to stop taking the drug, which usually clears up the trouble.

Muscle pain: Statins can cause muscle pain and tenderness, particularly at higher dosages. If you notice numbness or weakness in your muscles, be sure to tell your doctor. Lowering the dose or using a different statin can often relieve pain.

Fibrates

Fibrates lower blood triglyceride levels by reducing the liver's production of very low density lipoprotein—the triglyceride-carrying particle that circulates in the blood—and by speeding up the removal of triglycerides from the blood. Fibrates are usually prescribed in combination with statins. Fibrates include the following:

- Clofibrate (Abritate, Atromid-S)
- Fenofibrate (Tricor, Trilipix)
- Gemfibrozil (Lopid)

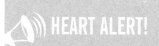

HEART ALERT!

Women of Child-Bearing Age
If you are pregnant or may become pregnant, make sure your doctor is aware of this fact. The safety of many cholesterol-lowering drugs has not been established for pregnancy or the fetus.

Side effects of fibrates can include the following:

- Fever, chills, or sore throat
- Muscle pain
- Unusual fatigue or weakness

Fenofibrate appears to have a lower risk of side effects than the older genfibrozil.

Resins (Bile Acid Sequestrants)

Resins reduce the amount of fat and cholesterol absorbed by your intestines. They can lower LDL levels by 15 percent to 30 percent and can raise HDL cholesterol levels by 3 percent to 5 percent. Here are some examples of resins:

- Cholestyramine (Questran, Questran Light)
- Colesevelam (Welchol)
- Colestipol (Colestid)

Side effects of resins can include the following:

- Muscle aches or pain
- Diarrhea
- Severe stomach pain with nausea and vomiting

Cholesterol Absorption Inhibitors

Cholesterol absorption inhibitors block the absorption of lipids in the intestines. They lower LDL cholesterol by 18 percent to 20 percent. Currently, ezetimibe (Zetia) is the only drug in this class that the U.S. Food and Drug Administration has approved. However, ezetimibe has not yet been shown to lower the risk of heart attacks. Side effects of Zetia include unexplained muscle pain, tenderness, or weakness (although some of these may relate to the statin therapy that is often used).

This drug is most commonly prescribed with statins. The combination of a statin and Zetia or the combination pill Vytorin (simvastatin and ezetimibe), reduces LDL cholesterol by as much as 50 percent to 60 percent. However, ezetimibe has not been shown to lower the risk of heart attacks. Side effects of Zetia include unexplained muscle pain, tenderness, or weakness (although some of these may relate to the statin therapy that is often used).

Niacin (Nicotinic Acid)

Niacin, also known as vitamin B3 or nicotinic acid, can raise HDL cholesterol by 20 percent to 35 percent, the most of currently available agents. Niacin also decreases LDL by 15 percent to 20 percent and decreases triglycerides by 30 percent to 60 percent. Niacin appears to slow the breakdown of triglycerides in the liver, in turn preventing fat storage and decreasing LDL production. Although niacin is widely available without a prescription, this is at a much lower dose (100 milligrams). To lower cholesterol, you need at least 1,000 mg and ideally

—⩗— WHAT'S NEW:

JUPITER Results Justify Statins

In chapter 9, we discussed a new test called the high-sensitivity C-reactive protein (hs-CRP) test, which measures inflammation in the blood vessels. When the results of this test are high (generally higher than 2 mg/L), patients are at higher risk of developing a heart attack, having a stroke, or even dying.

A new study called JUPITER (Justification for the Use of Statins in Primary Prevention: An Intervention Trial Evaluating Rosuvastatin) found that in patients without a high LDL cholesterol (but with a high hs-CRP), use of a strong statin (rosuvastatin, Crestor) led to a 44 percent reduction in major cardiovascular events (cardiovascular death, myocardial infarction, stroke, unstable angina requiring hospitalization, or need for angioplasty or bypass surgery).

What is the impact of the study? The JUPITER trial provides clinical evidence for the benefits of statin therapy in preventing heart attack, stroke, and death. It appears that a new group of patients, those with elevated hs-CRP levels but not increased LDL cholesterol, will have clinicians thinking about which patients should be tested, and whether they should be initiated on statin therapy. The trial also reinforces that statins are well tolerated and provide significant benefits.

Tips for Lowering Cholesterol

- Get less than 7 percent of your total daily calories from saturated fats (found in cholesterol-rich animal foods, such as fatty meats, egg yolks, and whole-milk dairy products) and less than 200 mg per day of cholesterol (the equivalent of one large egg).
- Make sure your total fat intake is less than 25 to 35 percent of your calorie intake each day.
- Include ½ teaspoon (2 g) per day of plant stanols and sterols, found in small quantities in many fruits, vegetables, nuts, seeds, cereals, legumes, and other plant sources, and 2 tablespoons (20–30 g) per day of soluble or viscous fiber (concentrated in oats, barley, soybeans, dried beans and peas, and citrus fruit).
- Eat lots of omega-3 fatty acids, found in cold-water fish such as salmon and mackerel, and some nuts such as walnuts, or take one gram per day in capsule form.
- Stay away from trans fats, which are used in margarines and many snack foods. They increase your total LDL cholesterol and lower your HDL cholesterol.
- Add soy foods such as tofu, miso soup, soy nuts, and meat substitutes to your diet. These products help block cholesterol absorption from the intestines.

2,000 mg. Thus, you should use niacin only under your physician's supervision. The trade name for niacin is Niaspan.

The red face of flushing is the most common side effect of niacin. Flushing can usually be reduced by gradually increasing the dose (with your physician's supervision) and by taking aspirin fifteen to twenty minutes before taking niacin.

Other side effects of niacin can include the following:

- Skin rash
- Headache
- Indigestion

TESTS AND DIAGNOSIS OF HIGH CHOLESTEROL

High cholesterol does not cause symptoms, so we have to rely on tests to determine whether it is a potential problem for patients. Your doctor will order a blood test called a fasting lipoprotein profile, also

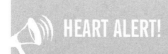
called lipid panel or lipid profile. A full lipid profile measures total cholesterol, LDL, HDL, and triglycerides. Your doctor will look over all of these measurements, along with other risk factors you may have for heart disease such as your age and whether you are diabetic, to determine your risk for heart disease.

CHOLESTEROL MEASUREMENTS

Cholesterol levels are measured in milligrams (mg) of cholesterol per deciliter (dL) of blood in the United States and some other countries. Canada and most European countries measure cholesterol in millimoles (mmol) per liter (L) of blood. You should consider the following general guidelines when you get your lipid panel (cholesterol test) results back to see whether your cholesterol falls in optimal levels.

CHOLESTEROL EXPLAINED

Cholesterol is a waxy type of fat (lipid) that is carried in your bloodstream, along with triglycerides, another type of fat. Your body uses cholesterol to make cell membranes and certain hormones. Your liver makes all the cholesterol your body needs. But some people's livers make too much cholesterol if they eat the wrong types of foods or because they have a family history that causes their livers to produce much more cholesterol than their bodies need.

Why is cholesterol such a culprit when it comes to heart disease? High cholesterol can cause fatty deposits, called plaques, that in effect gunk up your blood vessels, a condition called atherosclerosis.

Triglycerides also circulate in your blood and can contribute to atherosclerosis. Both cholesterol and triglycerides are carried to and from cells by lipoproteins, including the infamous LDL and famous HDL. If too much LDL collects in your blood, the result is plaque and atherosclerosis. If a tear develops on the plaque, a blood clot forms at the plaque site, and it blocks the artery, leading to a heart attack (see chapter 2) or stroke (see chapter 7).

HDL, on the other hand, is good cholesterol. It carries cholesterol out of the plaque, into the bloodstream, and then to the liver, where it exits your body. A high level of HDL protects you from building up too much plaque; if you have a low level, you are at greater risk for heart disease.

TOTAL CHOLESTEROL (UNITED STATES AND SOME OTHER COUNTRIES)	TOTAL CHOLESTEROL* (CANADA AND MOST OF EUROPE)	
Lower than 200 mg/dL	Lower than 5.2 mmol/L	Desirable
200–239 mg/dL	5.2–6.2 mmol/L	Borderline high
240 mg/dL and higher	Higher than 6.2 mmol/L	High
LDL CHOLESTEROL (UNITED STATES AND SOME OTHER COUNTRIES)	**LDL CHOLESTEROL* (CANADA AND MOST OF EUROPE)**	
Lower than 70 mg/dL	Lower than 1.8 mmol/L	Optimal for people at very high risk of heart disease
Lower than 100 mg/dL	Lower than 2.6 mmol/L	Optimal for people at risk of heart disease
100–129 mg/dL	2.6–3.3 mmol/L	Near optimal
130–159 mg/dL	3.4–4.1 mmol/L	Borderline high
160–189 mg/dL	4.1–4.9 mmol/L	High
190 mg/dL and higher	Higher than 4.9 mmol/L	Very high
HDL CHOLESTEROL (UNITED STATES AND SOME OTHER COUNTRIES)	**HDL CHOLESTEROL* (CANADA AND MOST OF EUROPE)**	
Lower than 40 mg/dL (men) Lower than 50 mg/dL (women)	Lower than 1 mmol/L (men) Lower than 1.3 mmol/L (women)	Poor
50–59 mg/dL	1.3–1.5 mmol/L	Better
60 mg/dL and higher	Higher than 1.5 mmol/L	Best
TRIGLYCERIDES (UNITED STATES AND SOME OTHER COUNTRIES)	**TRIGLYCERIDES* (CANADA AND MOST OF EUROPE)**	
Lower than 150 mg/dL	Lower than 1.7 mmol/L	Desirable
150–199 mg/dL	1.7–2.2 mmol/L	Borderline high
200–499 mg/dL	2.3–5.6 mmol/L	High
500 mg/dL and higher	Higher than 5.6 mmol/L	Very high

*Canadian and European guidelines differ slightly from U.S. guidelines. These conversions are based on U.S. guidelines.
Source: MayoClinic.com

Q. & A. with Dr. Cannon

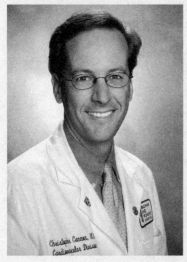

Q. I know there are different kinds of cholesterol. Which ones do I need to worry about?

A. There are several kinds of cholesterol; the bad cholesterol is called low-density lipoprotein (LDL) cholesterol that can build up inside the arteries. LDL is the most important one. The good cholesterol is high-density lipoprotein (HDL) cholesterol, which actually can help remove cholesterol from the plaque in the artery. Triglycerides are the "other bad" cholesterol and the first to carry cholesterol after you eat. The total cholesterol is calculated by adding all three (the exact formula is Total Cholesterol = LDL + HDL + 1/5 Triglycerides).

Q. What is a cholesterol ratio?

A. This is the ratio of your total cholesterol divided by your HDL. If this measure is high (greater than 5 has been a traditional cut point), it means your bad cholesterol is very high, your good cholesterol is low, or both. However, since our treatment focuses on the individual types of cholesterol, we tend to look more at the exact numbers of LDL and HDL (and then also the triglycerides).

Q. My neighbor said she had a new heart blood test at her cholesterol check last month that supposedly predicts heart attacks. What is that, and should I get one?

A. A new test is growing in use—C-reactive protein, or CRP. I do recommend getting this blood test. It has been shown in hundreds of studies to help predict heart attacks. The higher the CRP is, the higher the risk of heart attack. One guideline notes that less than 1 mg/L is excellent, 1–3 is borderline, and greater than 3 is high. Another study split the difference and found that if it is greater than 2, patients are at high risk and would benefit from aggressive treatment with statin drugs.

chapter 12:

CONTROLLING HIGH BLOOD PRESSURE

HIGH BLOOD PRESSURE

℞ THE PRESCRIPTION

Your major goal is to get your blood pressure down to as close to normal as possible. To accomplish this, your doctor will first counsel you to modify your lifestyle. Unhealthy habits and hypertension are strongly linked as cause and effect.

Use of blood-pressure lowering drugs is the next step. There are several; which one is used is tailored to each patient's history. Most patients require more than one anti-hypertensive medication.

THE FACTS ABOUT HIGH BLOOD PRESSURE

You are told you have high blood pressure (hypertension), yet you have no symptoms, which is characteristic of this dangerous condition. As the adage goes, "There are times when silence has a loud voice," and a diagnosis of hypertension is one of these times. High blood pressure can damage your heart, circulatory system, brain, and kidneys.

Because hypertension has no symptoms, it is important to have your blood pressure checked at least every two years, or you could be among the 60 million Americans with high hypertension—many of whom don't know it. If you have high blood pressure, you are not alone. About one in three adults in the United States has hypertension.

PREHYPTERENSION

Blood pressure is the force exerted on your artery walls as blood flows through your body. Slightly elevated blood pressure is known as prehypertension. Left untreated, prehypertension will likely turn into high blood pressure. Both prehypertension and high blood pressure increase your risk of heart attack, stroke, and heart failure.

A blood pressure reading has two numbers. The first, or upper, number measures the pressure in your arteries when your heart beats (systolic pressure). The second, or lower, number measures the pressure in your arteries between beats (diastolic pressure). Prehypertension is a systolic pressure from 120 to 139 millimeters of mercury (mm Hg) or a diastolic pressure from 80 to 89 mm Hg.

HEART FACT:

Over Age Forty

As a general rule, if you are over forty years of age, each 20 mm Hg increment in systolic blood pressure—or 10 mm Hg increment in diastolic pressurel—above normal doubles your risk of heart disease.

HEART ALERT!

Avoid These Foods on a Low-Sodium Diet

A low-salt diet means giving a red light (and police siren) to a number of food types, including the following:

- Frozen TV dinners
- Prepared foods
- Snack foods
- Chinese, Japanese, and other regional food types
- Fast food
- Cured foods (such as bacon and ham)
- Foods packed in brine (such as pickles, pickled vegetables, olives, and sauerkraut)
- Condiments (such as MSG, mustard, horseradish, ketchup, and soy, teriyaki, and barbecue sauces)
- Processed cheese (e.g., American cheese)

Low-Salt Nutrition Tips

- Remember: Limit your sodium intake to 2 g (or 2,000 mg) per day. A rule of thumb: One teaspoon of table salt has about 2,300 mg of sodium.
- Get into the habit of reading labels for sodium content. For example, the sodium content of processed foods (usually high in salt) is listed on the product labels.
- As a general rule, processed and restaurant foods break the sodium barrier. (To their credit, many restaurants now publish the ingredients of their foods.)
- Fresh fruit, vegetables, chicken, and fish are usually low in sodium. Many frozen vegetables are low in sodium.
- Many tasty condiments masquerade as flavor enhancers, but are really vehicles for lots of salt. Examples are bouillon, grated parmesan or Romano cheese, salad dressing, ketchup, soy sauce, and Worcestershire sauce. Again, be sure to read the labels for salt content.
- Do not use salt when you cook and prepare food. Try using pepper, garlic powder, chili powder, Italian seasoning, or other spices.
- Try magnesium chloride or potassium chlorine, sold as salt replacements.
- Beware of sodas and other drinks; many have hidden salt.
- Rinse canned foods, such as tuna, to remove some sodium.

You can't see or feel prehypertension, but there's plenty you can do about it. Losing weight, exercising, and making other healthy lifestyle changes can often control prehypertension—and set the stage for a lifetime of better health.

If your blood pressure exceeds 140/90 mm Hg (and this reading has been confirmed on multiple occasions), you have hypertension. If you have diabetes mellitus or kidney disease, your blood pressure is considered high if it is 130/80 mm Hg or higher. Such readings spell trouble for your heart (and brain); reducing your blood pressure should be a number-one priority.

LIFESTYLE CHANGES TO STOP AND REVERSE HYPERTENSION

The more lifestyle changes you make, the greater the payoff for your cardiovascular system. Even a small, persistent reduction in blood pressure can reverse the development of heart disease. Small improvements in lifestyle also have been shown to prevent type 2 diabetes, which often goes hand in hand with hypertension. You can take several positive steps to stop and reverse hypertension.

Eat a Heart-Healthy Diet

To manage blood pressure with diet, low salt is the name of the game. Consuming too much salt increases the amount of sodium in your blood and causes water retention, which increases demands on your heart. You should limit your sodium intake to 2 g, or 2,000 mg, per day. (See "Low-Salt Nutrition Tips" for practical guidelines to cut your salt intake.)

THE DASH EATING PLAN FOR HYPERTENSION

The DASH (Dietary Approaches to Stop Hypertension) eating plan has been proven to lower blood pressure in studies sponsored by the National Institutes of Health. The diet is based on two studies supported by the National Heart, Lung, and Blood Institute (NHLBI). Its results showed that blood pressures were reduced with an eating plan that is low in saturated fat, cholesterol, and total fat and that emphasizes fruits, vegetables, and low-fat dairy foods. This eating plan—known as the DASH eating plan—also includes whole-grain products, fish, poultry, and nuts. It is reduced in red meat, sweets, and sugar-containing beverages. It is rich in magnesium, potassium, and calcium, as well as protein and fiber. See www.nhlbi.nih.gov/hbp/prevent/h_eating/h_e_dash.htm for a rundown of the plan.

Get Lots of Exercise

A good general guideline is to exercise aerobically (such as walking briskly) for twenty to thirty minutes, five times per week. You should consult your cardiologist before starting any exercise program and slowly build up both the time and the frequency of exercise. (For more information on developing an exercise plan, see chapter 14.)

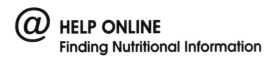

HELP ONLINE
Finding Nutritional Information

A good website for finding nutritional data—including sodium content—for fresh foods, processed foods, and many fast food restaurants is www.nutritiondata.com.

The DASH Sample Plan

The DASH sample plan is based on 2,000 calories per day.

Grains and grain products: 7 to 8 servings, such as 1 slice of bread or ½ cup (82 g) of cooked rice

Vegetables: 4 to 5 servings, such as 1 cup (20 g) of raw leafy greens, ½ cup (100 g) of cooked vegetables, or 6 oz (180 ml) of vegetable juice

Fruits: 4 to 5 servings, such as 6 oz (180 ml) of fruit juice, 1 medium fruit, or ½ cup (100–200 g) of fresh, frozen, or canned fruit

Low-fat or fat-free dairy foods: 2 to 3 servings, such as 8 oz (235 ml) of milk, 1 cup (245 g) of yogurt, or 1.5 oz (28–42 g) of cheese

Meats, poultry, and fish: 2 servings or less, such as 3 oz (50 g) of cooked meats, poultry, or fish

Nuts, seeds, and dry beans: 4 to 5 servings per week, such as ⅓ cup (45 g) of nuts; 2 tablespoon (17 g) of seeds, or ½ cup (125 g) of cooked dry beans or peas

Fats and oils: 2 to 3 servings, such as 1 teaspoon of soft margarine, 1 tablespoon (14 g) of low-fat mayonnaise, 2 tablespoon (28 g) of light salad dressing, or 1 teaspoon of vegetable oil

Sweets: 5 servings per week, such as 1 tablespoon (12 g) of sugar, 1 tablespoon (20 g) of jam or jelly, ½ oz (15 g) of jelly beans, or 8 oz (235 ml) of lemonade—sweets should be low in fat.

Lowering Blood Pressure

The lower your blood pressure, the better it is, as long as you have no symptoms such as dizziness or lightheadedness. As a general rule, your blood pressure should be 120/80 or lower, but it should not drop lower than 90/60. Some people, especially runners, will have low blood pressure in general, which is good. Once your blood pressure is at the normal level (about 120/80), there is no advantage to getting it even lower.

Positive lifestyle changes have proven to be highly successful for reversing hypertension *for people who take control of their unhealthy habits and work at changing them.* We are well aware that *it is work* to change a lifetime of unhealthy habits, which is the task for many people with hypertension.

When lifestyle modifications are not effective in lowering blood pressure, physicians recommend medication. In many cases, doctors prescribe both.

Don't Smoke

The nicotine and other chemicals in cigarette smoke raise blood pressure and make the heart beat faster. In the first year after the cessation of smoking, blood pressure falls and the risk of developing coronary heart disease drops sharply. (See chapter 14 for tips on quitting smoking.)

Maintain a Healthy Weight

Maintain normal body weight, losing weight if you need to. Losing as few as ten pounds can help decrease blood pressure. In fact, with every three pounds you lose, your systolic pressure drops about 2 mm Hg. (For information on diet and nutrition, see chapter 14.)

If You Drink Alcohol, Do So Moderately

Heavy drinking can lead to high blood pressure. Drink alcohol only in moderation—an average of one to two drinks per day for men and one drink per day for women.

MEDICATIONS TO LOWER BLOOD PRESSURE

If you have tried lifestyle changes but they have not reduced your blood pressure enough, the next step is to take an antihypertensive medication. These medications must be taken continually to work. If stopped, blood pressure rises again. The most common antihypertensive drugs are diuretics, beta blockers, calcium-channel blockers, angiotensin-converting enzyme (ACE) inhibitors, or angiotensin-receptor blockers (ARBs). Your doctor may prescribe these medicines alone or in combinations. The good news is that there are lots of different options for medications. Most have been around for years and are available as generic (and thus, low-cost) drugs.

Diuretics Help Reduce Fluid

Diuretics stimulate the kidneys to remove water and sodium from your body, which decreases the total volume of blood your heart has to pump. Diuretics prescribed to treat hypertension include the following:

- Acetazolamide (Diamox)
- Eplerenone (Inspra)
- Furosemide (Lasix)
- Hydrochlorothiazide (HCTZ HydroDiuril)
- Indapamide
- Metolazone (Zaroxolyn)

Potassium-sparing diuretics
- Spironolactone (Aldactone)
- Torsemide (Demadex)
- Triamterene (Dyrenium)

The main side effects of diuretics are increased urination and loss of potassium. Your doctor will monitor your potassium levels and may prescribe a potassium supplement. Eating foods such as bananas, which are high in potassium, can also help. Some diuretics block other hormones (e.g., aldosterone)

When Eating Out and Shopping

When eating out, ask how foods are prepared. Request that they be prepared without added salt, MSG, or salt-containing ingredients. Most restaurants are willing to accommodate requests.

- Know the terms that indicate high sodium content: *pickled, cured, soy sauce, broth.*
- Take the salt shaker off the table (or just don't use it).
- Limit condiments, such as mustard, ketchup, pickles, and sauces with salt-containing ingredients.
- Choose fruits or vegetables instead of salty snack foods.

When shopping, read the label. Here is a list of phrases that describe sodium content:

- Sodium free or salt free: less than 5 mg per serving
- Very low sodium: 35 mg or less of sodium per serving
- Low sodium: 140 mg or less of sodium per serving
- Low sodium meal: 140 mg or less of sodium per 3.5 oz (100 g)
- Reduced or less sodium: at least 25 percent less sodium than the regular version
- Light in sodium: 50 percent less sodium than the regular version
- Unsalted or no salt added: no salt added to the product during processing

and thus do not lead to low potassium and in fact can increase potassium levels. Either way, you usually will be asked to check your blood chemistry about a month or two after starting a diuretic or after increasing the dose, just to make sure your potassium is at a normal level.

Beta Blockers Calm the Heart

These drugs prevent the effects of hormones that stimulate the heartbeat and constrict arteries. Commonly used beta blockers include the following:

- Atenolol (Tenormin)
- Bisoprolol (Zebeta)
- Carvedilol (Coreg)
- Metoprolol (Lopressor, Toprol XL)
- Timolol (Blockadren)

Potential side effects of beta blockers include slowing the heart rate excessively, worsening heart failure, and rarely, confusion, depression, and impotence (erectile dysfunction can occur).

Calcium-Channel Blockers Dilate Vessels

Calcium-channel blockers cause blood vessels to dilate (open more widely), which lowers blood pressure. Although they once were thought to be not as protective as beta blockers or ACE inhibitors, recent studies have found that they do help protect against heart attacks and strokes.

These medicines include the following:

- Amlodipine (Norvasc)
- Felodipine (Plendil)

WHAT'S NEW:

Two Pills in One for High Blood Pressure and Cholesterol

The pharmaceutical company Pfizer has combined two of its widely used medicines into one pill that lowers both cholesterol and high blood pressure. The medicine, Caduet, merges the effects of Lipitor and Norvasc.

How does Caduet work? Statins lower cholesterol by blocking an enzyme in the liver that the body uses to make cholesterol. When less cholesterol is made, the liver uses more of it from the blood, which results in lower cholesterol levels. Lipitor has been clinically proven to lower bad cholesterol levels by 39 percent to 60 percent, when diet and exercise aren't enough (the average effect depends on the dose). Norvasc relaxes blood vessels, allowing blood to flow more freely. It lowers blood pressure

for up to twenty-four hours and may also be prescribed to relieve symptoms of angina.

What are the risks? Caduet is not for people with liver problems, nor for women who are nursing, pregnant, or may become pregnant. If you take Caduet, tell your doctor if you feel any new muscle pain or weakness. This could be a sign of rare but serious muscle side effects. Your doctor should conduct blood tests to check your liver function before and during treatment, and may adjust your dose. The most common side effects are edema, headache, and dizziness; they tend to be mild and often go away. Avoid drinking alcohol, which can be damaging to the liver.

- Idradipine (DynaCirc)
- Nicardipine (Cardene)
- Nisoldipine (Sular)

Calcium-channel blockers can have side effects and are used with caution in patients with pulmonary arterial hypertension and congestive heart failure. Many of the calcium-channel blockers cause headache and swelling in the ankles and feet.

ACE Inhibitors

These medications lower blood pressure by inhibiting substances in the kidneys (angiotensin II and aldosterone) that constrict blood vessels.

Many ACE inhibitors are available, including the following:

- Benazepril (Lotensin)
- Captopril (Capoten)
- Enalapril (Vasotec)
- Fosinopril (Monopril)
- Lisinopril (Prinivil, Zestril)
- Quinapril (Accupril)
- Ramipril (Altace)
- Trandolapril (Mavik)

ACE inhibitors are usually tolerated well, but side effects can include a chronic nonproductive cough and sudden swelling of the lips, face, and cheek areas. Stopping the ACE inhibitor should end the cough, and use of an ARB (discussed next) is usually recommended instead. ACE inhibitors can also increase levels of potassium and in some patients lead to worsening kidney function. Thus, your doctor will ask you to have your blood chemistries checked a month or two after starting an ACE inhibitor.

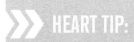

HEART TIP:

At-Home Measurement

If you have hypertension, monitoring your blood pressure at home with a portable cuff is a great way to keep track of your progress. Available in most drug stores, portable cuffs run from about $20 to $100, depending on features such as digital readout and sophistication of design.

Monitoring at home will help you measure your true blood pressure and can provide your doctor with a log of blood pressure measurements over time. This is helpful in diagnosing and preventing potential health problems. Also, be sure to take your home monitor to your doctor's office and compare the reading on your monitor with the pressure reading on your doctor's equipment to ensure accuracy between the two systems.

HEART HELP:

Preparing for Your Blood Pressure Test

You can do several things to make sure you get an accurate blood pressure reading in your doctor's office:

- Do not drink a caffeinated drink thirty minutes before your blood pressure check. Caffeine raises blood pressure.

- The same is true for smoking.

- Try not to rush. Be on time and be as relaxed as possible. Hurrying and anxiety raise blood pressure.

ARBs

Like ACE inhibitors, ARBs help to dilate the arteries, making it easier for the heart to pump blood. These drugs are relatively new and are still being studied. Currently available ARBs include the following:

- Candesartan (Atacand)
- Irbesartin (Avapro)
- Losartin (Cozaar)
- Telmisartin (Micardis)
- Valsartan (Diovan)

ARBs have very few side effects. Rarely, they can interfere with or worsen kidney function. Thus, as for ACE inhibitors, your doctor will ask you to have your blood chemistries checked a month or two after starting the medication. Several other classes of antihypertensive medications exist including (prazosin), vasodilators (hydralazine), and centrally acting agents (clonidine).

TESTS AND DIAGNOSIS OF HYPERTENSION

Measuring Blood Pressure

Blood pressure is measured with an inflatable cuff, called a sphygmomanometer, and a stethoscope. (Some blood pressure cuffs have built-in stethoscopes.) To measure blood pressure, a practitioner wraps the cuff around your upper arm and places the stethoscope near the inside of your elbow. The cuff is inflated until a gauge on the cuff reads at least 30 mm Hg higher than the expected systolic blood pressure. When the cuff is inflated, the blood flow (and pulse) is cut off in the arm. The cuff is then slowly deflated and the practitioner can hear the pulse, which then stops briefly and comes back.

⋀⋀⋀ WHAT'S NEW:

Renin Inhibitor Aliskiren (Tekturna)

How does Tekturna work? This medication may help lower your blood pressure by targeting an enzyme in your body called *renin*, which may contribute to high blood pressure. Renin is produced in the kidneys and it's part of the renin system, a chemical system that works throughout your body. It plays a role in the rising and falling of blood pressure. Renin starts a chemical process that narrows the blood vessels. In some people, the renin

system is inappropriately activated. By inhibiting renin, Tekturna helps to target the beginning of a process that may raise blood pressure.

What are the risks? Tekturna can be used alone or in combination with other antihypertensive drugs. It is often used with diuretics and an ARB. This medication should not be used during pregnancy.

HEART FACTS:

Blood Pressure and Aging

Blood pressure tends to rise with age. If you don't have high blood pressure by age fifty-five, you have a 90 percent chance of developing it at some point in your life, according to the NHLBI. Following a healthy lifestyle helps some people delay or prevent this rise in blood pressure.

Systolic pressure occurs when the pulse is first heard. This is the point when the pressure in the arteries is at its peak at the beginning of the pumping cycle.

The diastolic pressure is the point when the pulse is not audible. This is the resting phase between the beats of the heart's pumping cycle. Blood pressure values are typically reported in millimeters of mercury (mm Hg) despite the fact that many modern vascular pressure devices no longer use mercury. Blood pressure numbers are usually written with the systolic number above or before the diastolic number, such as 120/80 mm Hg.

If your blood pressure reading is high, your doctor will order additional tests to determine whether organ damage has occurred because of hypertension. These tests include the following:

- Blood analysis
- Echocardiography
- Electrocardiogram
- Urine analysis

HIGH BLOOD PRESSURE EXPLAINED

Blood pressure is literally the pressure inside the blood vessels of your body. It translates into the amount of force your blood makes on the walls of your blood vessels as it circulates through your body. The more blood your heart has to pump such as during stress or exercise and the narrower your arteries, the higher the force against your arterial walls and therefore the higher your blood pressure.

Doctors define high blood pressure as either primary hypertension (also known as essential hypertension) or secondary hypertension. The distinction between the two types is that primary hypertension has no known cause, whereas secondary hypertension is caused by another health condition.

HYPERTENSION SEVERITY	SYSTOLIC PRESSURE	DIASTOLIC PRESSURE
Normal	Lower than 120 mm Hg	Lower than 80 mm Hg
Prehypertension	Between 120 mm Hg and 139 mm Hg	Between 80 mm Hg and 89 mm Hg
Stage I	Between 140 mm Hg and 159 mm Hg	Between 90 mm Hg and 99 mm Hg
Stage II (Severe)	Greater than 160 mm Hg	Greater than 100 mm Hg

Fully 90 percent to 95 percent of all cases of hypertension are primary. This type of blood pressure develops gradually during adulthood and usually runs in families. It is also the type of hypertension that is linked to unhealthy lifestyle habits such as a high-salt diet and stress.

Secondary hypertension usually strikes suddenly and causes higher spikes in blood pressure than essential hypertension. The most common cause of secondary hypertension is kidney failure. Other causes are tumors of the adrenal gland, and taking certain medications (including birth control pills, acetaminophen [Tylenol], cold remedies, and some prescription drugs). Some illegal drugs such as cocaine and amphetamines can also cause high blood pressure.

Regardless of the type, high blood pressure is a major risk factor for strokes, heart attacks, heart failure, enlarged hearts, eye damage, and arterial aneurysm and is a leading cause of chronic kidney failure. Even blood pressure that is slightly high can shorten life. People with severe high blood pressure—which is defined as blood pressure that is at least 50 percent higher than average—can expect to live no more than a few years if they do not get treatment.

Q. & A. with Dr. Cannon

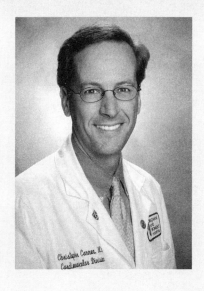

Christopher Cannon, M.D.
Cardiovascular Division

Q. I have "white coat" high blood pressure. What is that?

A. White coat hypertension is a subset of patients who have higher blood pressure measurements when they are in for a doctor's visit (i.e., when the blood pressure is taken with the doctor [in his or her white coat] overseeing the measurement). The idea is that the added stress and nervousness of a doctor's visit raise your blood pressure. By contrast, when patients are at home and more relaxed, if they take their blood pressures with a home device the readings are frequently lower. This is a common and real finding. Anxiety and stress do increase blood pressure.

Q. Do I have to worry about risks if I only have "white coat" hypertension?

A. Yes—it is a real finding. It says that although your blood pressure may be normal at some times of the day (e.g., when you are relaxed at home), at other times of the day when you have stress (which we all do) your blood pressure will sometimes get too high.

Q. What causes hypertension?

A. Interestingly, even after all these decades, we don't really know what causes hypertension in most patients. As noted in this chapter, some patients have secondary hypertension due to specific issues in the kidneys or adrenal glands, but for most people we still just consider it essential hypertension. Fortunately, even though we don't fully understand the cause, we have many different treatments.

Q. If my blood pressure is back to normal do I need to think about anything else?

A. Yes. Two recent studies have found that people with high blood pressure are at increased risk of having other ardiac risk factors. Thus, you need to ask your doctor to check your cholesterol, blood sugar, and other risk factors and control them if they are elevated.

Q. A friend with high blood pressure was just started on a cholesterol-lowering medication. Why?

A. Because the risk of heart attack increases with the number of risk factors you have, we tend to treat patients who have higher risk more aggressively. Thus, if you have one or more other risk factors, we tend to be more aggressive in lowering cholesterol. There are several studies of patients with high blood pressure (as their "main" problem) with average levels of cholesterol where taking a statin medication led to about a 40 percent lower risk of developing a heart attack, stroke, or dying.

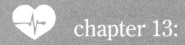 chapter 13:

DIABETES AND METABOLIC SYNDROME

DIABETES

℞ THE PRESCRIPTION

According to the American Diabetes Association (ADA) and the American College of Cardiology, the following actions have been proven to decrease heart attacks and other heart disease events in people with diabetes:

➡ Quitting smoking

➡ Treating high blood pressure and high cholesterol using medications such as angiotensin-converting enzyme (ACE) inhibitors and statin drugs

➡ Control of glucose levels has been the centerpiece of treatment aiming for a hemoglobin A1C test result of less than 7 percent. However, control of all cardiovascular risk factors are now emphasized.

DIABETES

You have diabetes, a disease in which damaging amounts of sugar accumulate in your blood. The buildup is caused by your body not being able to produce (type 1) or use (type 2) the hormone insulin, which it needs to convert the food you eat into energy. You know you must keep your blood sugar levels from skyrocketing or plummeting. Healthy eating, exercise, and blood glucose testing are important to manage your disease.

Did you also know that if you have diabetes, you are at high risk for developing heart disease and should take measures to prevent it? At least 65 percent of people with diabetes die from heart disease or stroke.

If you were not aware of the diabetes/heart disease connection, you are not alone. According to a recent American Diabetes Association (ADA) survey, more than 65 percent of diabetic patients do not consider heart disease to be a serious complication of diabetes, and only 18 percent of people with diabetes believe they have an increased risk for heart disease.

If you have diabetes, you can take a number of actions to reduce your risk of heart disease.

TREATING HYPERTENSION

Treating hypertension if you have diabetes can help save your heart and cardiovascular system. According to the U.S. Centers for Disease Control and Prevention (CDC), controlling blood pressure reduces the risk of heart disease or stroke for people with diabetes by 33 percent to 50 percent and the risk of small blood vessel problems (eye, kidney, and nerve diseases) by approximately 33 percent.

 HEART FACTS:

Facts on Heart Disease and Diabetes:

- Heart disease and stroke account for about 65 percent of deaths in people with diabetes.

- Adults with diabetes have heart-disease death rates about two to four times higher than people without diabetes.

- About 73 percent of adults with diabetes have blood pressure greater than or equal to 130/80 millimeters of mercury (mm Hg), which is higher than that recommended for people with diabetes, or use prescription medications for hypertension. And the prevalence of hypertension in the diabetic population is one and one-half to three times higher than that of nondiabetic age-matched groups.

- From 70 percent to 97 percent of people with diabetes have high levels of fat in their blood (a condition known as dyslipidemia).

- People with diabetes are two to three times more likely to have atherosclerosis than people without diabetes.

- The risk of death from heart disease is three times higher for men with diabetes than for men without diabetes.

- Diabetic patients who have not had a previous heart attack have as high a risk of a heart attack as nondiabetic patients *with* a previous heart attack.

Source: American Diabetes Association (ADA)

If you are diabetic, your goal is to keep your blood pressure lower than 130/80 to help prevent problems. (Blood pressure values are typically reported in mm Hg, despite the fact that many modern blood pressure devices no longer use mercury. Blood pressure numbers are usually written with the systolic number above or before the diastolic, such as 120/80 mm Hg. For information on how blood pressure is measured, see chapter 12.)

Lifestyle Changes to Reduce Hypertension

If your systolic blood pressure is between 130 mm Hg and 139 mm Hg or you have a diastolic blood pressure between 80 mm Hg and 89 mm Hg, your doctor may recommend that you make lifestyle changes for at least three months to lower your hypertension. These changes include restricting the amount of salt in your diet, losing weight, increasing physical activity, not smoking, and moderating how much alcohol you consume. For information on these lifestyle changes, see chapters 12 and 14. If after three months of lifestyle changes your blood pressure is still higher than 130 mm Hg systolic or 80 mm Hg diastolic, your doctor may recommend drug treatment to reduce your hypertension.

If you are diabetic and your blood pressure is equal to or higher than 140/90 mm Hg, your doctor is likely to recommend that you start pharmacological treatment right away and that you also make lifestyle changes to lower your hypertension.

Medications to Reduce Hypertension

Blood pressure medications must be taken continually to work. If stopped, blood pressure rises again. The most common antihypertensive drugs are diuretics, beta blockers, calcium-channel blockers, ACE inhibitors, and angiotensin-receptor blockers.

Your doctor may prescribe these medicines alone or in combinations. For information on these medications see chapter 12 and appendix III.

TREATING HYPERLIPIDEMIA

What is hyperlipidemia? *Lipid* is the scientific term for fats such as high-density lipoprotein (HDL), low-density lipoprotein (LDL), and triglycerides in the blood, and the term *hyperlipidemia* means high lipid levels in the blood. Hyperlipidemia usually means you have high cholesterol and triglyceride levels.

Lipid problems go hand in hand with diabetes and can greatly raise your risk for heart attack and stroke. If you are diabetic, the danger zone for your lipid levels is as follows:

- LDL levels equal to or higher than 130 mg/dL
- HDL levels lower than 35 mg/dL for men and 45 mg/dL for women
- Triglyceride levels equal to or higher than 400 mg/dL

(Lipid levels are measured in milligrams [mg] of cholesterol per deciliter [dL] of blood in the United States and some other countries. Canada and most European countries measure cholesterol in millimoles [mmol] per liter [L] of blood. For information on LDL cholesterol, HDL cholesterol, and triglycerides, see chapter 11.)

If you are diabetic, your goal is to do the following:

- Have LDL cholesterol levels lower than 100 mg/dL if you have no known heart disease

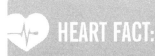

- Have LDL cholesterol levels lower than 70 mg/dL if you have heart disease
- Have HDL cholesterol levels higher than 45 mg/dL if you are a man and 55 mg/dL if you are a woman
- Have triglycerides lower than 150 mg/dL

Treating Hyperlipidemia with Lifestyle Changes

Your prescription for treating high lipid levels begins with eating a healthy diet and exercising (see chapter 14). If you are overweight, your doctor will encourage you to take pounds off and may prescribe a specific diet.

Statin Therapy

The ADA recommends that all people with diabetes take a statin drug to lower cholesterol, especially if their LDL cholesterol is higher than 130 mg/dL. Several large research trials have shown a reduction in heart attack, stroke, and death with statin treatment.

Aspirin Therapy

The ADA recommends taking enteric-coated aspirin daily (81–325 mg/day) to prevent heart disease, particularly for high-risk patients (those with a family history of heart disease, who smoke, who have hyperlipidemia, hypertension, or albuminuria [more than the normal amount of the protein albumin in the urine], or who are older than forty years of age). However, a recent large study cast doubt on the cardiac benefits of low-dose aspirin.

Japanese researchers found that low-dose aspirin did not significantly reduce the risk of cardiovascular events in people with type 2 diabetes, but there was a trend in that direction. In addition, some people should not take aspirin if they are at high risk for bleeding problems. Be sure to discuss the "aspirin issue" with your doctor before adding aspirin to your daily regimen.

MANAGING DIABETES

Managing your diabetes to stay healthy not only helps minimize the disease process, but also can ward off heart problems that often accompany the condition. There are similarities and differences in the management of type 1 and type 2 diabetes. For example, daily dietary habits are important for managing both types; however, the recommended nutritional guidelines for the two forms differ greatly. Carbohydrates play a central role in a healthy type 1 diet, whereas restricting calories is the name of the game for a type 2 diet. The need to exercise regularly, coordinated with monitoring blood sugar levels and diet, are keys to managing both types of diabetes.

Dietary Guidelines for Type 1 Diabetes

People with type 1 diabetes must carefully control the amount of carbohydrates they consume daily because carbohydrates greatly affect blood sugar levels and the amount of insulin an individual needs. However, there is no specific type 1 diet. If you have type 1 diabetes, you can try any healthy nutritional program as long as you follow two basic principles:

- Keep track of and control the amount of carbohydrate you eat.
- Eat the same amount of food with the same proportion of carbohydrates, proteins, and fats at the same time every day.

Your physician or a licensed nutritionist can help you develop a nutrition plan that fits your daily needs. As a general rule, you can have 45–60 grams of carbohydrate at each meal. (There are about 15 grams of carbohydrate in one small piece of fresh fruit or one slice of bread.) Once you know how many carbohydrates you will be having at your meals, you can choose your foods accordingly, being sure to include a lean protein and healthy fat.

Dietary Guidelines for Type 2 Diabetes

Because 80 percent to 90 percent of people with type 2 diabetes are overweight, weight reduction is the top goal when planning a nutrition program. At the same time, it is important to control the amount of carbohydrates consumed at each meal to control blood sugar levels. Therefore, the basic premise for people with type 2 diabetes is to eat a low-calorie diet with fewer carbohydrates.

Taking Insulin

If you have type 1 diabetes you'll have to inject insulin to survive. (Some people with type 2 diabetes

 HELP ONLINE:

Tracking what you eat can help you manage your diabetes and prevent the onset of heart disease. MyFoodAdvisor is a free online calorie-and-carbohydrate-counting tool developed by the ADA. Check it out at www.diabetes.org.

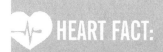 **HEART FACT:**

Diabetes and Other Conditions

Studies have shown that up to 60 percent of adults with diabetes have high blood pressure and nearly all have one or more lipid abnormalities, such as increased triglycerides, low HDL cholesterol, or elevated LDL cholesterol.

Source: American Diabetes Association (ADA)

also have to inject insulin.) It is important to inject the correct dosage or your blood glucose levels can swing out of control. There are two methods for taking in insulin: by injection with a needle or by injection with an insulin pump. Your insulin intake must be carefully balanced with the foods you eat and the amount of exercise you get.

Checking Your Blood Sugar

Testing your blood sugar levels regularly is an important part of managing your diabetes. Blood glucose meters (glucometers) can tell you whether your concentrations are in a normal range, are too high, or are too low. At least twenty-five different meters are available for purchase. With all types of meters, you prick your finger and dab a small drop of blood onto a disposable test strip, which the meter then interprets in mg/dL or mmol/L. If you have type 1 diabetes you should test your levels three or four times per day.

Exercise

Regular physical activity can help maintain blood sugar levels and reduce the risk of heart disease.

People with diabetes have to carefully balance exercise with their meals and insulin to avoid hypoglycemia (low blood sugar) or hyperglycemia (high blood sugar). This is an important issue to discuss with your health care team, who will help you develop an exercise plan.

TESTS AND DIAGNOSIS OF HEART DISEASE IN PEOPLE WITH DIABETES

THE ABCs OF DIABETES TESTS

Diabetes far too often leads to medical problems related to the small and large blood vessels of the circulatory system, including heart disease, blindness, kidney problems, peripheral artery disease, stroke, nerve problems, and amputations. If you have diabetes, there are three tests you should have on a regular basis so that you can take action to lower the risk and lessen the impact of these problems. The tests and their recommended results are called the ABCs of diabetes management:

A: A1C (blood glucose) less than 7 percent
B: Blood pressure less than 130/80 mm Hg
C: Cholesterol (LDL) less than 100 mg/dL

The Hemoglobin A1C Test

This test monitors blood glucose levels over time (i.e., the prior three months). If diabetes is not controlled, eventually glucose attaches to the protein hemoglobin within red blood cells. The level of hemoglobin to which sugar has bound, called *glycosylated hemoglobin*, correlates with blood sugar levels that have occurred in the past two to three months. The higher the hemoglobin A1C level, the less controlled the blood glucose has been over the past three months. Ideal numbers should be less than 7.0.

Medications for Type 2 Diabetes

Your doctor may prescribe medication to control your type 2 diabetes. Different groups of medications may be used with insulin.

Some common types of medication include the following:

- Alpha-glucosidase inhibitors (such as acarbose) decrease the absorption of carbohydrates from the digestive tract to lower after-meal glucose levels.
- Biguanides (Metformin) decrease the production of glucose in the liver. The result is an increase of glucose levels in the bloodstream. This agent is now generally the first medication to be used.
- Injectable medications (including exenatide and pramlintide) can lower blood sugar.
- Meglitinides (including repaglinide and nateglinide) trigger the pancreas to make more insulin in response to the level of glucose in the blood.
- Oral sulfonylureas (such as glimepiride, glyburide, and tolazamide) trigger the pancreas to make more insulin.
- Thiazolidinediones (such as pioglitazone) help insulin work better at the cell site. They increase the cell's sensitivity (responsiveness) to insulin. Rosiglitazone may increase the risk of heart problems.
- DPP-4 inhibitors (sitraplipton) are once-daily oral therapies that do not cause hypoglycemia, a common side effect seen with many diabetes medications. These drugs lower blood sugar levels by blocking an enzyme known as dipeptidyl peptidase IV (DPP-4).

(Source: Adapted from *Medline Plus Medical Encyclopedia*)

The ADA recommends the following A1C testing guidelines:

- Four times each year if you have type 1 or type 2 diabetes and use insulin
- Two times each year if you have type 2 diabetes and do not use insulin

Blood Pressure Tests

As we mentioned earlier in this chapter, if you have diabetes your blood pressure should be 130/80 or lower. For information on how blood pressure is measured, see chapter 12.

Lipid Tests

Lipid profiles should be taken at least annually. In children two years of age or older, lipid profiles should be taken after diagnosis of diabetes and when glucose control has been established. If values are in the low-risk category and there is no family history of heart disease, lipid profiles should be repeated every five years. As we mentioned earlier in this chapter, keep your bad cholesterol (LDL) level lower than 100 (and lower than 70 if you have known heart disease) and your triglycerides lower than 150 mg/dL.

TESTS FOR PEOPLE WHO HAVE PREDIABETES

Two tests are used to diagnose prediabetes: the fasting glucose test (IFG) and the glucose tolerance test (GTT). The GTT test checks your blood sugar two hours after a specific glucose load. If your blood sugar level is between 140 mg/dL and 199 mg/dL, you have prediabetes. The IFG test is taken in the morning before breakfast. If your blood sugar levels fall between 100 and 125 mg/dLt, you have prediabetes.

The U.S. Department of Health and Human Services (HHS) and the ADA recommend that doctors screen overweight people age forty-five and older for

WHAT'S NEW:

The Diabetes Crisis

The burgeoning number of people with diabetes is causing a global health care crisis. In the United States, diabetes affects nearly twenty-four million people, an increase of more than three million in approximately two years, according to 2007 estimates by the CDC. This means nearly 8 percent of the U.S. population has diabetes.

Worldwide, the number of people with diabetes is expected to almost double in thirty years, from 2.8 percent of people of all ages in the year 2000 to 4.4 percent of the worldwide population in 2030. The number of people affected is projected to increase from 171 million in 2000 to 366 million by 2030, according to an analysis published in Diabetes Care.

Some of the increase in diabetes rates is due to new understanding among the medical profession and the public of just how common the disease is today and what symptoms to look for. More people are aware that they have the disease, which is a good thing.

prediabetes during regular office visits using either one of these tests.

The HHS and ADA also recommend that physicians consider screening adults younger than age forty-five if they are significantly overweight and have one or more of the following risk factors:

- Family history of diabetes
- Low HDL cholesterol and high triglycerides
- High blood pressure
- History of gestational diabetes or gave birth to a baby weighing more than 9 lbs (4 kg)
- Belong to a minority group (African Americans, American Indians, Hispanic Americans/Latinos, and Asian American/Pacific Islanders are at increased risk for type 2 diabetes)

DIABETES EXPLAINED

The hallmark of diabetes is that your blood sugar levels are often higher than they should be. Because excess sugar in your blood can damage your blood vessels, if you have diabetes you are at high risk for heart disease and other vascular problems.

What is diabetes? *Diabetes mellitus*, commonly referred to as diabetes, is a group of diseases caused by high levels of blood sugar and problems with either the production of the hormone insulin or the body's ability to respond to insulin, which regulates blood glucose. Diabetes is a chronic condition; once it strikes it lasts throughout life.

About seventeen million people in the United States (8 percent of the population) have diabetes. Another twelve million people have diabetes and don't know it.

The Benefits of Controlling Your ABCs

Studies in the United States and United Kingdom have demonstrated the following benefits of controlling the ABCs of diabetes:

- Intensive glucose control reduces the risk of heart attack, stroke, or death from heart disease by 57 percent.
- In general, every percentage point drop in A1C blood test results (e.g., from 8.0 percent to 7.0 percent) reduces the risk of microvascular (small blood vessel) complications (eye, kidney, and nerve diseases) by 40 percent.
- Blood pressure control reduces the risk of heart disease among persons with diabetes by 33 percent to 50 percent and the risk of diabetic kidney, eye, and nerve disease by about 33 percent. In general, for every 10 mm Hg reduction in systolic blood pressure, the risk for any complication related to diabetes is reduced by 12 percent.
- Improved control of cholesterol or blood lipids (e.g., HDL, LDL, and triglycerides) can reduce heart disease complications by 20 percent to 50 percent.

Source: The HHS National Diabetes Education Program

There are three major types of diabetes. Another condition called *prediabetes* is closely linked to type 2 diabetes.

Types of Diabetes

People who have type 1 diabetes no longer produce insulin. Their immune systems have destroyed their pancreatic beta cells, which make the hormone insulin. They must take in insulin by injection or a pump. Type 1 diabetes usually strikes during childhood, and for this reason it was previously called juvenile diabetes. (Type 1 diabetes was also previously called insulin dependent diabetes mellitus.)

Although rare, some people develop type 1 diabetes later in life. This disease is called latent autoimmune diabetes in adults.

Five percent to ten percent of all diagnosed cases of diabetes are type 1 diabetes. Scientists do not know what causes the disease.

Although the immune system plays a role, type 2 diabetes is not an autoimmune disease as type 1 is. In type 2 diabetes, patients still produce insulin, but their bodies do not respond to it as they should. This insensitivity to insulin is called *insulin resistance.*

Type 2 diabetes was previously called non-insulin-dependent diabetes mellitus or adult-onset diabetes. It is the most common form of diabetes. Ninety percent to ninety-five percent of all diagnosed cases of diabetes are type 2 diabetes.

The risk factors for this form of diabetes are obesity, physical inactivity, a family history of diabetes, older age, having had gestational diabetes, and certain ethnicities. Here are some facts about these risk factors:

- Lifestyle plays a key role in the development of the disease. About 80 percent of people with type 2 diabetes are overweight or obese. Because of the obesity epidemic among today's youth, type 2 diabetes is increasingly being diagnosed in children and adolescents.
- Type 2 diabetes is more common in certain ethnic groups. Ten percent of African Americans have the disease. The same percentage holds for Asian Americans. The prevalence for Hispanics is 15 percent, and in certain Native American communities, 20 percent to 50 percent have the condition. Six percent of Caucasians have type 2 diabetes.
- Aging is a risk factor for Type 2 diabetes. Twenty percent of people between the ages of sixty-five and seventy-four have the disease.
- Diabetes occurs much more frequently in women who have had gestational diabetes.

Symptoms for type 2 diabetes include fatigue, increased thirst and hunger, frequent urination, weight loss, blurred vision, and wounds or sores that do not heal. The symptoms of type 2 diabetes emerge gradually, and some people have no symptoms.

Prediabetes

If you have prediabetes, your blood glucose levels are higher than they should be but not at the level for a diagnosis of diabetes. The condition is usually silent; you can have prediabetes but not be aware of it. The disease is a precursor to type 2 diabetes and increases the risk of heart disease by 50 percent. It's estimated that fifty-seven million people in the United States have prediabetes, most of whom do not know it.

Research supported by the HHS shows that most people with prediabetes are likely to develop diabetes within a decade unless they make changes in their diet and level of physical activity, which can help them reduce their risks and avoid the debilitating disease.

The HHS's Diabetes Prevention Program, a major clinical trial involving more than 3,000 people, showed that prevention efforts can be stunningly effective. The Diabetes Prevention Program found that diet and exercise resulting in a 5 percent to 7 percent weight loss lowered the incidence of type 2 diabetes by 58 percent. Participants lost weight by cutting fat and calories in their diet and by exercising at least thirty minutes per day, five days per week.

Gestational Diabetes

Gestational diabetes strikes 1 percent to 3 percent of pregnant women. It usually develops in the second trimester of pregnancy. Gestational diabetes usually goes away when the pregnancy ends. However, 5 percent to 10 percent of women with gestational diabetes discover that they actually have type 1 or type 2 diabetes.

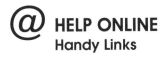

HELP ONLINE
Handy Links

American Heart Association (AHA):
> www.americanheart.org

American Diabetes Association (ADA):
> www.diabetes.org

National Diabetes Information Clearinghouse:
> www.diabetes.niddk.nih.gov

Gestational diabetes causes a lifelong risk for diabetes. Women who have had gestational diabetes have a 40 percent to 60 percent chance of developing one of the permanent forms of diabetes in five to ten years.

METABOLIC SYNDROME

Do you have a large waist? High triglyceride levels? High blood pressure? You might have a condition called *metabolic syndrome*, a clustering of risk factors associated with being overweight or obese. According to the National Heart, Lung, and Blood Institute (NHLBI), about 85 percent of people who have type 2 diabetes also have metabolic syndrome. Whether you are diabetic or not, if you have this condition you are at high risk for heart disease.

The following group of risk factors pertains to metabolic syndrome:

- Central obesity (a large waistline)—This is the "apple shape" where fat accumulates around the waist. Too much fat in the middle is a greater risk factor for heart disease than excess fat in the hips or other parts of the body.
- A high triglyceride level in the blood (or you're on medicine to treat high triglycerides)
- A lower than normal level of HDL cholesterol in the blood (or you're on medicine to raise HDL)—Low levels of HDL increase your chances of heart disease. High levels of HDL protect you against heart disease.
- Higher than normal blood pressure or you're on medicine to treat high blood pressure.

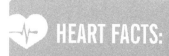
- Higher than normal fasting blood sugar (glucose)—or you're on medicine to treat high blood sugar. Mildly high blood sugar can be an early warning sign of diabetes.

According to the National Cholesterol Education Program, if you have three or more of these five risk factors you have metabolic syndrome.

The risk factors for metabolic syndrome are cumulative. The more risk factors you have, the greater your chance of developing heart disease or diabetes or of having a stroke. According to the NHLBI, if you have metabolic syndrome you are twice as likely to develop heart disease and five times as likely to develop diabetes as someone without metabolic syndrome.

THE PRESCRIPTION FOR METABOLIC SYNDROME

Your primary goal is to cut your risk for heart disease by making lifestyle changes including lowering your weight, being active and exercising, and following a heart-healthy diet. A second step is to take the appropriate medicines to control your risk factors, such as statins for high LDL levels, beta blockers for high blood pressure, and oral medicines (such as metformin) and/or insulin injections to control blood sugar levels.

Weight Loss

The NHLBI recommends that if you have metabolic syndrome and you are overweight or obese, you reduce your weight by 7 to 10 percent during the first year of treatment. After the first year, you should continue to lose weight, with a long-range target of lowering your body mass index (BMI) to less than 25. To learn how to calculate your BMI, see chapter 14.

Heart-Healthy Eating

To manage metabolic syndrome with diet, you should follow a heart-healthy diet. If blood pressure is a concern, you should also follow the DASH eating plan, which we describe in chapter 12. The bottom line is that you should limit your sodium intake to 2 g, or 2,000 mg, per day.

Increased Physical Activity

The NHLBI recommends that if you have metabolic syndrome, you should keep up a moderate level of activity, such as brisk walking for at least thirty minutes, at least five days per week. The ultimate goal is to maintain at least a moderate level of physical activity for sixty minutes per day for at least five days per week.

Quit Smoking

Among other known harmful effects on your heart, smoking raises your triglyceride level and lowers your HDL cholesterol.

Medicines

Your doctor may recommend a statin drug or other medicines to help treat unhealthy cholesterol levels and high blood pressure. High blood sugar is treated with oral medicines (such as metformin), insulin injections, or both. Your doctor may also prescribe aspirin to reduce the risk of blood clots, which are common for people with metabolic syndrome.

TESTS AND DIAGNOSIS OF METABOLIC SYNDROME

To be diagnosed with metabolic syndrome, you must have at least three out of five of the following risk factors:

- A waist measurement of 35 inches (89 cm) or more if you are a woman and 40 inches (102 cm) or more if you are a man
- A triglyceride level of 150 mg/dL or higher
- An HDL cholesterol level lower than 50 mg/dL if you are a woman and lower than 40 mg/dL if you are a man.
- A blood pressure of 130/85 or higher. If only one of your two blood pressure numbers is high, you still could have metabolic syndrome.
- A fasting blood sugar of 100 mg/dL or higher (prediabetes or diabetes)

METABOLIC SYNDROME EXPLAINED

About one in four American adults (forty-seven million people) have metabolic syndrome, and the proportion and number are increasing. In fact, the NHLBI asserts that in the future, metabolic syndrome may overtake smoking as the leading risk factor for heart disease.

Scientists have not yet pinpointed the exact cause of metabolic syndrome. They know that like type 2 diabetes, two major factors that can lead to the condition are being overweight and inactive. A third factor is insulin resistance, a condition in which your cells become resistant to the effects of insulin, the hormone that your body requires to remove and use glucose from your blood. They also know that aging, a family history of diabetes, and a personal history of diabetes (including gestational diabetes) are linked to the disease, but genetic and environmental factors are also probably involved.

Q. & A. with Dr. Cannon

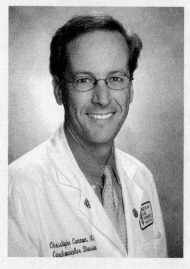

Christophe Cannon, M
Cardiovascular Division

Q. My doctor tells me that in addition to watching my sugar, I also have to be careful about my cholesterol and take a statin pill. Is that necessary?

A. Yes. It is critical if you have diabetes to take care of all of your risk factors for coronary artery disease. The reason is that not only does the diabetes damage your arteries but so do all the other factors such as cholesterol and high blood pressure, and the damage is cumulative. Thus, in patients with diabetes, we are extra careful to fully control all other risk factors.

Q. I have heard conflicting studies on the news about whether it helps to strictly control my blood glucose. Does it help?

A. Three large studies have looked at whether strict control of diabetes is better than loose control, and only one of the three showed a benefit in reducing heart attacks, strokes, or death with strict control. All three, however, showed that more strict control helped prevent kidney damage and damage to the eyes. Thus, most diabetes experts and the ADA have reaffirmed the guideline that the target for hemoglobin A1C is less than 7.0.

Q. My doctor keeps saying I need to exercise. Does it really matter?

A. *Yes*! There are actually a growing number of randomized trials of exercise, and there are clear benefits in better controlling diabetes. The HgbA1c is much better controlled in patients who exercise. It doesn't matter whether you do aerobic exercise or lift weights; both help, and mixing it up has been shown to control diabetes best. In addition, the general cardiovascular benefit of these forms of exercise exists as well.

chapter 14:

LIFESTYLE CHANGES TO HEAL YOUR HEART

LIFESTYLE CHANGES

℞ THE PRESCRIPTION

Cardiologists and other medical professionals have long known that lifestyle changes can greatly improve heart health. This chapter covers the top five changes that anyone interested in preventing or reversing heart disease should pay attention to:

➡ Maintaining a heart-healthy diet

➡ Controlling your weight

➡ Exercising regularly

➡ Not smoking

➡ Reducing stress

Our lifestyles greatly impact our heart health and longevity. From 1981 to 2006, researchers conducting the Physicians' Health Study evaluated the lifestyles of 2,357 men. Of them, 970 (41 percent) survived to at least ninety years of age. The results of the study showed that in the absence of smoking, diabetes, obesity, hypertension, and a sedentary lifestyle, the probability of surviving from age seventy to ninety was 54 percent. This probability fell from 36 percent to 22 percent for the men who had two of these bad habits and only 4 percent for those who had five risk factors. Regular exercise was associated with a nearly 30 percent lower mortality risk.

EAT A HEART-HEALTHY DIET

The prescription for a heart-healthy diet is twofold: Eat the nutritious, tasty foods that will not choke your arteries, and stay away from the empty calories, high-fat food, and salt that can choke your arteries. To accomplish this goal, you will have to follow some guidelines, but they are not rocket science and the result can save your heart. The guiding principles we describe in this chapter jibe with heart-healthy diets proposed by the American Heart Association (AHA), the Harvard School of Public Health, and the American Dietetic Association. They also draw on the popular Mediterranean diet.

Balanced diets include produce (vegetables and fruits); whole-grain foods; plant oils; nuts and legumes; fish, poultry, and eggs; and low-fat dairy products. The following sections provide guidelines on these foods.

Produce (Vegetables and Fruits)

Vegetables and fruits are the cornerstones of a nutritious diet. Men should eat nine servings of fruits and vegetables a day, and women should eat seven

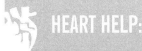

HEART HELP:

For a Healthy Diet

- Eat a well-balanced variety of wholesome foods.

- Eat one good source of omega-3 fatty acids every day.

- Limit your cholesterol intake.

- Eliminate refined and processed foods as much as possible.

- Limit salt.

- If you drink alcohol, do so in moderation.

servings. If you eat a fruit or vegetable of every color a couple of times per day, you will get the full range of value from produce and will be more likely to eat the recommended servings of vegetables and fruits every day. Salads, stir fries, and casseroles are great ways to combine produce of every color.

Whole-Grain Foods

Whole grains are good-for-you carbohydrates that your body uses for energy. Along with fruits and vegetables, they are the foundation of heart-healthy diets. Whole grains contain all the essential parts of the grain's seed, lots of fiber, and complex carbohydrates. Try to eat them at most meals. Examples of whole-grain foods and flours are amaranth, barley (lightly pearled), brown and colored rice, buckwheat, bulgur, corn and whole cornmeal, kamut, millet, oatmeal and whole oats, popcorn, quinoa, spelt, triticale, whole rye, whole or cracked wheat, wheat berries, and wild rice.

HEART FACTS:

The Power of Fruits and Vegetables

- Eating fruits and vegetables can help prevent heart disease and other chronic health problems.

- Because they are high in fiber, fruits and vegetables are great for your digestive system.

- Because they are generally low in calories, fruits and vegetables are great for weight control.

- Because they have no fat, fruits and vegetables do not increase lipid levels in blood.

- Because they have no salt, fruits and vegetables do not increase blood pressure. In fact, a diet high in fruits and vegetables can help reduce blood pressure.

- Complex carbohydrates, such as fruits and vegetables, give the body what it needs for energy.

- Fruits and vegetables are high in phytochemicals that are thought to reduce your risk of heart disease, cancer, and other diseases.

Nutritional Fats

- Fats provide much-loved flavor to foods. They also give us the feeling of fullness that helps us feel satisfied long after the last bite.

- Essential fatty acids are the building blocks of fats. Fatty acids supply our bodies with the raw materials that help control inflammation, blood pressure, blood clotting, and other key body functions. Our bodies do not produce them; we must obtain them from food.

- You should limit the amount of total fat in your diet to less than 30 percent.

Stay away from food products made with "white" flour. When you eat breads and other food products made with white flour, you are essentially eating empty calories that do not provide any nutritive value.

Plant Oils

Plant oils are essential to your diet, but they must be heart-healthy. Trans fats, animal fats, palm, palm kernel, and coconut oils should all be on your do-not-eat list. Eating too much of these fats is directly linked to heart disease. Replace them with olive or canola oil. Flaxseed and nut oils are also great for your heart and for fighting inflammation. Fried foods are also on the forbidden list, along with margarines unless they contain an ingredient called sitostanol, a plant sterol that lowers cholesterol absorption. Benecol, Take Control, and other margarine-like spreads contain this ingredient.

Good Fats

Unsaturated fats help to lower blood cholesterol if used in place of saturated fats. There are two types: monounsaturated and polyunsaturated.

Monounsaturated fats are good fats because they lower levels of bad cholesterol and raise levels of good cholesterol. Monounsaturated fats are liquid at room temperature but may solidify in the refrigerator. Foods high in monounsaturated fat include olive, peanut, and canola oils.

Polyunsaturated fats are essential nutrients for the human body. However, our bodies cannot produce them; we have to get them from what we consume. They are found in safflower, sunflower, corn, and soybean oils.

We require two types of polyunsaturated fats to live: omega-3s and omega-6s. Both produce hormones that either lead to or diminish inflammation; omega-6's hormones create inflammation, whereas omega-3's hormones quiet inflammation. Unfortunately, it is much harder to find and consume the omega-3s than the omega-6s:

- Omega-6s are found in oils from certain seeds and the fat of animals fed on grains.
- Omega-3s are in oily fish from cold waters, leafy greens, certain seeds and nuts, flax, hemp, certain vegetable oils, and sea vegetables.

Bad Fats

Saturated fats are the tasty nutritional culprits that can lead to high levels of low-density lipoprotein (LDL). Saturated fats are found in animal products such as butter, cheese, whole milk, ice cream, cream, and fatty meats. They are also found in some plant oils such as coconut, palm, and palm kernel oils.

The AHA recommends that you limit your saturated fat intake to 7 to 10 percent of total calories each day. Less is even better. The American College of Cardiology recommends keeping saturated fat levels at 7 percent or lower.

Trans-fatty acids result from turning liquid vegetable oil into a solid, a procedure called hydrogenation. In the process, the fats are changed from being mostly unsaturated (and good for you) to being mainly saturated (and bad for you). Trans fats raise the level of LDL and lower the level of high-density lipoprotein (HDL). They are found in fried foods, commercially baked goods (donuts, cookies, and crackers), processed foods, and margarines.

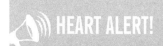

HEART ALERT!

Western Diet = Greater Heart Attack Risk

The ground-breaking INTERHEART study of 16,000 participants in fifty-two countries, led by Dr. Salim Yusuf of Canada's McMaster University, found that the risk of heart attack correlates strongly with a Western diet that is high in salty snacks, fried foods, and meat.

The study showed the risk is 30 percent higher for people who eat a Western diet than for those who follow a "prudent diet" rich in fruits and vegetables. Researchers concluded that the higher the regular intake of fried and salty foods, the higher the risk of heart attack, regardless of the region of the world in which one resides. The results of the study were consistent from region to region.

A study by the Harvard School of Public Health found that women in the United States with the highest levels of trans fat in their blood had three times the risk of heart disease as those with the lowest levels.

Limit the trans fat in your diet to less than 1 percent of your total calories. The government requires that the amount of trans fat in foods be listed on product labels.

Nuts and Legumes (Beans)

Nuts are high in heart-healthy fat and are recommended as part of the DASH diet (see chapter 12).

HEART FACTS:

The Magic of Nuts

A one-year study of 1,224 older men and women living in Spain and at high risk of heart disease randomly assigned participants to one of three groups:

- A control group that was advised to follow a low-fat diet

- A group that was given advice to follow a Mediterranean diet and to use virgin olive oil in place of the refined olive oil they were using

- A group that was given advice to follow a Mediterranean diet and to eat about two table-spoons (28 g) of mixed nuts (½ walnuts, ¼ almonds, and ¼ hazelnuts) each day

All three groups were allowed to eat as much food as they wanted and were not told to get more exercise. None of the participants lost weight over the one-year period. But among patients who were at increased risk of heart disease due to metabolic syndrome, those in the nut group were 70 percent more likely to have reversal of the disease.

The study was conducted at the University of Rovira i Virgili in Reus, Spain. A Mediterranean diet consists of abundant vegetables and beans, fresh fruit, olive oil, dairy products (principally cheese and yogurt), fish, and poultry. It includes four eggs or fewer per week, small amounts of red meat, and wine consumed in low to moderate amounts.

The FDA recommends eating up to 1.5 ounces (40 g) of nuts daily. (A 1.5-ounce serving is equivalent to about ⅓ cup of nuts.)

Legumes are low in fat, are high in protein, and have many nutrients that are important to prevent heart disease. They are also high in complex carbohydrates, fiber, vitamins, and minerals.

For a complete protein, eat lentils with whole-grain rice. There are many classes of dry beans, including black, black eye, chickpea, cranberry, Great Northern, kidney, lima, navy (pea), and pinto.

Fish, Poultry, Eggs, and Low-Fat Dairy

These foods are great sources of lean protein. The best choices are fish, shellfish, lean chicken or turkey (with the skin off), low-fat or fat-free dairy (skim milk, low-fat cheese), egg whites (not the yolk), and egg substitute. Eat these foods one to three times daily.

Stay away from high-fat meats, such as hamburgers and marbled steaks, and high-fat dairy products such as butter and anything with the word *cream* in the title (ice cream, sour cream, and plain-old cream).

Omega-3 Fatty Acids and Fish

Omega-3s decrease inflammation, prevent irregular heartbeats, reduce plaque in artery walls, and decrease blood clotting, blood fats, and blood pressure. Researchers at the National Academy of Sciences have established a minimum daily requirement for them: 0.04 ounces (1.1 grams) for women and 0.06 ounces (1.7 grams) for men. The AHA urges everyone to eat at least two (3-ounce [85-gram]) servings of fish per week. The AHA also advises people who already have heart disease to consume 0.04 ounces (1.1 gram) of omega-3 fatty acids daily. For most, this

The Proportion of Fats in Common Foods

OILS	AMOUNT	SATURATED FAT	MONOUNSATURATED FAT	POLYUNSATURATED FAT	TRANS FAT
Canola	1 T (15 ml)	1 g	8 g	4 g	0
Canola for frying (partially hydrogenated)	1 T (15 ml)	1 g	10 g	2 g	4 g
French fries (McDonald's)	1 medium serving	3 g	8 g	5 g	4 g
Margarine spread	1 oz (28 g)	3 g	5 g	6 g	1 g
Margarine (hard)	1 T (15 ml)	2 g	5 g	3 g	3 g
Olive oil	1 T (15 ml)	2 g	10 g	1 g	0 g
Chocolate-cream cookies	1	—	1 g	—	1 g
Safflower	1 T (15 ml)	1 g	10 g	2 g	0 g
Saltines	1 C crushed	1 g	5 g	1 g	3 g

Source: NutritionData.com; USDA National Nutrient Database for Standard Reference, Release 18.

means taking a supplement. If you are concerned about mercury and other contaminants in seafood, you might consider getting your omega-3s from plant oils such as flax, walnuts, or canola oil.

A recent observational study, the Cardiovascular Health Study involving 4,263 people, found that over an eleven-year period, participants who ate broiled or baked fish at least twice per week, compared with those who ate it less than once per month, lowered their odds of dying from a heart attack by up to 8 percent. (Fried fish and fish sandwiches were not protective.) The study was conducted by a team of researchers led by cardiologist Dariush Mozaffarian, M.D., DrPH, of Brigham & Women's Hospital and Harvard Medical School in Boston.

 HEART ALERT!

"Zero" Doesn't Mean None

According to the U.S. Food and Drug Administration (FDA), a product claiming to have zero trans fat can contain up to half a gram. (Canada set a different standard of zero as less than 0.2 grams.) That means if you eat two servings, you are actually taking in a gram of trans fat. Check the ingredient list of any food you are purchasing, even if it claims to have no trans fat, for "partially hydrogenated vegetable oil" and "vegetable shortening," which means the product does contain some bad fats.

Limit Cholesterol Intake

Cholesterol is a waxy, fatlike substance that occurs naturally in your body. But although it is essential to life, if you have too much cholesterol in your blood it attaches to the walls of your arteries as plaque, leading to atherosclerosis and heart disease. To prevent this from happening, the American College of Cardiology recommends eating less than 200 mg per day of cholesterol. To prevent cholesterol buildup, they also recommend adding 2 gm/day of plant stanols/sterols (found in many fruits, vegetables, nuts, seeds, cereals, legumes, and other plant sources) to your diet and at least 10 gm per day of soluble or viscous fiber (concentrated in oats, barley, soybeans, dried beans and peas, and citrus fruit).

Eliminate Refined and Processed Foods

Refined flour, rice, and sugar are all empty calories; this means they provide no nutritive value and can lead to unwanted pounds. Food processing has stripped refined foods of their nutrients, and often fat, sugar, sodium, additives, and preservatives are added. In addition, eating refined sugar causes spiked increases in blood sugar, which, over time, raises the risk of diabetes and heart disease.

Examples of processed or refined foods are frozen meals, prepackaged meals, fried foods, cakes, cookies, canned biscuits, chips, breakfast bars, toaster treats, white flour, white bread, white rice, white pasta, sodas, juice with sugar, margarine, mayonnaise, and foods containing trans fats. As a general rule, save processed foods for special treats and eat them infrequently.

Limit Salt

The AHA recommends that healthy American adults should eat less than 2,300 mg of sodium per day. This is about one teaspoon (4.9 ml) of sodium chloride

WHAT'S NEW:

The Benefits of Fish Oil

What's so good about fish oil? The omega-3 fatty acids in fish oil have been shown to help reduce triglyceride levels, raise HDL levels, and slightly reduce blood pressure. The FDA has approved a prescription for fish oil (Lovaza), which your doctor can prescribe for high cholesterol. Fish oil tablets are also available over the counter. The recommended dosage is 1 to 4 g once daily or in divided doses.

What are the risks? Fish oil supplements can cause upset stomach and diarrhea. A fishy aftertaste is also common. You can reduce these side effects if you take the oils with meals and if you start low and gradually increase the dosage. You also might want to try freezing the capsules before taking them to prevent "fish burps." These effects may vary with different preparations.

(salt). However, for people with heart failure, recommended sodium intake is no more than 2,000 mg per day. For more information on how to reduce your salt intake and on the DASH eating plan for reducing blood pressure with a heart-healthy low-fat diet, see chapter 12.

About Alcohol: The Good and the Bad

Research has shown that drinking alcohol can be both good and bad for your cardiovascular system. Studies have revealed the following:

- Moderate alcohol consumption decreases the risk of sudden cardiac death in men compared to those who never or rarely drank.
- Moderate alcohol consumption has a beneficial effect on the rate of coronary artery disease and heart attack (myocardial infarction).
- Moderate drinking may protect the heart against congestive heart failure and the risk of having a heart attack.
- Light to moderate alcohol consumption appears to reduce various risks in patients with high blood pressure, including decreasing the risk of heart attack and death.
- Substances in red wine have been found to help guard against blood clotting and to relax blood vessels, helping to increase blood flow.

However:

- Heavy drinking (more than three drinks per day) increases the risk of sudden cardiac death and irregular heart rhythms (arrhythmias).
- Excessive alcohol consumption weakens the heart muscle and prevents it from pumping efficiently, a condition called *alcoholic cardiomyopathy*.

- People who drink three or more drinks daily are much more likely to have elevated blood pressures compared to nondrinkers.

The bottom line is that drinking alcohol in more than moderate amounts is bad for not only your liver and brain, but also your heart. In the United States, one "drink" is 12 ounces (355 ml) of beer, 5 ounces (150 ml) of wine, or 1.5 ounces (42 ml) of

HEART HELP:

How Much Is a Serving?

Apples, raw 1 medium

Orange juice, ¾ cup (177 ml)

String beans, cooked ½ cup (50 g)

Broccoli, cooked ½ cup (35 g)

Fluid milk, 1 cup (235 ml)

Cheese, 1½ oz (40 g)

White bread, 1 slice

Rice, cooked ½ cup (82 g)

RTE cereals, 1 oz (28 g),
   (pre-sweetened cereals)

Pasta, cooked ½ cup (25 g)

Muffins, 1 oz (28 g)

Beef steak, cooked 1 oz (28 g)

Ham, cured cooked 1 oz (28 g)

Eggs, fried 1 large

Dry beans, cooked ½ cup (50 g)

hard liquor. The latest recommendations for alcohol consumption are no more than one drink per day for women and no more than two drinks per day for men. (These guidelines are from the U.S. Department of Agriculture and the FDA's Dietary Guidelines for Americans.)

CONTROL YOUR WEIGHT

If you are like two-thirds of the adults in the United States, you are overweight or obese, which means you are high risk for high blood pressure, heart disease, diabetes, metabolic syndrome, and related problems. Getting your weight under control should be a priority for your heart health.

How do you tell whether you are overweight or obese? The obvious answer is that if you look and feel fat, you probably are. You can also use two key measures—body mass index (BMI) and waist circumference—to judge whether you are overweight or obese.

BMI

Use the BMI tables on the next page to estimate your total body fat. The BMI score means the following: Find your height in inches in the left-hand column labeled "Height." Move across to your weight (in pounds). (Pounds are rounded off.) The number at the top of the column is the BMI at that height and weight.

WHAT'S NEW:

Healthy Diets on the Upswing

Eating a heart-healthy diet is catching on. According to a 2008 survey of 783 U.S. adults by the American Dietetic Association, participants increased their intake of the following top five foods or nutrients during the past five years:

- **Whole grains:** 56 percent are eating more whole grains.

- **Vegetables:** 50 percent are eating more vegetables.

- **Fruits:** 48 percent are eating more fruit.

- **Low-fat foods:** 48 percent are eating more low-fat foods.

- **Omega-3 fatty acids:** 38 percent have boosted their consumption.

Meanwhile, participants decreased their intake of the following top five foods or nutrients during that same time frame:

- **Trans fat:** 56 percent are cutting back on foods containing trans fat.

- **Beef:** 41 percent are eating less beef.

- **Pork:** 33 percent are eating less pork.

- **Dairy:** 23 percent are cutting back on dairy products.

- **Low-sugar foods:** 20 percent say they've cut back on sugary foods.

BMI Ratings

	BMI
Underweight	Lower than 18.5
Normal	18.5–24.9
Overweight	25.0–29.9
Obese	30.0 and higher

BMI Calculation table

BMI (kg/m²)	19	20	21	22	23	24	25	26	27	28	29	30	35	40
HEIGHT (in)	WEIGHT (lb)													
58" (4 ft 10)	91	96	100	105	110	115	119	124	129	134	138	143	167	191
59" (4 ft 11)	94	99	104	109	114	119	124	128	133	138	143	148	173	198
60" (5 ft 0)	97	102	107	112	118	123	128	133	138	143	148	153	179	204
61" (5 ft 1)	100	106	111	116	122	127	132	137	143	148	153	158	185	211
62" (5 ft 2)	104	109	115	120	126	131	136	142	147	153	158	164	191	218
63" (5 ft 3)	107	113	118	124	130	135	141	146	152	158	163	169	197	225
64" (5 ft 4)	110	116	122	128	134	140	145	151	157	163	169	174	204	232
65" (5 ft 5)	114	120	126	132	138	144	150	156	162	168	174	180	210	240
66" (5 ft 6)	118	124	130	136	142	148	155	161	167	173	179	186	216	247
67" (5 ft 7)	121	127	134	140	146	153	159	166	172	178	185	191	223	255
68" (5 ft 8)	125	131	138	144	151	158	164	171	177	184	190	197	230	262
69" (5 ft 9)	128	135	142	149	155	162	169	176	182	189	196	203	236	270
70" (5 ft 10)	132	139	146	153	160	167	174	181	188	195	202	207	243	278
71" (5 ft 11)	136	143	150	157	165	172	179	186	193	200	208	215	250	286
72" (6 ft 0)	140	147	154	162	169	177	184	191	199	206	213	221	258	294
73" (6 ft 1)	144	151	159	166	174	182	189	197	204	212	219	227	265	302
74" (6 ft 2)	148	155	163	171	179	186	194	202	210	218	225	233	272	311
75" (6 ft 3)	152	160	168	176	184	192	200	208	216	224	232	240	279	319
76" (6 ft 4)	156	164	172	180	189	197	205	213	221	230	238	246	287	328

Tips for Effective Weight Loss

- Consider keeping a daily food diary. In a recent Kaiser Permanente Center for Health Research study, dieters who kept track of what they ate in a daily food diary showed double the weight loss of those who didn't. The more food records people kept, the more weight they lost. The study included 1,700 overweight or obese adult participants. They followed the Dietary Approaches to Stop Hypertension (DASH) diet, which is high in fruits and vegetables and low in fat, attended weekly group sessions, and exercised at moderate intensity levels for at least thirty minutes per day. After six months, the average weight loss among the nearly 1,700 participants was 13 lb (5.9 kg). Participants who kept a daily food diary lost an average of 18 lb (8.2 kg) compared to 9 lb (4.1 kg) for those who didn't.

- One pound (0.5 kg) of body weight is equal to 3,500 calories. If you eat 500 fewer calories per day than the amount you need, you will lose 1 lb (0.5 kg) per week. The same rule applies to exercise. If you exercise to the equivalent of another 500 calories per day— such as exercising on an elliptical machine for thirty minutes—in addition to eating 500 fewer calories per day, you will lose 2 lb (0.9 kg) per week.

- Set realistic goals that won't jeopardize your health. Losing 1–2 lb (0.5–0.9 kg) per week is realistic. Losing 5 lb (2.3 kg) per week is losing too much too fast and is hard on your heart and overall health.

- Don't cut too far back on calories. Eating too few calories depletes your body of the nutrition it needs to maintain health. Men and very active women may need up to 2,500 calories daily. Inactive men and women need only about 2,000 calories daily. A safe plan is to eat 300 to 500 fewer calories per day to lose 1–2 lbs (0.5–0.9 kg) per week.

- Beware of fad diets that call for eating a lot of one type of food and no food from major food groups such as fruits or grains. These diets do not work for long-term weight loss and will not give you the nutrients you need daily.

- Beware of diet pills that are sold over the counter or that you buy over the Internet. The FDA recently identified twenty-eight diet pills sold in the United States that contain potentially harmful ingredients that should be available only by prescription. For example, some contained sibutramine, an appetite suppressant found in Meridia, prescribed for the medical management of obesity. It should be used only under a doctor's supervision because it can cause heart attacks, strokes, and heart palpitations, particularly in those with a history of high blood pressure or heart problems.

  If you do use over-the-counter diet pills or buy them on the Internet, make sure they are FDA-approved and do not take more than the recommended dose. Taking too much could cause high blood pressure and other problems.

High BMIs, High Risk

New research suggests that the higher your BMI is, the higher your risk for heart disease. In a study of 54,783 healthy, middle-aged men and women, scientists in Denmark and the United States found that for every point increase in BMI, the risk of developing acute coronary syndrome (ACS) increased by 5 percent to 7 percent, *regardless of healthy behaviors.* (ACS is inadequate blood supply to the heart.)

Even among the top 8 percent of study participants who reported the healthiest lifestyle—exercising regularly, not smoking, eating a healthful diet, and drinking alcohol in moderation—those who were obese demonstrated a two-and-a-half-fold increase in risk of ACS, and those who were overweight had a 65 percent higher risk of ACS, compared with people who maintained a healthy weight.

Waist Circumference

A large waist increases the risk of early death. Scientists studied about 360,000 Europeans from nine European countries. They found that people with the most belly fat had about double the risk of dying prematurely as people with the least amount of belly fat. And the risk of death increased with waist circumference, even for participants who were not overweight.

Determine your waist circumference by placing a measuring tape snugly around your waist. The risk is increased in men with a waist measurement of more than 40 inches (1 m) and more than 35 inches (88.9 cm) in women.

The table on the next page tells you whether your BMI and waist circumference increase your risk for developing type 2 diabetes, dislipidemia, hypertension, and heart disease.

The Only Way to Lose Weight

There is no way around it. The only way to lose weight is to take in fewer calories than you use. This means stepping up exercise and/or stepping down the number of calories you consume, a prospect that most people dread. Many diet plans are available that promote weight loss, all of which have to follow this basic premise to work. It is important that any diet you choose match up with the heart-healthy guidelines we wrote about earlier in this chapter. And of course, before you start a weight-loss program, talk to your doctor.

GET REGULAR EXERCISE

Exercise strengthens the heart and helps to control weight. It also reduces stress, improves circulation and blood pressure, reduces bad cholesterol, increases good cholesterol, and reduces inflammation of the artery walls. There is no doubt that exercise should play a central role in a heart-healthy lifestyle. But many people are unsure which exercises are best and how much they should do. The American College of Sports Medicine and the U.S. Centers for Disease Control and Prevention (CDC) provide national guidelines on physical activity and public health which are straightforward and easy to follow. The AHA endorses and supports these recommendations.

The guidelines for healthy adults age eighteen to sixty-five are as follows:

- Moderate-intensity aerobic physical activity for a minimum of thirty minutes, five days each week, *or* vigorous-intensity aerobic physical activity for a minimum of twenty minutes, three days each week—moderate-intensity aerobic activity can be compared to a brisk walk that accelerates your heart rate.

An example of vigorous activity is jogging, which causes rapid breathing and a substantial increase in heart rate.

- The daily guidelines can be met in three 10-minute segments of moderate exercise.
- Moderate and vigorous activity can be combined to meet the guidelines. For example, you could walk briskly for thirty minutes twice during the week and then jog for twenty minutes on two other days.

In addition to exercise guidelines, the agencies recommend activities that maintain or increase muscular strength and endurance for a minimum of two days each week:

- Eight to ten exercises on two or more nonconsecutive days every week using the major muscle groups—to maximize strength development, use a resistance (weight) that allows eight to twelve repetitions of each exercise, resulting in volitional fatigue. (*Volitional fatigue* is the point in the repetitions where you can't continue without cheating, such as using momentum or leaning way back.)

Muscle-strengthening activities can include a progressive weight-training program, weight-bearing calisthenics, stair climbing, and similar resistance exercises that use the major muscle groups. For a demonstration on how to strengthen your major muscle groups, check out About.com's exercise page at http://exercise.about.com.

Classification of Overweight and Obesity by BMI, Waist Circumference, and Associated Disease Risks

	BMI (kg/m^2)	DISEASE RISK* RELATIVE TO NORMAL WEIGHT AND WAIST CIRCUMFERENCE	
		MEN 40 in (102 cm) OR LESS WOMEN 35 in (88 cm) OR LESS	MEN GREATER THAN 40 in (102 cm) WOMEN GREATER THAN 35 in (88 cm)
Underweight	Lower than 18.5	—	—
Normal	18.5–24.9	—	—
Overweight	25.0–29.9	Increased	High
Obese	30.0–34.9	High	Very high
	35.0–39.9	Very high	Very high
Extremely obese	40.0 +	Extremely high	Extremely high

* Disease risk for type 2 diabetes, dislipidemia, hypertension, and heart disease
+ Increased waist circumference can also be a marker for increased risk even in persons of normal weight.
Source: National Heart, Lung, and Blood Institute

Activities and Intensity levels

Higher-intensity activities require less time to gain cardiac benefits. Lower-intensity activities require more time but are equally good for the heart.

Light-intensity activities include the following:

- Walking slowly
- Golfing, powered cart
- Swimming, slow treading
- Gardening or pruning
- Bicycling, very light effort
- Dusting or vacuuming
- Conditioning exercise, light stretching, or warm-up

Moderate-intensity activities include the following:

- Walking briskly
- Golfing, pulling or carrying clubs
- Swimming, recreational
- Mowing lawn, power motor
- Playing tennis, doubles
- Bicycling 5–9 miles (8–14 km) per hour, level terrain, or with a few hills
- Scrubbing floors or washing windows
- Weight lifting, Nautilus machines, or free weights

Vigorous-intensity activities include the following:

- Race walking, jogging, or running
- Swimming laps
- Mowing lawn, hand mower
- Playing tennis, singles
- Bicycling more than 10 mph, or on a steep uphill terrain
- Moving or pushing furniture
- Circuit training

Another way to measure the intensity of exercise is to apply the "talk test." If you are active at a light intensity level, you should be able to sing while doing the exercise. If you are active at a moderate intensity level, you should be able to carry on a conversation comfortably while exercising. If are too winded or too out of breath to carry on a conversation, the activity is *vigorous.*

JUST DON'T SMOKE

Why is smoking so lethal? Among other things, when you draw the chemicals in tobacco smoke into your lungs and circulatory system, they cause your heartbeat to speed up and become more forceful. Your blood vessels also narrow. The result is high blood pressure. Smoking also lowers levels of high-density lipoprotein (the good cholesterol) and increases the risk of atherosclerosis and thrombosis (blood clots blocking a blood vessel), raising the risk of a heart attack or stroke.

The good news is that even if you have a long-standing habit, within just a few years of quitting your risk of dying from a smoking-related disease drops dramatically. In the Nurses' Health Study, which included about 105,000 American women, researchers found that within five years of quitting smoking, study participants had reduced their risk for heart disease by 47 percent and their risk of having a stroke by 27 percent. Within twenty years of quitting, the risk of dying among former smokers was similar to that of people who never smoked.

Five Keys for Quitting Smoking

Studies have shown that these five steps from the CDC will help you quit smoking for good. You have the best chances of quitting if you use them together.

- Get ready.
- Get support.
- Learn new skills and behaviors.
- Get medication and use it correctly.
- Be prepared for relapse or difficult situations.

Get Ready

- Set a quit date.
- Change your environment if you can until you have some "quit" time behind you.
- Get rid of all cigarettes and ashtrays in your home, car, and place of work.
- Don't let people smoke around you.
- Review your past attempts to quit. Think about what worked and what did not.
- Once you quit, don't smoke—not even a puff!

Get Support and Encouragement

Studies have shown that you have a better chance of being successful if you have help. You can get support in many ways:

- Tell your family, friends, and co-workers that you are going to quit and want their support. Ask them not to smoke around you or leave cigarettes out where you can see them.
- Talk to your health care provider (e.g., doctor, dentist, nurse, pharmacist, psychologist, or smoking cessation coach or counselor).
- Get individual, group, or telephone counseling. Counseling doubles your chances of success.
- The more help you have, the better your chances are of quitting. Programs are available at local hospitals and health centers for free. Call your local health department for information about programs in your area.

Learn New Skills and Behaviors

- Try to distract yourself from urges to smoke. Talk to someone, go for a walk, or get busy with a task.
- When you first try to quit, change your routine. Use a different route to work. Drink tea instead of coffee. Eat breakfast in a different place.
- Do something to reduce your stress. Take a hot bath, exercise, or read a book.
- Plan something enjoyable to do every day.
- Drink a lot of water and other fluids.

Get Medication and Use It Correctly

When used according to directions, medications can help reduce nicotine cravings.

Nearly everyone who is trying to quit can benefit from using a medication. However, if you are pregnant or trying to become pregnant, nursing, under age eighteen, smoking fewer than ten cigarettes per day, or have a medical condition, talk to your doctor or other health care provider before taking medications to quit smoking.

MEDICATIONS TO HELP YOU QUIT

If you are going to give up cigarettes, there are seven medications or devices available to help you quit. All of these approaches will double your chances of quitting and quitting for good.

Varenicline (Chantix)

Taking varenicline takes the "fun" and pleasure out of smoking. The drug alters nicotine's effect in the brain, which blocks the relaxing pleasure of smoking. It also lessens withdrawal symptoms. Varenicline is available by prescription only.

Varenicline's potential side effects are serious enough that the FDA has issued a Public Health Advisory about the drug, and the Federal Aviation Administration has banned pilots and air traffic controllers from using it. Dangerous side effects include changes in behavior, agitation, depressed mood, suicidal ideation, and actual suicidal behavior.

You should start taking varenicline one week prior to the day you quit smoking. You may smoke during the first week. Take the drug after eating and with an 8 oz (237 ml) glass of water. For the first three days, take one white tablet. On days four through seven, take one white tablet in the morning and one in the evening. On day eight through the end of treatment (usually twelve weeks), take a blue tablet twice per day. (The blue tablet is a higher dosage than the white tablet.)

Bupropion SR (Zyban)

Bupropion was originally marketed as an antidepressant drug under the name Wellbutrin. In 1997, the FDA approved bupropion to be used as a smoking cessation aid and marketed it as Zyban. Bupropion is often used along with the nicotine patch, nicotine gum, or other smoking cessation aids. It is available by prescription only.

Common side effects of Zyban include:

- Dry mouth
- Dizziness
- Insomnia
- Change in appetite
- Agitation
- Headaches

More serious side effects, such as seizures, although rare, can occur.

Don't take bupropion if any of the following applies to you:

- You are taking Wellbutrin or Wellbutrin SR (both are bupropion HCl).
- You are taking any other medicine containing bupropion HCl.
- You have or have had a seizure disorder.
- You have or have had an eating disorder.
- You are abruptly discontinuing use of alcohol or sedatives (including benzodiazepines).
- You are currently taking or have recently taken a monoamine oxidase inhibitor.
- You are allergic to bupropion HCl.
- You are pregnant or nursing.

Your doctor will prescribe bupropion in a dose less than 300 mg/day. (Dosages higher than 300 mg/day have been associated with the risk of seizures.) You can start the medication before you quit smoking and eventually reach a quit date. You can take the drug for as long as you and your doctor feel necessary after you have quit smoking.

Nicotine Gum (Nicoderm/ Nicorette and Nicotinell)

Chewing nicotine gum releases nicotine into the tissues of your mouth and bloodstream (and not into your lungs), reducing the craving for getting the stimulant into your system through smoking cigarettes. Nicotine gum is currently available for adults over the counter in Europe, the United States, and elsewhere. Popular brands include Nicoderm/ Nicorette and Nicotinell.

Nicotine gum has a peppery taste and causes tingling in your mouth. Common side effects during the first few days of using the medication are mouth sores, jaw muscle aches, increased saliva production, indigestion, and headache. These side effects go away as you continue to use the gum. Do not use nicotine gum if you are pregnant or nursing.

Use nicotine gum only after you have stopped smoking. Do not eat or drink for fifteen minutes before using, or while chewing the gum (some foods and beverages can reduce its effectiveness).

Pop a piece of gum into your mouth when you have a craving to smoke. Nicotine gum is not chewed like most other gum. Instead, use the "chew and park" method. Chew the gum until you notice a tingly sensation and/or peppery taste, and then park it between your cheek and your gum and leave it there until the tingling stops. Then chew the gum again, parking the gum in a different place in your mouth. Continue this process until all of the nicotine has been released from the gum (about thirty minutes). Note: If you chew the gum without parking it, the nicotine will end up in your stomach rather than your bloodstream, causing a stomachache *and* a craving for nicotine.

For most people, nicotine gum contains enough nicotine to take the edge off a craving to smoke. The over-the-counter gum is available in 2 mg doses (for people who smoke twenty-four or fewer cigarettes per day) and 4 mg doses (for those who smoke twenty-five or more cigarettes per day). Do not chew more than twenty-four pieces per day. Your use of the gum should decrease as you get used to not smoking.

Nicotine Inhaler (Nicotrol)

The nicotine inhaler is a plastic cylinder and cartridge that delivers nicotine into your mouth (and not your lungs). The device imitates the puffing characteristics of smoking, but does not deliver nicotine to the lungs. The nicotine inhaler is available only by prescription. Side effects of the inhaler include irritation of the throat and mouth, runny nose, stomachache, and coughing. The effects will dissipate after awhile.

Users puff on the inhaler when they have a craving for a cigarette. Eighty puffs roughly equal the amount of nicotine delivered by one cigarette. Each nicotine inhaler cartridge delivers up to 400 puffs of nicotine. Use no more than sixteen cartridges per day for up to twelve weeks.

Nicotine Nasal Spray (Nicotrol NS)

The nicotine nasal spray is a device that is used to squirt a nicotine-containing mist into the nose. Many heavy smokers who are trying to quit prefer the spray because it is quickly absorbed by the nasal membranes and delivers a nicotine "hit" faster than the inhaler, patch, or other nicotine replacement therapies. It is available by prescription only.

The most common side effects from nicotine nasal spray are irritation of the nose and throat, watery eyes, sneezing, and coughing. These negative reactions usually go away after the first week of use.

Users generally inhale one to two doses per hour. (One spray to each nostril constitutes a dose.) Spray no more than five doses per hour, or forty doses per day. The spray can be used for up to eight weeks, and then should be stopped during the following four to six weeks.

Nicotine Patch (Habitrol, Nicoderm CQ, Nicotrol)

Nicotine patches are similar to adhesive bandages, but when applied to the skin they release a small but constant amount of nicotine into your body. Patches are a relatively slow method of nicotine delivery; the nicotine takes up to three hours to pass through the layers of skin and into the bloodstream.

Nicotine patches are available in different shapes and sizes. Larger patches deliver more nicotine through the skin. Using a nicotine patch may cause headache, dizziness, lightheadedness, drowsiness, stomach upset, nausea, or flushing for the first few days as your body adjusts to the medication.

Apply the patch to a clean, dry, nonhairy area on your trunk or upper arm. Press firmly for ten to twenty seconds to make sure the patch stays in place. Be sure the edges are held firmly to the skin. Wash your hands after applying the patch.

The length of time the patches are left on the skin varies from twenty-four hours per day to during waking hours only. Apply each new patch to a different area of the skin to prevent irritation.

Nicotine Lozenge

This method of nicotine delivery is a hard candy that releases nicotine as it dissolves in your mouth. The most common side effects are sore teeth and gums, indigestion, and an irritated throat. These side effects usually go away quickly.

Do not eat or drink for fifteen minutes before using the lozenge or while you are using it. Put the lozenge in your mouth and let it dissolve. Do not bite into or chew the lozenge. Each lozenge is one dose and will last about twenty to thirty minutes Do not use nicotine lozenges for longer than twelve weeks, and you should taper off your use of the lozenges during the twelve-week period until you are nicotine-free. Do not use more than twenty lozenges per day. Because the lozenge looks like candy, be sure to keep it away from children.

Be Prepared for Relapse or Difficult Situations

Most relapses occur within the first three months after quitting. Don't be discouraged if you start smoking again. Remember, most people try several times before they finally quit. The following are some difficult situations you may encounter:

Alcohol: Avoid drinking alcohol. Drinking lowers your chances of success.

Other smokers: Being around smoking can make you want to smoke.

Weight gain: Many smokers will gain some weight when they quit, usually less than 10 lbs (4.5 kg). Eat a healthy diet and stay active. Don't let weight gain distract you from your main goal: quitting smoking. Some smoking cessation medications may help delay weight gain.

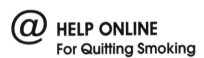

HELP ONLINE
For Quitting Smoking

Smokefree.gov can help you or someone you care about quit smoking. You will find the following on the website:

- An online step-by-step cessation guide
- Local and state telephone "quit lines"
- The National Cancer Institute's national telephone quit line
- The National Cancer Institute's instant messaging service
- Publications which you can download, print, or order

Check it out at www.smokefree.gov.

Bad mood or depression: There are a lot of ways to improve your mood other than smoking. Some smoking cessation medications also lessen depression.

If you are having problems with any of these situations, talk to your doctor or other health care provider.

REDUCE STRESS

Stress is bad for your heart. Acute stress occurs in response to an often-dramatic episode such as a fire at home, a firing at the office, or a physical assault such as surgery; chronic stress is a long-term grinding anxiety or tension. Both types of stress raise your heart rate and blood pressure and release stress hormones, such as epinephrine, into your system. They can cause a heart attack, heart failure, or arrhythmias (abnormal heart rhythms). They can also cause increased oxygen demand and spasms of the coronary blood vessels.

Although there is tremendous variability among individuals, if you are feeling stress you may have one or more of the following symptoms:

- Feeling pressured and hurried
- Sadness and depression
- Worrying and anxiety
- Irritability and moodiness
- Difficulty concentrating and making decisions
- Physical symptoms such as stomach problems, headaches, or chest pain
- Allergic reactions, such as a skin rash or asthma

- Problems sleeping
- Feeling overwhelmed and helpless
- Drinking too much alcohol, smoking, or misusing drugs
- Eating too much or not enough

Stress, a Huge Factor

To test the effects of stress on the heart, British scientists kept track of 6,576 men and women who did not have heart disease (ages thirty-seven to sixty-four). Over a period of seven years, 223 cardiovascular events such as heart attacks occurred. The scientists found that those participants who reported being tense and upset were 54 percent more likely to suffer a stroke, develop heart failure, or undergo bypass surgery or angioplasty than those free from stressful feelings. And 65 percent of the increased risk was attributed to smoking, physical inactivity, and other lifestyle factors. The study results and editorial comment are published in the December 16/23, 2008 issue of the *Journal of the American College of Cardiology.*

It is important for your heart health to curb stress as much as you can and when you can. From meditation to yoga, many techniques can help you reduce stress. Guidance and instruction on these approaches to stress reduction are available through your local community center, hospital, religious organization, or educational institutions.

Q. & A. with Dr. Cannon

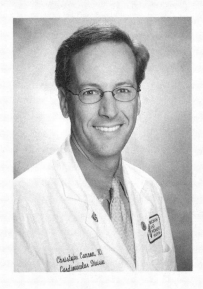

Q. I have high cholesterol and want to avoid taking medications by changing my diet. Can it work?

A. Sometimes it can work. Reducing fat intake, eating a balanced diet, and losing weight can all have a beneficial effect in reducing your cholesterol. A good diet can result in 5 percent to 25 percent lower cholesterol. For many people with borderline high cholesterol, that may be enough. Others will need both dietary changes and medication. This is especially true if you have had a heart attack; you will need to take a statin medication both for its benefit in lowering cholesterol and for its help in preventing heart attacks.

Q. Are there differences among diets as to which one is better for the heart?

A. Surprisingly, not as much as you would think. A study just published in the *New England Journal of Medicine* compared low-fat and low-carb diets, finding that all had similar beneficial effects on cardiovascular risk factors. The biggest factor associated with benefit was the amount of weigh lost, so the key is to find a diet that you can stick with for the long term.

Q. How much exercise do I need to do to stay healthy?

A. The current guidelines recommend exercising five times per week for thirty minutes per day. But they also note that more is better—so if you can aim for every day that is even better. Vigorous exercise has been seen to have better effects on risk factors such as good cholesterol (HDL), but any exercise is good. I generally try to fit in exercise every day, but miss one or two times, so end up at five times per week. In talking with my patients, I see what they like to do, and encourage more of that. If you have a dog, it is excellent exercise to walk the dog. Maybe go five or ten minutes longer each day. Your dog will love it, and it will help you too!

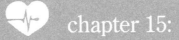

chapter 15:

WOMEN AND HEART DISEASE

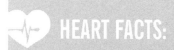

HEART FACTS:

The Numbers

- 8 million women in the United States have heart disease.

- 435,000 American women have heart attacks annually, of which 83,000 are younger than sixty-five years of age.

- 267,000 women in the United States die each year from heart attacks, which is six times the number of women who die from breast cancer.

- 8.6 million women worldwide die from heart disease each year, accounting for one-third of all deaths in women; this includes three million who die from stroke each year.

- Women develop heart problems later in life than men—typically seven or eight years later. However, by about age sixty-five, a woman's risk is almost the same as a man's.

- The age-adjusted rate of heart disease for African American women is 72 percent higher than for white women.

- 38 percent of women and 25 percent of men will die within one year of a first recognized heart attack; women are twice as likely as men to die within the first few weeks after having a heart attack.

- Women comprise only 24 percent of participants in all heart-related studies.

THE SOBERING FACTS FOR WOMEN

Many people believe that cancer is the leading cause of death for women, but the truth is that heart disease has this dubious distinction. Coronary heart disease (CHD), which causes heart attack, is the leading cause of death for American women over the age of sixty-five. Nearly twice as many women in the United States die of heart disease, stroke, and other cardiovascular diseases as from all forms of cancer, including breast cancer.

When it comes to diagnosing and treating heart disease, there is a gender gap. Heart disease in women is often under-recognized and undertreated, which is one of the reasons women are less likely to survive heart attacks than men. Another reason could be that women's smaller hearts and blood vessels are more easily damaged. Several studies showed that the death risk for women was one-and-one-half to twice that of men, when adjusted for age, size, and other factors.

The most common symptom of a heart attack in both men and women is some type of pain, pressure, or discomfort in the chest. Often, women do not experience severe pain during a heart attack, but rather describe their chest pain as pressure, tightness, or an ache. They are also less likely to report pain than men.

"Atypical" Symptoms Are Common

Women are more likely than men (twice as likely in one study) to experience so-called "atypical" symptoms such as back, neck, or jaw pain, shortness of breath, nausea or vomiting, indigestion, weakness, fatigue, and dizziness. The term *atypical* appears to be a misnomer as these symptoms are actually relatively common for women.

Shortness of breath appears to be a particularly important symptom and may precede or occur at the same time as chest pain. Sweating is less common in women than men. One study of nearly 18,000 men and women (40 percent were women) showed that those who experienced shortness of breath were three to five times more likely to die from heart disease than those who did not have this symptom.

Women commonly experience *preheart attack* or *prodromal* symptoms, meaning symptoms that occur before a heart attack, generally from about four to six months to one week before the event. A study of 515 women who had heart attacks showed that 78 percent experienced at least one preheart attack symptom for more than one month, either daily or several times per week, with the most common symptoms being unusual fatigue (about 71 percent) and sleep disturbance (about 50 percent).

The lack of awareness, even among doctors, of the subtle signs of heart attacks in females can lead to delays in diagnosis and treatment. Many lifesaving heart attack treatments, such as clot-busting drugs and balloon angioplasty, work best if given within the first few hours after a heart attack begins. Women tend to wait longer than men to seek medical help when they are having a heart attack.

This delay can result in death or long-lasting heart damage, and is an important reason why women tend to experience worse outcomes after a heart attack than men. If you are a woman, recognize the serious threat of heart disease and become familiar with the wide variety of symptoms you may experience both before and during a heart attack. This will help you to quickly get the treatment you need and could save your life.

Carla's Story

For the past four weeks, Carla has felt short of breath while doing simple tasks such as washing her kids' clothes or unloading the car. She has also been more tired than usual and is spending more time lying on the couch watching TV after coming home from work. Carla is a bit overweight, and knows she should eat better, but has little time for cooking at home or exercise.

As the wife of a local business dealer who has been struggling lately amid the global financial crisis, and a mother of two young kids, Carla has myriad responsibilities in addition to her stressful job as an accountant. Having read about heart disease in women, she decides to take a day off from work to visit her doctor. Her doctor dismisses her worries and tells her that at age forty-five, she is "too young" to have heart disease, and if anything, her husband needs to worry more about heart disease than she does. He mentions anxiety and stress as the cause of her symptoms and sends her home with a prescription for Ativan to "calm her nerves."

Two weeks later, as Carla is lying in bed after a tiring day, she develops burning pain in her upper belly. She dismisses the pain as heartburn, pops an antacid, and falls asleep. Carla wakes up at three o'clock in the morning and the pain is still there, and she also feels short-winded. Carla wakes up her husband who calls 9-1-1 and she is brought to the emergency room of the nearest hospital. After all kinds of blood tests and an electrocardiogram, Carla is told that she has suffered a "heart attack."

THE PRESCRIPTION FOR WOMEN WITH HEART DISEASE

Treatment plans for heart disease in women can differ from those for men. Women have unique concerns, and several important biological and socioeconomic gender differences need to be addressed when formulating treatment plans. Although the medicines and special procedures are generally the same as in men, there are some important guidelines and distinctions.

Risk Factors for Women Are Different Than Those for Men

The risk factors (factors which increase your risk of developing a disease) for heart disease are different for men and women. As a woman, it is extremely important for you to control certain risk factors such as obesity, smoking, and diabetes, which can cause more heart damage in women than men. Women also are known to have higher levels of C-reactive protein (CRP), a known marker of cardiovascular risk.

Studies have shown that metabolic syndrome—a combination of abdominal obesity, increased blood pressure, elevated blood glucose, and triglycerides—has a greater impact on women than on men. Women lose much more than men if they smoke; one recent study found that women who smoke have heart attacks about fourteen years earlier than women who don't smoke, whereas male smokers have heart attacks about six years earlier than men who don't smoke.

WHAT'S NEW:

Reynolds Risk Score for Women

The oft-used Framingham risk score has been found to underestimate the risk of heart disease in women. The new Reynolds risk score was developed in a study of almost 25,000 initially healthy American women (forty-five and older) who were followed for ten years, and is designed especially for women.

What's different about this score? The Reynolds score utilizes a new formula that in addition to your age, blood pressure, cholesterol levels, and whether you currently smoke (factors used to calculate the Framingham risk score) also uses information from two other risk factors: a blood test called hs-CRP (high-sensitivity CRP, a mea-sure of inflammation) and whether either of your parents had a heart attack before they reached age sixty (a measure of genetic risk). The new score measures your risk of having a heart attack or stroke, dying of heart disease, or needing a heart procedure such as bypass surgery or angioplasty within the next ten years.

How can I calculate my score? Like the Framingham risk calculator, the Reynolds risk score does not work for women who already have heart disease. To calculate your Reynolds risk score, go to www.reynoldsriskscore.org.

Drinking Alcohol

Recent research suggests that moderate drinkers are less likely to develop heart disease than people who don't drink any alcohol or who drink too much. However, if you drink alcohol, do so only in moderation; for women, *moderate drinking* is defined as no more than one drink per day. Alcohol can increase the risk of breast cancer, however; talk to your doctor to weigh the benefits and risks. If you are pregnant or planning to become pregnant, you should not drink.

Stress and Depression/Anxiety

It is important to recognize mental stress and depression in women, as these conditions can affect women's hearts more than men's. Many women are balancing the challenge of raising children with other family obligations or working in high-stress careers. Unmanaged stress can lead to high blood pressure, heart attack, irregular heart rhythms, and a weakened immune system.

Depression is twice as common in women as in men and it increases your risk of heart disease by two to three times, compared with those who aren't depressed. About one in five women who has had a heart attack, bypass surgery, or stroke or has been hospitalized with heart failure has evidence of depression. Women generally experience more symptoms of depression than men after a heart attack or bypass surgery.

Depression makes it difficult to maintain a healthy lifestyle and follow recommended treatment. Many, but not all, studies have found that depression increases the risk of dying from a heart-related cause within the first year of a heart attack. In a study of people who underwent bypass surgery, depression was a stronger predictor of lack of functional improvement for women than men.

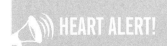

HEART ALERT!

Panic Attack or Heart Attack?

Heart disease in women is often mistaken for panic attack. Chest pain, shortness of breath, anxiety, palpitations, and indigestion are common symptoms in both.

If you have any of these symptoms and they last for more than two to three minutes or if the pain leaves and then returns it could be heart disease. You need to call 9-1-1 and get to the ER right away. Your doctor will perform an ECG and other tests to determine whether the pain is coming from your heart.

New research suggests that older women who experience panic attacks might have an increased risk for having heart attacks or heart-related death.

Anxiety is also more common in women than in men after a heart attack or bypass surgery. Anxiety after a heart attack does not appear to increase your risk of dying, but one small study found that people with higher anxiety levels forty-eight hours after their heart attack were five times more likely to have heart rhythm and blood-flow problems. Another study of heart attack patients found that anxiety did not increase the risk of dying from a heart-related cause after one year in females, but it slightly increased the risk of dying for males with very high anxiety levels.

MEDICAL TREATMENTS FOR WOMEN WITH HEART DISEASE

Before taking any heart pill, be sure to tell your doctor if you are pregnant, may become pregnant, are breast-feeding, if you are taking birth control pills, or if you are taking any over-the-counter or alternative medicines or dietary supplements.

Anticlotting Medicines

A recent, large study called the Women's Health Study looked at the role of aspirin to prevent heart disease in women. Approximately 40,000 healthy women forty-five years of age or older were given 100 mg of aspirin or a dummy pill to take every other day. After ten years, aspirin did not reduce the risk of having a heart attack, but did reduce the risk of having a stroke by 17 percent. On the other hand, studies in healthy men have shown that aspirin leads to a 32 percent reduction in heart attack risk, but does not lower the risk of stroke.

The reason for these gender differences is not clear, but researchers believe women experience more strokes than heart attacks, in contrast to men, who experience more heart attacks and are more likely to encounter aspirin resistance, a condition in which the body is resistant to the blood-thinning effects of aspirin.

Of note, in this study women over the age of sixty-five did benefit with a lower risk of heart attack, stroke, or death from taking low-dose aspirin. In general, if your risk of heart disease is high (i.e., you are older or have one or two risk factors), we would more likely recommend taking aspirin. If you have already had a heart attack, a stroke, or a heart procedure, we will definitely recommend aspirin. We usually prescribe low-dose aspirin of 81 mg/day for long-term use; 325 mg is frequently prescribed in the hospital and in the early months after heart procedures.

There are several other blood-thinning medicines that have important differences in the way they act in women versus men. Adding clopidogrel to aspirin was shown in a recent study to be equally effective in reducing the risk of heart attacks in both women and men; similarly, the risk of major bleeding was increased in both men and women. Anticoagulants such as heparin (given in the hospital for acute heart problems) can cause more bleeding problems in women than men. Warfarin should not be used during pregnancy as it can lead to birth defects and cause serious bleeding in the fetus.

Thrombolytics or Clot Busters

Despite equal benefits from clot-busting drugs for heart attacks in women and men, multiple studies have found that women are less likely to receive these clot-busting medications than men. These drugs work best when given within twelve hours after symptoms of a heart attack begin. They are not recommended for everyone who is having a heart attack, and the decision to administer these drugs is based on ECG findings. Women who are having heart attacks tend to wait longer than men before heading to the ER, and when they do arrive, the hospital staff takes longer to administer the drugs or don't administer them at all, even though the women might be ideal candidates, according to a new study from the American Heart Association's (AHA's) "Get with the Guidelines" program.

A study conducted in the state of Washington found that among 1,078 females who were screened for eligibility for clot-busting drugs, as many as 39 percent were considered too old (although current guidelines do not have any age limit), 59 percent had nondiagnostic ECGs (meaning absence of the specific pattern seen on the ECG that qualifies one for these drugs), and 30 percent came to the hospital too late for the drugs to be effective. Overall, only 16 percent of the women screened were considered eligible, compared with 25 percent of men, and, of the eligible women, 55 percent received the drug, compared with 78 percent of men.

Studies have shown that clot-busting medications can reduce the risk of a woman dying within thirty-five days of a heart attack by 12 percent; the benefit is slightly less than in men. Although the reason is not clear, significantly more women treated with clot busters die or have a stroke, compared to men.

Caution: Blood Pressure Drugs

Research suggests that this large group of drugs work equally well in men and women. However, angiotensin-converting enzyme inhibitors should not be used during pregnancy; these have received a black box warning from the U.S. Food and Drug Administration, implying that the drugs carry a significant risk of serious or even life-threatening effects as they greatly increase the chance of delivering babies with congenital malformations. Angiotensin-receptor blockers are also contraindicated during pregnancy.

Older aldosterone blockers such as spironolactone can block hormone receptors and cause excessive hair growth in women. Some early studies found that calcium-channel blockers could increase the risk of many types of cancer, including breast and uterine cancer, but later studies showed that this is most likely not true.

Cholesterol-Reducing Drugs: Statins

Some research indicates that women are less likely than men to be screened for high cholesterol or treated with appropriate medication. In a study of people with heart disease, 35 percent of women received cholesterol-lowering medications, compared to 55 percent of men. This is despite several studies showing the statins to be equally effective and safe in men and women with heart disease.

The question of whether statins can prevent heart attacks and death in women who do not have heart disease was answered by a recent landmark study, the JUPITER trial. Investigators found that healthy women older than sixty years of age (comprising around 38 percent of the total population) with normal cholesterol levels but high levels of CRP had fewer cardiovascular events and fewer deaths when they took 20 mg of the statin rosuvastatin (Crestor). This massive study provides strong evidence that statins work as well to prevent heart attacks and death in women who do not have heart disease as they do in men. CRP, measured by a simple blood test that costs about $25, detects levels of inflammation in your body and can be used to identify women for whom statins would be a smart addition to a prevention program that includes a healthy diet and increased exercise.

Menopausal Hormone Therapy

Women tend to develop heart disease ten to fifteen years later in life than men. This delay is thought to be largely due to the protective effects of estrogen. It was widely believed for decades that boosting estrogen levels after menopause could ward off heart disease, and hormone replacement therapy was universally recommended. Then a study came out in 2002 called the Women's Health Initiative that totally changed our practice.

This study of more than 16,000 healthy post-menopausal women found that the combination of estrogen plus progestin provided no protection,

Birth Control Pills

- Don't mix smoking and "the pill." Cigarette smoking boosts the risk of serious health problems from birth control pill use, especially the risk of blood clots. The risk is particularly high if you are over the age of thirty-five.

- If you are a diabetic or have a close relative who is a diabetic, you should have regular blood sugar tests because the levels of blood sugar can sometimes change dramatically with birth control pill use.

- Your blood pressure may go up after taking these pills. If it increases to 140/90 mm Hg or higher, ask your doctor about changing pills or switching to another form of birth control.

- If you have heart disease, birth control pills may not be a safe choice. Be sure your doctor knows about these or other serious health conditions before prescribing birth control pills.

and in fact it increased the risk of heart disease, stroke, breast cancer, and blood clots. Many women in this study started taking hormone therapy more than ten years after menopause began.

A 2007 analysis of the Women's Health Initiative showed that for women who started taking hormone therapy between ages fifty and fifty-nine, the risks of developing heart disease or of dying from any cause

were actually slightly lower than women taking a dummy pill. Ongoing trials are exploring the possibility of whether hormone therapy can reduce heart disease risk in younger women, particularly if it is taken in the first five years after menopause.

For now, do not take hormone therapy to prevent heart disease. And if you already have heart disease and are on hormone therapy, consider stopping it after consulting your doctor. If you experience severe menopausal symptoms such as hot flashes, mood swings, or vaginal dryness, use the lowest effective dose for the shortest amount of time needed to treat your symptoms. In addition, plenty of alternative therapies are available to treat your symptoms; consult your doctor for more information on these.

Hormone therapy does prevent osteoporosis, but the risks of taking this long-term to prevent bone loss outweigh the benefits. Other treatments are available to prevent osteoporosis that don't come with these risks, such as the drugs alendronate (Fosamax) and raloxifene (Evista).

SPECIAL PROCEDURES FOR TREATING WOMEN WITH HEART DISEASE

Coronary Angioplasty and Stents

Women are less likely to be referred for cardiac catheterization than men. However, once they undergo cardiac catheterization, they are just as likely as men to be treated with angioplasty or stents.

Women are more likely to die after angioplasty or stent placement than men. These procedures are in general riskier and trickier to perform in smaller blood vessels, and there is an increased risk of tearing the artery. Women have smaller blood vessels than men even after adjusting for their smaller body size. Additionally, women are more prone to bleeding problems arising from the procedure itself, as well as from the blood-thinning medications that are often used simultaneously. However, the good news is that women who survive the initial hospital period do as well as men in the long term.

Coronary Artery Bypass Surgery

Women are more likely to die in the hospital than men after bypass surgery. Women are generally older at the time of bypass surgery and are more likely to have additional health problems such as heart failure and diabetes. They also have smaller blood vessels, making the surgery more difficult and putting them at a higher risk of complications after surgery. In one study of 6,630 subjects, the death rate for women was significantly higher in all age groups; four women undergoing bypass surgery died for every man in the 40–49-year group, and three women died for every man in the 50–59-year group.

After bypass surgery, women are more likely than men to require blood transfusions and generally have to stay in the hospital longer. Women have a slower physical recovery, experience more physical symptoms, and have more severe adverse mood effects after surgery than men. Starting at about six weeks after surgery, both women and men are less anxious and less depressed than they were before surgery. One study found that even though both women and men improved after surgery, after one year women had more symptoms of depression and scored lower on tests of physical and social functioning than men.

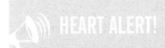

HEART ALERT!

Pitfalls of Coronary Angiogram

Just because your arteries appear clear on an angiogram, it does not mean you are not at risk of heart disease. A study by the National Institutes of Health, called the Women's Ischemia Syndrome Evaluation, indicated that as many as three million women previously diagnosed with healthy arteries could actually have an increased risk of heart attack.

This study found, among other things, that the gold-standard test for assessing coronary artery disease (CAD)—the coronary angiogram—may not spot the form of heart disease called *coronary microvascular syndrome*, in which plaque spreads evenly throughout the walls of very small arteries, rather than building up in a larger, main artery. These diffuse plaques might not be treatable using traditional methods such as angioplasty and stenting, and drug treatment might be a better option.

If you are told that you have a "normal" angiogram but continue having chest pain or other symptoms, ask your doctor whether you might have a problem with the functioning of your small arteries. To find out, your doctor may administer a questionnaire called the Duke Activity Status Index that measures how easily you can perform everyday tasks and can help to predict your heart attack risk. The prognosis is generally excellent, but it is reasonable to get a clear diagnosis.

Pacemaker and AICD

Women appear to live longer than men after getting a pacemaker implanted. In one study of about 6,500 people, women lived an average of two years longer than men, despite being older when they had their pacemaker implanted. In another study of nearly 1,600 people older than eighty, women were 30 percent less likely to die in the years following their pacemaker implantation than men.

Automatic implantable cardioverter defibrillators (AICDs) are less successful at correcting fast heartbeats in women than in men and have a higher rate of complications. Although an AICD should slow the heartbeat, in one study women were three times more likely to have their heart rate further increased by AICDs, compared to men. When it comes to preventing sudden cardiac death, AICDs seem to work equally well in both men and women. A recent study published in the *Journal of the American Medical Association* showed that women are two to three times less likely than men to receive an AICD, even when tests showed they might need them.

TESTS AND DIAGNOSIS OF HEART DISEASE IN WOMEN

Heart disease is often misdiagnosed in women, especially younger women. One study that looked at more than 10,000 patients (48 percent were women) who went to the ER with chest pain or other heart attack symptoms found that women younger than fifty-five years of age were seven times more likely to be misdiagnosed than men of the same age. The consequences of this were enormous: Being sent away from the hospital doubled the chances of dying. One major factor that contributes to women being misdiagnosed is the persistent myth that heart disease is a man's disease. The only way to reduce the rate of heart disease misdiagnoses in women is to increase the awareness of this problem by health care providers and women themselves.

Heart Attack Tests

Heart attack tests include creatine kinase (CK), CKMB, and troponins T and I. They are equally accurate in men and women and should be ordered in any woman with symptoms suggesting a possible heart attack. Interestingly, even among patients coming to the hospital with chest pain or a heart attack, women less often have positive troponin tests (and more often have the newer blood risk markers such as CRP elevated). Thus, this new research suggests use of additional blood tests that measure the newer risk markers might be important for women.

CRP

If your CRP level is high, you have a higher risk of developing heart disease. However, the general cutoffs for high and low CRP set by the AHA and CDC may not be accurate in women, since research shows that women have higher levels of CRP to begin with than men. A study conducted in Dallas that involved nearly 2,750 people aged thirty to sixty-five years—of which more than half were women—found that CRP levels were almost twice as high in women than in men (3.3 mg/L versus 1.8 mg/L). Factors such as hormone therapy, pregnancy, and birth control pills can raise CRP levels, whereas cholesterol-lowering statin drugs and anti-inflammatories such as aspirin and ibuprofen may lower CRP levels. Even after accounting for these and other factors, white women were 60 percent more likely and black women were 70 percent more likely to have high CRP levels than white men. Being overweight or obese was very strongly associated with high CRP levels—more so in women than men.

ECG and Exercise ECG

ECG results are less accurate in women than in men; women are more prone to inconclusive tests, meaning the results aren't clearly positive or negative. Similarly, exercise ECG is less accurate for diagnosing heart disease in women, compared to men. The test can be affected by the phase of the menstrual cycle and by oral contraceptive use, implicating sex hormones as a factor. Women are prone to *false positive tests* (meaning the test shows a problem but in reality there isn't one) and inconclusive tests; in these cases, you might be sent for further testing such as echocardiography or a nuclear stress test. A negative test, on the other hand, is just as reliable in women as in men.

Echocardiogram (Echo)

Echocardiography has similar accuracy in men and women. Women with a negative (normal) rest or stress echo have a low risk for developing future problems such as a heart attack and a less than 1 percent annual risk of death. If you have a positive (abnormal) echo, you are at increased risk of experiencing heart problems or dying from a heart attack. If you are obese or have large breasts, the images produced by echocardiography may appear fuzzy, making it difficult to interpret. This test does not involve radiation, and hence, it is safe to undergo during pregnancy.

Nuclear Stress Test

Although this test is highly accurate, if you are obese or have large breasts, the images may have artifact changes, leading to a false positive result (meaning the test indicates a problem but in

HEART HELP:

Know the Warning Signs and Act Quickly

- Women experience different symptoms of heart attack than men. Although chest pain is the most common symptom in both women and men, women are more likely than men to have atypical symptoms, such as discomfort in other areas of the upper body (one or both arms, neck, back, or stomach), shortness of breath, nausea or vomiting, lightheadedness, and unusual fatigue.

- If you think you or someone else may be having a heart attack, you must act quickly to prevent disability or death. Wait no more than a few minutes—five at most—before dialing 9-1-1.

- Although it is frustrating that some doctors don't take women's concerns seriously, don't be afraid to speak up for what you need—or bring someone who can speak up for you. Ask for tests that can determine whether you are having a heart attack.

- Don't let anyone tell you at the hospital that your symptoms are "just indigestion" or that you're "overreacting." You have the right to be thoroughly examined for a possible heart attack.

reality there is none). Modern computer programs can correct for some of the blurring and muffling, and timing the pictures for when the heart is moving the least (called ECG-gating) improves the quality of the images further. When these techniques are used, nuclear stress testing has a similar accuracy in men and women. Some, but not all, studies suggest that women with a positive (abnormal) test have a higher risk of dying or having a heart attack than men with an abnormal test, particularly when the test is severely abnormal.

Cardiac Catheterization

Research on women undergoing cardiac catheterization has had varied results. A 1987 study of more than 80,000 heart disease patients found that women were less likely than men to undergo cardiac catheterization. If this is the case, it is debatable whether the disparity reflects gender bias or because women do not need this test as often as men. Up to 40 percent of women are found to have no significant blockages in their arteries upon cardiac catheterization, compared with 20 percent of men. More recent

WHAT'S NEW:

Test for Sleep Apnea

New research suggests that sleep apnea may increase your risk of heart disease. Specifically, it can increase your risk of high blood pressure and possibly heart failure, stroke, an abnormal heart rhythm (atrial fibrillation), and heart attack. The test for sleep apnea is called *polysomnography* or *sleep study*, which is usually performed overnight in a sleep center.

Facts about Sleep Apnea:

- More than eighteen million Americans suffer from sleep apnea, of which six million are women.

- Up to 90 percent remain undiagnosed.

- An analysis of questionnaire responses from more than 2,700 patients seen at a sleep laboratory showed that men were more likely to have traditional apnea symptoms, such as snoring, and women were more likely to report sleep disturbances, longer delay until falling asleep, and greater difficulty sleeping.

- The diagnosis is often missed in women, as many doctors mistakenly believe that sleep apnea is rare in women.

- Although more common in obese middle-aged men, in women it becomes much more common after menopause.

- Other factors that increase the risk of developing sleep apnea include being overweight or obese, smoking, the use of alcohol or sleeping pills, and a family history of sleep apnea.

- Sleep apnea is common in obese women with polycystic ovarian syndrome and may worsen insulin resistance in such patients.

- One recent study showed that sleep apnea might decrease women's sexual function by reducing sexual desire, sensation, and lubrication.

research finds that if age and risk factors are taken into account, women are just as likely as men to undergo this test.

Calcium Scan or Electron Beam Computed Tomography (EBCT)

Calcium scans may be useful for detecting early signs of fatty plaque buildup in women with risk factors who have no symptoms of heart disease. Some studies suggest that the same calcium score may confer a higher risk for a woman than a man. A large study of more than 10,000 healthy men and women (40 percent were women) found that at every level of calcium score, women had a higher risk of dying within five years of the scan than men; the risk of dying was highest for women with an intermediate to high risk of heart disease and a calcium score greater than 400. Women's arteries are smaller than men's, so the same amount of calcium would be expected to block off more of the artery. Since this involves X-rays, you should not undergo this test if you are pregnant.

HEART DISEASE IN WOMEN EXPLAINED

The most common form of heart disease in women is Coronary Artery Disease (CAD), caused by a narrowing of the arteries that feed the heart (coronary arteries). Women are more likely than men to have "silent" heart attacks (especially in the presence of diabetes), which cause no symptoms, and are discovered days, weeks, or even months later during ECG testing.

The reason women don't develop obvious crushing chest pain during heart attacks but have subtler symptoms and signs could be due to their smaller arteries—or because in women, plaques erode, ex-

posing the inner layers of the artery, whereas in men the bulky, unstable plaques tend to burst open. Differences in symptoms may also be related to a condition called *endothelial dysfunction*. Endothelial dysfunction, in which the lining of the artery doesn't allow the artery to expand (dilate) properly to boost blood flow during activity, is more common in women and increases the risk of coronary artery spasm and sudden death. Ultimately, women tend to show up in ERs after much heart damage has already occurred, leading to poorer outcomes when compared to men.

Arrhythmia

Another common heart condition that women experience is arrhythmias, or abnormal heart rhythms. Palpitations are a significant source of discomfort and concern to female patients. Some women have an increased sensation of their heart pounding in the absence of any heart rhythm disturbance, a situation that has been dubbed *enhanced cardiac awareness*. Others have extra heartbeats such as premature atrial and ventricular beats, which can cause palpitations. Still others have atrial and ventricular arrhythmias, which can be serious. Women have a longer *QT interval* (the time required for depolarization and repolarization of your heart to occur) than men, and a rare genetic disease called congenital Long QT syndrome may lead to sudden death more frequently in young women than in men. Some women have monthly fluctuations in the occurrences of certain arrhythmias.

Stroke

Women are more likely to report unusual stroke symptoms than men. A study of 1,124 stroke survivors found that 28 percent of women had nontraditional stroke symptoms, compared to 19 percent of men. Nontraditional symptoms and signs that may indicate a stroke include sudden face, arm, or

HEART FACTS:

Stroke in Women

- Over the course of a lifetime, one in five women will suffer a stroke, versus one in six men. Each year, more than 370,000 women have a stroke—about 46,000 more women than men. This is largely because the risk of stroke increases with older age, and women live longer than men.

- One-year mortality after a first stroke is approximately 24 percent in women forty years or older and 21 percent in men, according to data from three large studies. Within five years of a first stroke, 51 percent of women and 47 percent of men will die, with an additional 22 percent of women and 13 percent of men experiencing another stroke. For women sixty to sixty-nine years of age, the average survival after a first stroke is 7.4 years (6.8 years for men).

- Women tend to have worse outcomes and are more disabled after a stroke than men. This is probably because women are older on average when they have strokes.

- Women seem to derive a larger benefit from tissue plasminogen activator (tPA), a clot-busting drug. In an analysis of nearly 1,000 women from three studies, women were more likely than men to benefit from tPA. Despite this, studies have shown that women who are eligible for tPA treatment are less likely to receive it than their male counterparts.

leg pain, nausea, tiredness, chest pain, shortness of breath, or a pounding or racing heartbeat.

Data from the Framingham Heart Study indicates that diabetes may have a greater impact on stroke risk in older women, compared with men, though the reasons for this are not clear. In addition to having an increased risk of stroke, people with diabetes who have a stroke often fare worse than nondiabetic stroke victims—especially women. One study found that 16 percent of stroke deaths in men and 33 percent in women were attributable to diabetes. Other stroke risk factors are unique to women. For example, women taking hormone therapy have a slightly increased risk of stroke as shown in the Women's Health Initiative study. Using birth control pills raises the risk of stroke by a small but significant amount. In healthy young women (nonsmokers younger than age thirty-five who do not have high blood pressure), the overall risk is low.

Stress Cardiomyopathy

You are struck by intense grief. Your beloved husband, battling for months with lung cancer, passed away this morning. You can't stop crying, and your daughter who is a nurse has been trying to console you all day. All of a sudden in the evening, you become breathless and start experiencing chest pain. Your daughter, concerned that you might be having a heart attack, calls 9-1-1 and you are brought to the ER of the hospital where she works. Luckily, the cardiologist still hasn't left for the day and he is asked to evaluate you. He decides to do an echocardiogram at your bedside. You hear the doctor and your daughter talking in hushed tones outside your room. A few seconds later, they both walk in, and the doctor informs you that you will have to be admitted to the hospital as the intense emotional trauma that you have experienced today has "broken" your heart and caused stress cardiomyopathy. (See the box at right for information on this condition.)

PREGNANCY AND HEART DISEASE

Pregnancy stresses your heart and circulatory system. During pregnancy, your blood volume increases by 40 percent to 50 percent to nourish your growing baby. The amount of blood your heart pumps each minute increases by 30 percent to 50 percent and your heart rate increases as well. All of these changes cause your heart to work harder.

If you have a cardiovascular disease such as congenital heart disease, CAD, a heart valve disorder, or high-risk factors such as high blood pressure or diabetes, pregnancy can pose serious concerns to you as well as your baby. You will need to have prepregnancy consultation with a cardiologist who has expertise in the field, and your obstetric care will have to be coordinated between your obstetrician and your cardiologist. You will need frequent testing throughout your pregnancy to monitor your health and that of your baby.

If you have congenital heart disease, you may have a higher risk of delivering a baby with some type of heart defect. Today, many women with different forms of heart disease safely deliver healthy babies. However, certain heart conditions carry a high risk of life-threatening complications for mother or baby, including severe pulmonary hypertension, severe cardiomyopathy, Eisenmenger's syndrome (a condition which develops in individuals with significant heart defects and is characterized by right-to-left shunting of blood in the heart, resulting in an

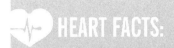

HEART FACTS:

Stress Cardiomyopathy—"Broken Heart Syndrome"

- Stress cardiomyopathy is a condition in which intense emotional or physical stress such as grief (e.g., the death of a loved one), fear, extreme anger, and surprise causes rapid and severe heart muscle weakness. It most commonly affects middle-aged or elderly women.

- You can have symptoms similar to a heart attack, including chest pain, shortness of breath, and dizziness. Typically, these symptoms begin just minutes to hours after you are exposed to a severe and usually unexpected stress.

- An echocardiogram, in many cases, reveals a peculiar type of heart muscle weakness, where the apex of your left ventricle balloons outward. Cardiac catheterization reveals fairly normal coronary arteries and no severe blockages, unlike in the case of a heart attack.

- The cause of stress cardiomyopathy is unknown, but it is believed that your heart muscle is overwhelmed by the large amount of stress hormones (e.g., adrenaline) that is produced in response to emotional trauma. Your heart muscle cells are "stunned" rather than destroyed as they would be if you had a heart attack.

- You can develop congestive heart failure, low blood pressure, or life-threatening heart rhythm abnormalities as a result of stress cardiomyopathy. Thankfully, the heart usually recovers within a couple of weeks, and there is no permanent damage. It is unusual for the syndrome to reoccur with future stressful situations.

inadequate oxygen supply to organs), and so forth. If you have one of these conditions, you might be advised against becoming pregnant.

Cardiac Abnormalities in Pregnancy

Because pregnancy has a profound effect on a woman's heart, some women with healthy hearts may experience cardiac abnormalities while they are pregnant. For example, you may develop a heart murmur, which you didn't have before. If so, although heart murmurs are usually harmless, your doctor will want to determine the cause and make sure your heart valves are functioning properly. Some women may develop irregular heartbeats called arrhythmias during pregnancy. Most often, they cause no symptoms and are noticed while taking the pulse. Occasionally, they can cause symptoms such as palpitations, dizziness, or lightheadedness, and in such cases your doctor may want to perform an ECG or have you wear a heart monitor for twenty-four hours to better understand your rhythm. You probably won't need treatment, but if you do, your doctor will advise you about how it will affect you and your baby.

High Blood Pressure during Pregnancy

Different kinds of high blood pressure disorders can occur during pregnancy. A woman who already has high blood pressure may become pregnant (chronic hypertension), she can develop high blood pressure during pregnancy (gestational hypertension), she can have a short-term rise in blood pressure that starts in mid-pregnancy and goes away after birth (transient hypertension of pregnancy), or high blood pressure that is a sign of a more serious syndrome can occur, which requires immediate medical attention (preeclampsia).

If your blood pressure is dangerously high (higher than 160/100 mm Hg) your doctor might prescribe blood pressure medicines. It is less clear if drug treatment of mild high blood pressure during pregnancy is any better than no therapy at all. Preeclampsia can be associated with rapid weight gain, swollen ankles, and protein in the urine. It is a serious complication of pregnancy and often necessitates preterm delivery. Some studies have demonstrated an increased risk of heart disease in preeclampsia survivors, compared to women with a history of normotensive (those with normal blood pressure) pregnancy. Thus, the presence of preeclampsia affords a screening opportunity to detect women at risk for future heart disease and to institute lifestyle changes that may help to avoid such consequences.

Diabetes and Pregnancy

Women with type 1 or type 2 diabetes have an increased risk of pregnancy complications such as birth defects or death for the baby. The higher the mother's blood glucose is, the greater the risk of these complications. Fortunately, proper care can greatly reduce the risk of problems for the baby, so if you have diabetes and are planning to become pregnant, it is extremely important to discuss this with your doctor.

Sometimes a woman who never had diabetes before develops high blood sugar during pregnancy (gestational diabetes). This occurs in 2 percent to 9 percent of pregnancies and usually disappears once the baby is born. Gestational diabetes can be harmful to the baby, causing macrosomia (big baby), but it does not carry the same cardiovascular risks (e.g., early death, heart disease, and in stroke) to the mother as type 1 or type 2 diabetes does. However, women who have gestational diabetes are at increased risk for developing type 2 diabetes later in life. Nearly all pregnant women (except those at very low risk) should be tested for gestational diabetes during the 24th to 28th weeks of pregnancy.

Stroke during Pregnancy

There are stroke concerns that are unique to pregnancy. Overall, stroke risk appears to increase 2.5-fold during and after pregnancy; approximately 90 percent of pregnancy-related strokes happen during birth or in the first six weeks after the baby is born. Between 25 percent and 45 percent of pregnancy-related strokes occur in women with preeclampsia or eclampsia, making it the most common cause of pregnancy-related stroke. One study found that the risk of blocked-vessel (ischemic) stroke was not increased during pregnancy, but was 8.7 times higher than normal in the first six weeks after the baby was born, whereas the risk of a bleeding stroke (intracerebral hemorrhage) was two to three times higher than normal during pregnancy, and twenty-eight times higher in the six weeks following delivery. Fortunately, the overall risk of a pregnancy-related stroke is still quite low.

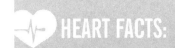 **HEART FACTS:**

Peripartum Cardiomyopathy

You are in your last trimester of pregnancy, and feel tired, breathless, and bloated. You have had four prior pregnancies. You give birth to twins and are discharged from the hospital. However, your symptoms worsen and you end up coming back. Your doctor orders an echocardiogram and the results are shocking: You have developed a mysterious form of heart failure called peripartum cardiomyopathy. This is a serious complication that often improves with six to nine months of treatment, but in up to one third of patients a weakened heart remains.

Doctors know little about the mechanisms behind this pregnancy-related heart failure, yet, peripartum cardiomyopathy complicates one in every 1,300 to 4,000 deliveries.

The risk of peripartum cardiomyopathy is greater in women older than age thirty who have had previous pregnancies, and in African American women. Risk factors also include obesity, a history of cardiac disorders such as myocarditis, smoking, alcoholism, and being malnourished.

Treatment includes the usual treatments for heart failure. Your heart might return to normal size within a few months, in which case the outlook is good. Some patients, however, get worse very quickly and may be candidates for a heart transplant.

If you have peripartum cardiomyopathy, you are at high risk of developing the same problem with future pregnancies and should discuss contraception with your doctor.

Q. & A. with Dr. Cannon

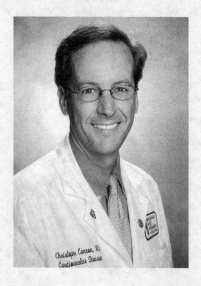

Q. If a woman comes to the hospital with chest pain at rest and blood tests don't show a heart attack, what testing should be done?

A. For patients with what we call unstable angina—chest pain coming at rest—the new American College of Cardiology/American Heart Association guidelines say that medical treatment and a stress test is the right approach. Some women will have a positive stress test and then will go on for a cardiac catheterization. But making all women undergo cardiac catheterization has recently been seen to be potentially harmful.

Q. If I have chest discomfort when I exercise a certain amount, should I get a stress test? If so, should it be a regular one, or one with nuclear imaging, or an echo?

A. Chest pressure (or pain or some type of discomfort) that comes on when you walk up a hill or go upstairs suggests pain coming from a blockage in the heart. It would be reasonable for your doctor to order a stress test. In general, a regular stress test (where only an ECG is done during the treadmill exercise) can be okay, but more women than men have false positive stress tests. Thus, many doctors will order additional imaging to see the heart better (either visualize the blood flow to your heart muscle via a nuclear stress test or see how well your heart muscle is moving by an echocardiogram).

Q. Should I get a 64-slice computed tomography scan to screen for a heart attack?

A. This is a big question in medicine today. Although very pretty pictures can be achieved from these scans, the test does involve a fair amount of radiation to see whether there are blockages in the heart arteries. Thus, these tests are not widely recommended for general screening but rather after some initial screening is done and your doctor wants to know whether there are blockages. (Of course, doing a stress test is another way to do that.) Another test—the calcium score—involves much lower radiation and can be a better initial screening test. It will say whether there is any sign of calcium in the arteries (which is a sign that cholesterol plaque buildup has started).

EPILOGUE:

INTO THE CRYSTAL BALL

ADVANCES IN UNDERSTANDING AND TREATING HEART DISEASE

Some of the most promising developments in understanding and treating heart disease surround the areas of stem cells, genetic tests, and devices to assist or replace a weak heart. Although our knowledge about stem cells and heart disease genes is relatively recent, research into the development of artificial hearts and ventricular assist devices (VADs) has been ongoing for decades. Those years of research are bearing fruit and bringing innovations within reach. In the next five to ten years, most of these experimental tests and treatments will become commonplace. This will allow us to detect at-risk individuals at very early stages and at the same time treat patients with advanced heart disease with greater success rates.

STEM CELLS IN TREATMENT OF HEART DISEASE

Normally, specialized cells in our body, such as nerve or muscle cells, do not readily divide and replenish themselves. Stem cells are unspecialized cells that have two unique properties that make them appealing:

- They can divide and renew themselves for long periods of time. Thus, when a stem cell divides, each new cell has the capacity to function as a stem cell.
- Given the right conditions, this cell can also be coaxed into becoming a more specialized cell, such as a beating heart cell, an insulin-producing pancreatic cell, or a conducting nerve cell.

Thus, we can potentially take a few stem cells, allow them to divide and create as many stem cells as required in the lab, and then induce them into becoming specialized cells (such as heart muscle cells) that can then be used to repair damaged organs (such as the heart).

The most unspecialized (and versatile) stem cells, called embryonal stem cells, are obtained from the embryo. Embryonal stem cells are pluripotent (i.e., they can potentially develop into any cell of the body) and are easy to multiply in the lab. A single parent stem cell can multiply several times to form a group of similar daughter stem cells, which share the same common origin and functions. This group would now be called a stem cell line, which is sort of an assembly line to produce individual stem cells. By growing stem cells with concoctions of growth factors, enzymes, and genes in the lab, it is possible to control their differentiation (specialization) into specific cell types. Basic "recipes" to produce specific cell types from these stem cells are known. However, using stem cells from embryos raises moral and ethical issues for many, as the embryo cannot mature further once these cells are harvested from it.

Adult stem cells are found in small numbers in various tissues of our body: the brain, bone marrow, blood, blood vessels, muscles, skin, and liver. Adult stem cells are somewhat more specialized, difficult to multiply under normal conditions, and can give rise only to the same cell types seen in their parent tissues. For example, brain stem cells will only form different types of brain cells, and blood stem cells will develop into various blood cells. But recently, scientists have found that some adult stem cells may be able to change and produce specialized cell types of other, completely different tissues (plasticity or transdifferentiation), again by using specific recipes. This has led to the possibility of using adult stem cells in the treatment of heart disease.

Hematopoetic stem cells are adult stem cells in the bone marrow that normally give rise to red blood cells, white blood cells, and platelets. They may be obtained directly from the bone marrow or in lesser numbers from the blood, usually from the patient (known as autologous stem cells). These are the most commonly studied stem cells for heart conditions.

Recently, stem cells have been found in umbilical cord blood and amniotic fluid (a fluid that surrounds the developing fetus in the womb).

Potential Uses for Heart Conditions

Heart muscle or valve cells cannot divide and hence cannot regenerate. For people with heart attacks, heart failure, or heart valve disease, stem cells may have significant uses in the future.

- In animals, when hematopoetic stem cells are transplanted into infarcted (dead) heart muscle after a heart attack or into dilated failing hearts, they survive, divide, and develop into heart muscle cells. They may be able to replace some of the dead tissue, repopulate the heart, and prevent further worsening of the pumping function of the heart. Similar effects can occur with other stem cells from the skeletal muscle, bone marrow, or the heart.

- In humans who have had a heart attack, initial studies using hematopoetic stem cells did suggest some benefit, but recent, better-designed studies have largely shown mixed results. Studies have shown that when these stem cells are injected (at the time of cardiac catheterization) into the blocked artery that caused the heart attack, they may have moderate beneficial effects in the short term, including reducing the extent of the heart muscle death (infarct size), accelerating the recovery of the pumping function (ejection fraction), and improving exercise capacity.

- In patients with heart failure due to a prior heart attack, studies have shown that directly injecting stem cells into the damaged heart muscle can improve the pumping function and enhance blood flow to the injured portion of the heart.

- Stem cells from bone marrow have been used to make "living" heart valve tissue in the laboratory. Stem cells are first induced to differentiate into heart valve cells in the lab, which are then placed on scaffolds made from the protein collagen so that a disc similar to a heart valve is obtained. These living valves may function much better than the current artificial replacements, and may eliminate the need for lifelong medication and periodic replacement. However, living valves are still in the initial phases of testing. How they perform in real-life conditions (in animal models) is yet to be studied. Human trials are still years away.

- Some studies have used muscle stem cells from the patient (autologous skeletal myoblasts). When directly injected into the areas of scar tissue, these cells have survived, multiplied, and integrated themselves into the heart muscle, increasing the heart's ejection fraction.

- Other studies are using stem cells that specifically enhance blood vessel formation. When injected into damaged heart muscle, these cells may potentially increase blood flow by giving rise to new blood vessels.

- Studies are also ongoing to see whether stem cells can be modified so that they would hone in on damaged heart tissue even when injected peripherally (in an arm or leg vessel) instead of directly (in and around the heart).

Reasons for Caution

Although several studies have shown varying amounts of benefit, a few others have failed to confirm these results. To justify stem cell use, the benefits have to be roughly predictable and worth the cost and risks involved.

We have not seen any significant impact on the two aspects that matter the most: prolonging life and reducing symptoms of heart disease. Thus, these findings are not consistent and may not be as relevant to patients as they are to researchers.

We are still not sure what types of stem cells work best and where or when and how they should be injected for maximal benefit. We still do not know the exact mechanism of benefit—some studies suggest that instead of differentiating into functioning heart tissue, stem cells may act by releasing signaling chemicals that may prevent existing heart cells from dying; they may cause blood vessel formation and greater blood flow; or they may activate existing cells in the heart to divide and form heart muscle. We also do not know whether stem cells are safe in the long run. To answer these questions, further research—in the lab, on animal models, and then in humans—is needed before we can use this investigational technique.

GENETIC TESTING FOR HEART DISEASE

It is well known that heart disease sometimes clusters in families. Having a parent or relative affected by heart disease increases the risk of developing this condition, especially if multiple relatives are affected and at younger ages.

Comparing Markers

A gene is the basic unit of heredity. It is, in effect, a stretch of our DNA (deoxyribonucleic acid) that has coded instructions to help us make certain proteins which perform essential functions in our body. Only small portions of our DNA function as genes (functional genetic code), interspersed with large stretches of inactive, nonfunctional genetic code.

The human genome is the full compilation of our genes; it forms the blueprint of our body. All genes are inherited in pairs, one from each parent, and therefore can carry certain traits which affect our heart disease risk. All genetic code is made of a specific sequence of subunits called nucleotides. Sometimes there are variations (called polymorphisms) in these sequences, which may give rise to different versions of functioning (genes) or nonfunctioning genetic code.

When two sequences of nucleotides differ from each other due to a change in just a single nucleotide, it is called a single nucleotide polymorphism (SNP). As most of our DNA consists of nonfunctional stretches of genetic code and only small portions function as genes, SNPs are mostly located between or near genes, rather than within them. However, SNPs tend be linked to their nearby genes, and are usually inherited together with these genes from one generation to the next. This allows us to use these SNPs as markers for nearby disease-causing genes. Every individual has a unique pattern of SNPs, based on the genes present in his or her genome.

In genome-wide association studies (GWASs), scientists analyze SNP patterns in the entire genome of a large number of people, and then compare the patterns of those who have heart disease to those who do not. In this way, they can detect differences between the SNP patterns of the two groups and determine a likely association between a specific SNP pattern and a risk-altering gene. The ultimate hope is that we would be able to predict whether an individual is at a greater or lesser risk of heart disease just by looking at his or her SNP pattern. Genetically high-risk persons could then be intensively followed and all their modifiable risk factors could be aggressively treated.

GWAS Studies Report Varied Results

A study in the British population compared the genome-wide SNPs of 2,000 CHD patients with 3,000 disease-free individuals. The study found one region (or locus) of DNA that was strongly associated with heart disease, and six that were moderately associated. More detailed analysis identified a total of nine loci that were thought to directly influence the development of heart disease. Subsequently, researchers used a German population to try to confirm whether the regions altered the risk of having a heart attack. They found three regions of DNA that increased heart disease risk in both populations. Interestingly, in both populations, the same locus (called chromosome 9p21) was most strongly associated with development of heart disease. By combining data from the British and German populations, researchers were also able to identify four additional loci that increased the risk of heart disease. Some of these regions increased the risk of heart disease by 20 to 40 percent. Also, around one-quarter to one-half of individuals of European descent (Caucasians) carried these loci in their DNA.

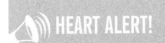

HEART ALERT!

Benefits of Genetic Testing

Coronary heart disease (CHD), diabetes, and hypertension have a multifactorial inheritance whereby many different genes affect the risk of developing heart disease by varying (usually small) amounts. By contrast, some diseases of the heart are monogenic, in which a single defective gene is sufficient to cause the disease.

In familial hypercholesterolemia, the body is unable to remove low-density lipoprotein (LDL) cholesterol from the bloodstream due to a gene defect. The LDL accumulates in the blood and high levels of LDL lead to development of atherosclerosis and heart attacks at a young age.

In familial hypertrophic cardiomyopathy, a portion of the heart muscle thickens without any obvious cause. In addition, the normal microscopic alignment of muscle cells is lost. This condition is one of the major causes of sudden cardiac death, especially in younger people.

Both diseases affect one in 500 people, and they are examples where genetic testing can be extremely beneficial. Using newly developed rapid screening tests to detect the variant genes, we can now easily identify patients with these conditions. Furthermore, screening can also be offered to apparently healthy relatives and family members who might develop symptoms from these conditions at a later date so that appropriate follow-up and treatment measures can be initiated.

Other genome-wide association studies have had interesting results:

- In a study examining DNA from 23,000 people, Canadian and U.S. researchers found that variation in a region on chromosome 9p21 increased the risk of having heart disease. They found that about one in four Caucasians carried two copies of this variant stretch of DNA and had a 30 percent to 40 percent higher risk of CHD. Half the people had one copy, and they had a 15 percent to 20 percent higher risk of heart disease. Of people getting early-onset heart disease (earlier than age fifty in men and age sixty in women), one-third carried this variant. African Americans did not carry this region of DNA.

- A separate group of researchers tested DNA from 17,000 people. They found that 21 percent of them had two copies of this variant DNA stretch on chromosome 9p21, and it gave them a 64 percent higher risk of having a heart attack. It also more than doubled the risk of having an early-onset heart attack. Of note, this stretch on 9p21 was found near two other regions that researchers had previously identified to be associated with type 2 diabetes. Although these subjects had heart disease, none of them had diabetes.

In all of these studies, marker SNPs were analyzed using gene chips or DNA microarrays for each participating individual. These gene chips can scan a person's entire genome for certain programmed SNPs. Some of these are now commercially available for use. However, several important issues need to be sorted out before we can use these gene chips in a safe and effective manner.

Treat Data with Caution

One recent study involving around 1,500 patients failed to find any significant association between eighty-five different genetic variants and heart disease. Although the variants tested came from older and smaller studies, some of them were incorporated into commercially available testing panels that are still available. This tells us that we must treat the recent data with caution until further confirmation from different research teams is available. All of these recent studies were in Caucasian populations, and the results might not hold for people of African American, Asian, and other ethnicities. Also, right now, we only know which regions of DNA increase the risk for heart disease. As SNPs are just markers for nearby genes, we are not certain which genes are actually responsible and how they affect our heart disease risk.

Association of some portions of DNA with increased heart disease risk does not implicate them as a cause of heart disease. CHD is multifactorial—there are several different commonly found genetic variations, which individually increase the risk of heart disease by only small amounts. However, when they are present together in greater numbers, their effect becomes significant. Any one variation in itself is not sufficient to cause disease. It is likely that certain individuals might have some genetic variations. But in absence of a large number of variations, their risk might not be affected to a great degree.

Other risk factors such as high cholesterol, high blood pressure, and smoking are far more important for reducing heart disease risk. Even in persons with all the "bad genes," heart disease might not occur if they control these other risk factors, which provide the all-important trigger for onset of disease. In the long term, we might see a component of genetic testing being incorporated into traditional risk assessment methods such as the Framingham risk score (see chapter 9). For that, we need more research to find out whether genetic tests can do a better job of predicting risk than these currently known risk factors.

We also need to know more about gene-gene interactions (Do the effects of all these variants simply add up, or is their effect on each other more complex?) and gene-environment interactions (Is having one gene on top of one risk factor worse than another gene-risk factor combination?)

Other issues that will come up include psychological and social issues (How will the knowledge that you are likely to develop heart disease affect your life? How will your friends and family deal with this information?), as well as the potential for misuse of this information by insurers and employers. To guard against the latter possibility, the Genetic Information Nondiscrimination Act was signed into law in 2008, making it illegal for health insurers and employers to discriminate against persons based on their genetic information.

DEVICES TO SUPPORT THE FAILING HEART

Ventricular Assist Device (VAD)

A VAD is a mechanical pump that works in concert with a weak, failing heart and helps it deliver blood to the rest of the body. VADs are typically used in patients with advanced heart failure in the following conditions:

- As a "bridge to transplant:" Although candidates for heart transplant are waiting for donor hearts to become available, they might experience a worsening of their condition due to their weak hearts. These devices can be used to support these patients until they undergo a heart transplant.

- As "destination therapy:" Some patients with chronic heart failure are not transplant candidates due to their advanced age or if they have other chronic conditions such as liver, kidney, or lung disease. In these patients, the devices are used on a permanent basis to extend life.

Sometimes VADs can also be used for temporary support in conditions that cause sudden weakness of the heart, such as after major heart surgery, after a massive heart attack, after severe myocarditis (inflammation of the middle layer of the heart wall), or when a transplanted heart is rejected by the recipient's immune system.

All VADs have a pump that helps move blood through the body, a controller (a computer that monitors device function and can adjust it according to the patient's circulatory demands), and a power source. Usually the power source and the controller stay outside the body, whereas the pump can be inside (implantable) or outside (external to) the body. An inflow tube carries blood from the ventricle to the pump through an inflow valve, while an outflow tube carries blood from the pump to a major artery through an outflow valve. There are three types of VADs:

- In a left VAD (LVAD), the pump is connected to the left ventricle and the aorta.
- In a right VAD (RVAD), the pump is between the right ventricle and the pulmonary artery.
- A biventricular VAD (BiVAD) combines both of the preceding functions.

Thoratec VAD

The Thoratec VAD is one of the most commonly used VADs. The pump is in the form of a flexible plastic sac that is compressed using air from an external console. The console has a built-in compressor that delivers pressure and vacuum to the pump in a pulse-like manner. This, in turn, leads to periodic emptying and refilling of the pumping sac. Because the pump is external, patients have limited mobility with this device and cannot be discharged from the hospital. It is used as a bridge to transplant and to temporarily support the heart after open-heart surgery. It is not intended for use as destination therapy on a permanent basis.

The Thoracic VAD is a very versatile device that can be used as an LVAD, RVAD, or BiVAD. Complications include bleeding, infection, and thromboembolism (where clots form in the device, break loose, and travel to other organs, causing complications such as strokes). Patients with these devices need to be on heparin, an anticoagulant drug that prevents clot formation. An implantable version of the Thoratec VAD has been approved by the U.S. Food and Drug Administration (FDA), which allows patients to return home while on the device.

Novacor LVAD

In the Novacor LVAD, the pump is implanted within the abdominal wall. It is about the size of a human heart and uses an electromagnet to compress a pouch that pumps the blood. The controller and the battery packs that keep the device working can be worn on a belt or carried in a shoulder bag, vest, or back pack or can be placed by a small bedside monitor (when the person is sleeping). The controller is connected to the pump by a percutaneous lead— a small tube that brings control and power wires through a tiny opening in the skin. This device is currently approved as a bridge to transplant and allows patients to have near-normal mobility due to its portability. It is currently undergoing clinical trials for use as destination therapy.

A newer version of the Novacor LVAD, which can also be used as an RVAD, is in animal trials. It claims to be smaller, simpler, quieter, more durable, and more easily implantable than the current form. Complications are similar to the Thoratec VAD and anticoagulation medicine in necessary.

HeartMate LVAD

The widely used HeartMate LVAD is available in two versions, depending on the pumping device: implantable pneumatic (IP) and vented electric (XVE). Both versions are FDA-approved as a bridge to transplant. The XVE version was recently also approved for destination therapy. The IP version has an air chamber that receives air from the controller to help drive blood flow, and the XVE version has an electric motor to pump the blood. Both versions of this device have a separate blood chamber with a unique textured surface, depending upon which cellular lining develops on the pump over time. This lining prevents blood clot formation, so no anticoagulation medication is required and thromboembolic risk is reduced. Although patients on the IP version can have some mobility within the hospital, the XVE version allows discharge from the hospital and a more normal lifestyle. Heart failure symptoms, exercise capacity, and measurements of cardiac performance all improve with this device. Interestingly, when patients receive the XVE device as a bridge to transplant as opposed to just the usual medications, they have improved results after the transplant. As a destination therapy, compared to medications alone, survival rates were doubled at the end of one year and almost tripled by two years, but rates were still

Pulsatile Flow versus Continuous Flow VADs

Pulsatile flow VADs mimic the natural pumping action of the heart and generate pulses of blood flow. However, these devices carry a higher risk of infection and device failure and have a large pump size. The pulsatile action also causes damage to the blood cells that pass through the pump (traumatic hemolysis) and patients may require blood transfusion as a result.

The newer continuous flow devices generate a continuous stream of blood flow instead of intermittent pulses. They are smaller, which makes their use possible in women, children, and men with small body sizes. As less space needs to be created in the body to house them, the implantation procedure is a lot simpler and bleeding and infection rates are reduced. They have simpler designs and fewer moving parts, which makes them quieter and may improve long-term durability and reliability.

lower compared to heart transplant in all except the lowest-risk patients.

HeartMate II

The HeartMate II is the first continuous flow device to be approved by the FDA as a bridge to transplant. The pump does not have a sac, bladder, or separate chamber for blood. Instead, it has a rotor assembly that is moved by a motor. This rotor helps propel blood through the circulation. Because it is made of clot-resistant material, only low-dose anticoagulation medication is required. Besides a base unit, it has a portable battery pack that can be worn around the waist and can support the pump for three hours. In one trial, three out of four people who received this device survived for at least six months, and two out of three were alive at the end of one year. Functional status, exercise capacity, and quality of life were also improved. Eventually, continuous flow devices such as the HeartMate II might be more suitable for long-term use as destination therapy.

Jarvik 2000 Pump

The Jarvik 2000 pump is the smallest and simplest of the VADs. It is a compact, continuous flow device about the size and shape of a C battery and roughly one-tenth the size of the HeartMate. Unlike prior devices, the Jarvik 2000 is placed directly into the left ventricle and does not have any valves or inflow grafts. It has only one moving part: an electrically powered rotor or impeller that maintains blood flow. Because this device is practically surrounded by the heart, the risk of infection is reduced. The lack of valves or inflow grafts, along with other design factors, also reduces the risk of clotting and hemolysis (the breakdown of red blood cells).

Unlike other VADs, the Jarvik 2000 is manually controlled by the patient. Using a five-speed controller, the patient can increase pump speed to increase blood flow during exercise or slow it down during sleep. An external battery pack is worn in a waist belt or a shoulder bag and is connected to the pump through a cable that enters through the abdomen (for bridge to transplant) or through the base of the skull (for destination therapy). It can support the device for eight to ten hours.

This VAD has been shown to improve heart performance and quality of life. However, it is approved by the FDA only as an experimental device and at present can be used only as part of a clinical trial.

Total Artificial Heart

A total artificial heart (TAH) differs from a VAD as it completely takes over the function of the natural heart instead of just assisting it. It is inserted in the location of the natural heart and therefore requires removal of the patient's own ventricles.

CardioWest TAH

The CardioWest TAH was previously known as the Jarvik-7 TAH. It is consists of two pumps which are attached to the atria, replacing each ventricle. Air pressure is used to drive a disc-shaped mechanism that pumps the blood in a pulselike manner. A large controller pumps in compressed air through drive lines into the device. This controller in turn needs to be connected to sources of electricity, vacuum and compressed air, although backup batteries and air tanks are present. A portable controller is also available (but not FDA-approved) that allows stable patients to be discharged and have more mobility. The CardioWest TAH is currently used only as a temporary bridge to transplant and not as a permanent replacement for heart transplant.

In a recent study among transplant-eligible patients with biventricular failure, almost eight out of ten people on this device survived until they received their heart transplant, and the device more than doubled overall survival at the end of one year. Complications include bleeding, infection, strokes, and dysfunction of the kidney, liver, and lungs.

Abiomed TAH

The Abiomed TAH is the world's first completely self-contained replacement heart. There is no external controller and no wires or tubes going through the skin. It has an internal pumping unit weighing around two pounds, with two artificial ventricles with corresponding valves. Instead of using air or mechanical energy, the Abiomed TAH uses a motorized hydraulic system to pump the blood. It has an internal emergency battery that can last for thirty minutes. For routine use, there is an external portable battery that powers the device and charges the internal battery using a transcutaneous system; power gets transmitted across the skin without wires when an external coil is placed over an implanted internal coil. An internal electronics system is implanted in the abdomen, which monitors and adjusts the device's function.

This device is currently undergoing clinical trials in end-stage biventricular heart failure patients who are not eligible for any other treatment options, including heart transplant. The Abiomed TAH may be approved by the FDA for wider use after results from initial trials confirm its benefits.

Q. & A. with Dr. Cannon

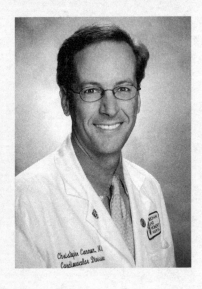

Q. If I am in a clinical trial of a new treatment, is there a danger of having DNA testing as part of the study?

A. No. Genetic testing done in the setting of a study has very strict privacy restrictions; your sample cannot be traced to you personally. It becomes coded as a number in the database, in which your personal information is not kept. Thus, if you participate in the study to help advance medicine, you can rest assured it won't hurt you and may help advance science.

Q. If I had genetic testing and was found to have a genetic marker associated with developing heart disease, what should I do?

A. Generally, treatment algorithms specific to patients with certain genetic defects have not been developed. If, however, you were seen to have a marker associated with higher risk of a heart attack, you should aim to do a better job in following all the standard recommendations (i.e., lowering cholesterol, exercising, eating right, etc.).

Q. Who should get evaluated with new devices?

A. New devices are usually tested in patients who don't have good alternatives. For example, the trials of the new aortic valves that are placed by catheters through the groin are being tested in trials where surgery is not an option.

Of note, new devices and drugs are tested in clinical trials with very specific eligibility criteria, where the researchers have tried to balance potential benefit with safety for the patients in the trial. This is also then reviewed by the FDA, as well as each hospital's Institutional Review Board (IRB), to again focus on safety for patients enrolled in the trial. Thus, the doctors will check that you are a candidate based on the study protocol and only then approach you for participation in the trial.

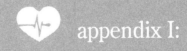 appendix I:

HOW TO SAVE A LIFE

KNOWLEDGE AND SPEED SAVE LIVES

Sudden cardiac arrest kills more than 250,000 people annually. The key to saving these lives is to know what to do when you find someone who is unresponsive. Responding quickly by calling for help and administering cardiopulmonary resuscitation (CPR) can save someone's life.

Cardiac arrest is not a single medical condition; it is the end result of a number of problems. Sometimes the cause will be obvious, such as in the case of a witnessed drowning. Or perhaps prior to collapse, the patient was having chest pain that he or she recognized as a heart attack. Whatever the cause, the effect of these conditions is that blood flow to the body is compromised. CPR is a series of techniques for supporting blood flow and oxygen delivery to the body to keep the victim alive.

BASIC PRINCIPLES OF ADULT CPR

Performing CPR is a learned skill. Many community organizations sponsor hands-on training in CPR, and we recommend you find a course near you for formal training. The American Heart Association (AHA; www.americanheart.org) and the American Red Cross (www.redcross.org) are good sources of information for finding a CPR training course in your area.

Good CPR involves many details, so it is useful to start with basic principles you can easily remember. We outline the basic steps to CPR in the section "Basic Life Support: The Steps to CPR" later in this chapter. As you arrive at the scene of an unresponsive victim, focus on the following three things.

Getting Help

Whether you witness a person collapse or arrive at the scene afterward, the first thing to do is to call 9-1-1 and enlist the help of bystanders at the scene. Even if you're not sure what happened, you should always call for help first and ask questions later.

Common mistake: Many responders are reluctant to leave the victim to call for help. Remember that the basic life support measures outlined in this appendix are intended to sustain life until professional health care providers arrive. CPR alone will not be sufficient—victims of cardiac arrest need to get to a hospital. Calling for help is the most important thing you can do and therefore should be the very first thing you do.

Using Automatic External Defibrillators (AEDs) to Save Lives

After calling for help, your next thoughts should turn to finding an AED. An AED is a device that shocks the heart back to a normal rhythm, which helps to restore the normal pumping of blood to the body. AEDs are becoming more commonplace in public settings, including airports, sporting events, and schools. If you are alone at the scene and know where you can quickly find an AED, you should retrieve it before performing CPR. Ideally, you should ask a bystander to call for help and retrieve the AED while you attend to the victim. Research has demonstrated that lifesaving efforts are most effective when a shock is delivered within five minutes of the cardiac arrest!

Common mistake: Sometimes people fail to think of the AED early. Most people know that chest compressions and rescue breaths are important parts of resuscitating an unresponsive victim, but people are much less familiar with AEDs. Remember: Early defibrillation is essential.

Providing Effective Chest Compressions

Providing effective chest compressions with minimal interruptions is the most important part of CPR for most victims.

Common mistake: Research has demonstrated that rescuers interrupt chest compressions too frequently. There are many reasons for this—the scene of a cardiac arrest can become very hectic with multiple distractions; transitions between chest compressions and rescue breaths (discussed on page 294) can be difficult to coordinate; and chest compressions are very tiring. Remember this: Some countries have begun recommending chest-compression-only CPR. Even the latest statement from the AHA says that chest-compression-only resuscitation is an acceptable alternative to standard (chest compressions + rescue breathing) CPR. If you can't remember the correct ratio between the number of chest compressions and rescue breaths, just remember that every second without chest compressions is a second without blood flow to the victim's brain.

BASIC LIFE SUPPORT: THE STEPS TO CPR

1. Survey the scene, assess for responsiveness, and get help—call 9-1-1, and retrieve AED if available.
2. Position the victim and assess for normal breathing.
3. Provide two rescue breaths.
4. Begin chest compressions with a 30:2 ratio of chest compressions to rescue breaths.
5. Use the AED as soon as possible.
6. Continue until help arrives.

Arrive at the Scene

Make sure the scene is safe. Putting yourself in harm's way is not recommended. Phone for a professional to help you.

Assess whether the victim is responsive. Ask "Are you okay?" and tap the victim on the shoulder to see whether he or she is able to talk to you. If the person can talk or make purposeful movements, the person's heart and lungs are working and he or she does not need CPR at that moment.

Get help. If you're the lone rescuer, remember that your first job is to call for help. If another person is with you to help, have that person call 9-1-1 while you attend to the victim. The emergency dispatchers will send trained emergency medical technicians to the scene. Also, the dispatchers will stay with you on the telephone to provide CPR instructions.

Position the Victim and Assess for Normal Breathing

For CPR, the victim should be lying on his or her back on a hard surface. Open the airway by tilting the head back and pulling the chin forward. This maneuver is essential to allowing airflow in and out of the chest.

Next, "look, listen, and feel" for signs of life. The recommendation is to spend no more than ten seconds determining whether the victim has normal breathing. Sometimes the victim might be making gasping movements—this should not be considered normal breathing.

Common mistake: Poor positioning of the victim can make it difficult to properly assess breathing, and also can make CPR ineffective. Even if a decision is made to not provide rescue breaths (discussed on page 294), opening the victim's airway with the head tilt is essential. Chest compressions create pressure changes in the chest cavity that move air in and out of the lungs—but only if the airway has been opened properly!

Provide Two Rescue Breaths

After appropriately positioning the head, tightly pinch the victim's nose. Establish a tight seal with your lips when providing mouth-to-mouth resuscitation. Take a normal breath prior to providing a rescue breath. The rescue breath need not be forceful—just provide enough air over one second to raise the chest wall of the victim. After the first two rescue breaths, begin chest compressions immediately.

You should provide two rescue breaths for every thirty chest compressions. If there are two rescuers, one should stay positioned near the victim's head to provide rescue breaths, and the other should stay near the chest to provide chest compressions.

Guide to Rescue Breathing

1. Perform the head tilt to open the airway and pinch the victim's nose.
2. Take in a normal breath.
3. Establish an airtight seal between the victim's mouth and yours.
4. Exhale over one second to provide a rescue breath. The victim's chest wall should rise.

Note: Mouth-to-mouth resuscitation is a safe technique for providing CPR. Nonetheless, many people, including some health care providers, are uncomfortable providing rescue breaths. If this is the case, there are two options. First, commercially available barrier devices help limit contact between the victim and the rescuer. If a barrier device is not available, the lay rescuer should provide CPR with chest compressions only.

Common mistake: Rescuers take too much time giving rescue breaths. Without blood pumping into the lungs to pick up the oxygen and carry it to the body, rescue breaths will not be effective. Studies have shown that the time spent providing rescue breaths is usually much longer than what is recommended. Give the breaths and begin providing chest compressions quickly. Again, every second without chest compressions is a second without blood flow to the brain.

Fully Release the Compressions

Compressing the chest wall around the heart increases pressure within the chest cavity, pumping a small amount of blood to the vital organs, including the brain. With full release of the chest compression, negative pressure is created in the chest, drawing venous blood into the heart and air into the lungs. Therefore, compression and full release of pressure are necessary for effective resuscitation.

First, position yourself kneeling next to the victim's chest. Find the sternum, the bone in the front of the chest between the nipples. Use the heel of one hand as the contact point with the mid-sternum, between the nipples. Place the heel of your other hand on top of the first hand for support.

Guide to Chest Compressions

- Chest compressions should be hard and fast.
- Provide 100 compressions per minute.
- Compress the chest 1.5 to 2 inches (3.8 to 5.1 cm).
- Fully release between compressions.
- The ratio of chest compression to rescue breaths is 30:2. In other words, perform 2 rescue breaths for every 30 chest compressions.
- Minimize time without chest compressions.
- Get others to take turns providing compressions.

Common mistakes:

- Proper chest compressions can be difficult to administer, even for trained health care providers. Almost one-half of chest compressions by lay rescuers do not compress the chest wall far enough. Compressing the chest is hard work! Consequently, rescuers quickly tire and the rate and depth of compressions suffer. Again, the most important aspect of CPR is to get help! In the hospital, physicians provide chest compressions in a rotation of two to three minutes. In many communities, EMS response times can be up to eight to ten minutes. If help is there, use it!

- Rescuers often focus too much on compressing without remembering to fully release between compressions. Allowing the chest wall to recoil to a resting position is essential for blood to fill the heart between compressions. It is not necessary to take your hands off the victim's chest, but do ensure that full chest-wall recoil was allowed.

- Too much time is spent transitioning between chest compressions and rescue breaths. If more than one rescuer is available, one person should provide rescue breaths while the second provides chest compressions. There should be no delay between providing chest compressions and rescue breaths.

USE THE AED AS SOON AS POSSIBLE

As discussed in the introduction to this appendix, cardiac arrest is not a single medical condition but rather the end result of a number of different problems. Most cardiac arrests that occur in the community setting are associated with ventricular fibrillation or related disorders.

Ventricular fibrillation is the medical term for disorganized electrical activity of the heart. The heart is an electrical organ, and organization of the electrical activity is necessary so that all the heart muscle cells beat in concert, creating a pumping action. When the electrical activity is disorganized, the heart cannot pump blood.

The treatment of ventricular fibrillation and related heart rhythm disorders is to provide a shock to the heart. This helps to reset the electrical system of the heart, much like unplugging a computer. The shock stops all electrical circuits, allowing the normal heart circuits to begin anew.

AEDs are user-friendly devices that can analyze the heart rhythm and tell you whether a shock would be appropriate as treatment. For some causes of cardiac arrest, electrical shocks can make the problem worse, which is why it is not recommended to shock every victim. AEDs are becoming common in public places and are marked with the AED symbol of a heart with a lightning bolt through it.

Remember:

- Early use of the AED is lifesaving! It is estimated that for every minute that passes until defibrillation, survival is reduced by almost 10 percent.

- Continue chest compressions while the AED is being set up. Again, every second without chest compressions is a second without blood flow to the brain.

HOW TO USE AN AED

Follow the instructions on the AED. Some AEDs use voice prompts to direct the rescuer.

Place the Defibrillation Pads on the Chest

Remove all clothing, medication patches, and so forth from the skin prior to placing the defibrillation pads. Also, make sure the victim is not lying in water and that the skin is dry prior to pad placement. Good contact with the skin is essential. One pad is placed to the right of the sternum, and the other is placed just lateral to the nipple on the left side of the victim's chest. The exact positioning is usually displayed in picture form on the pads or the AED itself. The pads form the electrical contacts with the body. The electrical current will flow between the pads, crossing through the heart.

Common mistake: Unless absolutely necessary, do not stop CPR as the pads are being applied. There is no electrical danger at this point.

Stand Clear

Say "clear" to make sure no one is touching the victim. Stop chest compressions just before you are ready to start the next step, rhythm analysis.

Analyze the Rhythm

Some AEDs will do this automatically, and others might ask you to touch the "analyze" button. During this time, the AED determines whether the heart rhythm is appropriate to shock.

Deliver the Shock

If appropriate, the AED will prompt you to deliver a shock. Double-check that everyone is "clear." After the shock is delivered, resume chest compressions and rescue breaths for two minutes before reanalyzing the rhythm. The victim might require multiple shocks.

Approach the Choking Victim

Abdominal thrusts, also known at the Heimlich maneuver, are a proven method for removing airway blockages in a choking victim. This procedure can be done only on a conscious person older than one year of age. If a choking victim is unconscious, CPR (including rescue breathing) is the appropriate resuscitation technique. As with all lifesaving procedures, it is always important to call for help!

Wheezing, coughing, and weak voice are all signs of choking. If a victim is unable to talk or cough, this is much more concerning. Act fast! Early intervention with abdominal thrusts can save a life. The purpose of the abdominal thrusts is to increase the pressure in the abdomen (belly). This increased pressure is transmitted to the chest, creating a strong cough that can expel the object blocking the airway.

Guide to Abdominal Thrusts

1. Position yourself behind the victim.
2. Wrap your arms around the victim's waist.
3. Position your hands just above the victim's belly button, below the ribs.
4. Clench one fist and place your other hand over the clenched fist.
5. Squeeze your hands into the victim's belly quickly. Repeat until the object is expelled or the victim collapses. If the victim collapses, begin CPR, including rescue breathing.

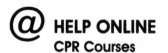

@ HELP ONLINE
CPR Courses

www.americanheart.org

www.redcross.org

CPR for Children

How does CPR differ when the victim is a child (age one to eight)?

Children are more likely to choke, drown, or have suffered an injury as the cause of cardiac arrest and less likely to suffer from deadly heart rhythm disturbances than are adults. As a result, clearing the airway of any obstructions and delivering rescue breaths are most critical in the resuscitation effort, even more important than early defibrillation in most cases.

Performing CPR on children is very similar to performing CPR on adults. As with adults, if you have help at the scene, send one person to call 9-1-1 and retrieve an AED while you assess for breathing and begin CPR. If you're the lone rescuer, assess for breathing, deliver two rescue breaths, and begin CPR before leaving the victim to call 9-1-1 and retrieve an AED. This is the main difference between CPR for adults and CPR for children.

It is recommended that you complete five cycles of CPR before leaving the victim to activate the EMS and retrieve an AED. For children, rather than compressing the chest 1.5 to 2 inches (3.8 to 5.1 cm), the guidelines say to compress the chest wall one-third to one-half the chest diameter to ensure effective compression. Position your hands as you would for an adult; however, if you do not require two hands for effective compressions, use one hand only. For rescue breaths, give enough air to make sure the chest wall rises. The ratio of chest compressions to rescue breaths is the same as with adults, as is the most important thing: Get help!

How does CPR differ when the victim is an infant (less than one year old)?

Infants are treated in a similar manner to children, with a few differences. Chest compressions need to be performed differently because of their small size. It is recommended that you use two fingers to compress the chest in the midline, below the nipples. As with children, ensure that the chest cavity is compressed one-third to one-half the diameter for adequate compressions. Rescue breathing can be difficult in infants as well. The important thing is to make sure the air seal is tight and that the chest wall rises. This might involve covering the infant's mouth and nose with your mouth or performing mouth-to-nose or mouth-to-mouth rescue breaths. The ratio of chest compressions to rescue breaths is the same as for adults. Finally, there is little evidence regarding the use of AEDs for infants, and therefore the guidelines make no recommendations for or against the use of AEDs for infants.

Check with Your Child's Doctor

Formal training in basic life support techniques for victims of all ages is always a good idea. If you have a child who has a medical condition that makes him or her predisposed to sudden death, be sure to ask your doctor about specific lifesaving techniques for your child. Some medical conditions require special instructions for rescuers.

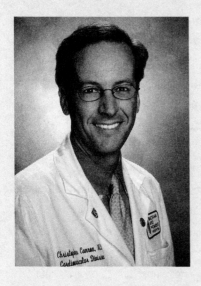

Q. My husband just had a heart attack. Should I try to learn CPR?

A. Yes. This is a good idea. Your husband hopefully will be well stabilized following the heart attack, but he will be at higher risk of having another heart attack or a life-threatening arrhythmia, so the CPR could be critical. There are lots of CPR courses; you can find them at the Red Cross, your local YMCA, or your local hospital.

Q. I have seen the AEDs at the airport. Do they work if a nonmedical person tries to use them?

A. Yes. They are designed to be used by anyone. The directions are simple, and the box usually also gives audible instructions on what to do, step by step. The key is time; the faster a patient in cardiac arrest is defibrillated, the greater his or her chance of survival—and this is measured in minutes. If the defibrillation is done in the first two or three minutes, the chance of survival is reasonable, but after ten minutes, chances are as low as 1 percent. So, if you have the chance to use one, go for it!

Q. If I see someone who collapsed and I try CPR, could I be sued if it doesn't work?

A. No. Essentially, all states have the Good Samaritan law, where if you are trying to help, you are not liable. A first step in this case would be to call 9-1-1, but if you can, also try to do CPR.

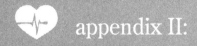 appendix II:

A REFERENCE OF TESTS TO DIAGNOSE HEART DISEASE

NEW TESTS CONFIRM HEART DISEASE

As technology advances, newer tests are being developed to improve a physician's ability to diagnose heart disease in a safe and efficient manner. As in other specialties of medicine, tests and procedures are becoming more commonplace in cardiology. Cardiac tests confirm the clinical diagnosis, aid in prognosis and clinical management decisions, and occasionally provide a therapeutic intervention. However, no test has replaced a thorough history and physical exam, which remain the first steps in making the diagnosis of heart disease.

Deciding which cardiac test is necessary for an individual patient can be difficult, and practice varies among experienced physicians. The newest tests might offer advantages over older tests, but less high-tech tests can often provide the same or even more useful information. In addition, tests that are considered the "gold standard," or the best tests available, are not always appropriate for every patient. For example, coronary angiography (a cath) is the gold-standard test for the diagnosis of coronary artery disease (CAD). However, for patients with stable CAD, sometimes the physician will decide to manage symptoms with medications, and not perform an invasive procedure such as a cardiac cath. The bottom line is that every patient is different, and decisions about the use of cardiac testing are made on a patient-by-patient basis.

ELECTROCARDIOGRAM (ECG or EKG)

The ECG documents the electrical activity of the heart. The heart is an electrical organ; signals are generated at the "pacemaker" part of the heart—the sinus node—which normally sets the heart rate. The electrical activity then travels through a specialized conducting system to the heart muscle cells.

When the muscle cells receive the electrical signal salt channels on the cell surface change, allowing calcium to rush into the cells. The calcium causes muscle cells to contract, and the organized contraction of the many muscle cells results in a heartbeat. After contraction, the muscle cells have to actively restore the levels of various salts to the resting concentration so that the cells will be ready to respond to the next electrical signal. The ECG monitors all of these processes by measuring electrical activity over different regions of the chest wall.

The ECG is most often used for diagnosis of a heart attack. When a heart attack has damaged an area of the heart, that area will have difficulty regulating the concentration of salts with every beat. That impairment is seen on the ECG as ST-segment changes. (This is where we get the terms ST-segment elevation myocardial infarction and non-ST-segment elevation myocardial infarction, which describe the two types of heart attacks, discussed in chapter 2.) The multiple ECG electrodes monitor the different regions of the heart, allowing the doctor to locate the damaged regions. Because the different branches of the coronary (heart) arteries supply different regions of the heart, the ECG can be used to predict which artery branches might be blocked during a heart attack.

ECGs Also Detect Previous Heart Attacks

Almost one in three heart attacks go unnoticed by the patient, so it is not uncommon for a doctor to diagnose previous heart attacks by the ECG in patients who have no recollection of past heart troubles. After a heart attack, the damaged muscle cells become scar tissue which is no longer electrically active. These areas are identified on the ECG as Q waves, the ECG sign of electrical activity moving away from scar tissue. In years past, heart attacks were described as Q-wave or non-Q-wave myocardial infarctions. This distinction is still meaningful, but has lost common use in current medical practice.

Heart Rhythm Disturbances and Other Conditions

The second most common use of the ECG is to diagnose heart rhythm disturbances. As mentioned earlier, the sinus node is the generator for the electrical circuits in the heart under normal circumstances. The electrical activity is usually very organized, activating the muscle cells in the atria first and then the muscle cells in the ventricle. Sometimes, however, areas other than the sinus node begin initiating the electrical activity (the medical term for this is enhanced automaticity). For instance, abnormal loops of electricity can form around scar tissue in the heart or in pathologically enlarged heart chambers. These heart arrhythmias are for the most part easily diagnosed via the ECG.

Although the diagnosis of heart attacks and rhythm disturbances is the most common purpose of the ECG, almost all forms of heart disease result in characteristic changes on the ECG. Therefore, the ECG can direct physicians toward a number of common and uncommon heart conditions and is a central diagnostic tool.

For example, if the heart muscle is thickened because it has had to pump against high blood pressures for years, it gives larger signals on the ECG. Even problems outside the heart can show up on the ECG. Common examples are obstructive lung diseases such as asthma and emphysema and blood-vessel problems such as a pulmonary embolism (a blood clot in the lung arteries).

STRESS TESTING

The stress test is really a group of different testing approaches physicians use to evaluate a heart's ability to accommodate increased metabolic demand. There are many different types of "stress" and many different types of "tests." The stress is often exercise, which can take many forms, including walking on a treadmill, bicycle riding, or performing arm exercises. The second type of stress is "chemical," which involves administering intravenous medicines that make the heart work harder or that dilate blood vessels in the heart. The type of tests used for stress testing includes ECGs and echocardiograms or even a highly technical PET scan (discussed shortly).

Chemicals Used for Stress Testing

Dobutamine: Dobutamine is an intravenous medication that causes the heart to pump harder. It is used in combination with imaging tests, such as the so-called stress echo. When the heart pumps harder, it requires more oxygen and nutrients. This metabolic stress can be helpful in diagnosing disease in the heart arteries or muscle. Dobutamine is used with caution in patients at risk for dangerous heart rhythms or in patients with critical CAD.

Adenosine or dipyridamole: Adenosine is a natural compound that dilates the heart blood vessels. Dipyridamole (brand name Persantine) is a chemical that causes an increase in adenosine in the heart. Both compounds function as vasodilators. The main difference between the two medications is how long the effect lasts. Both are used in combination with imaging tests such as SPECT or PET. If there is a blockage in an artery, less blood can get through under stress conditions, whereas when at rest enough blood can usually get past blockages. Caution is used when giving these medications to patients with reactive airway diseases such as asthma or emphysema, low blood pressure, or conduction disease in the heart.

Purpose of Stress Testing

Stress tests are most often used in patients with known or suspected CAD. In that setting, stress tests have a number of purposes:

Establish a diagnosis: Stress tests are a noninvasive way to demonstrate coronary heart disease.

Risk stratification: After a heart attack or a near-heart attack, stress tests are useful to classify patients into different risk groups. They can identify patients who are at high risk for a repeat event, or have a large area of heart muscle that has insufficient blood flow due to a blockage in the artery. In this setting, stress tests can be used to decide among different treatment strategies. For example, a stress test might help decide whether cardiac catheterization is needed to directly see the blockages.

Inform prognosis: For most medical conditions, the best measure of prognosis (i.e., how long a patient will likely live) is functional status, meaning how much exertion the patient is able to undergo at home. For instance, a patient with heart failure who can walk one mile without symptoms has a better prognosis than another patient who cannot walk to the bathroom without breathing difficulty. Exercise stress tests serve a similar purpose. A person who can walk for fifteen minutes on a treadmill stress test under standard testing protocols has less chance of dying from a heart attack over the next five years than a patient who can walk for only two minutes before developing chest pain.

Stress ECG

The exercise ECG is the most basic stress test. In most patients without contraindications, this is the test of choice for CAD evaluation.

Study details: The patient wears ECG electrodes while exercising. Most commonly, the patient is asked to walk on a treadmill that changes speed and incline in a set way, following a standardized protocol. Many aspects of the test are useful to the clinician—ECG changes, time of exercise, heart rate, blood pressure responses, symptoms, vital signs during recovery, and so on.

Contraindications: The patient's resting ECG cannot have certain abnormalities that would make the test uninterpretable. Also, many patients with bad arthritis or other illnesses that limit their ability to exercise would be better evaluated with a different test (i.e., a chemical stress test that makes the heart work without the patient having to exercise). For any exercise stress test to be useful, the patient much reach a heart rate goal that is age-specific.

Radionuclide Myocardial Perfusion Imaging

This diverse group of cardiovascular tests is generally referred to as a nuclear stress test. They involve injection of a radioactive agent (radionuclide) into the blood stream. (The radiation goes away after twelve to twenty-four hours. Although it is important to pay attention to the lifetime dose of radiation from various tests, the radiation exposure from stress testing is considered safe.)

The radionuclide goes to the different areas of the heart in proportion to blood flow (myocardial perfusion). Blood flow is assessed by imaging under rest and stressed conditions, and differences in blood flow between rest and stress can diagnose CAD. The stresses used are the same as those used for other stress tests—exercise or chemical stresses.

SPECT and PET Tests

Different radionuclides are used with various imaging techniques, and the testing protocol and diagnostic capabilities of the stress test vary among tests. Common radionuclides used include radioactive forms of technetium (Tc), thallium, rubidium, and nitrogen. These radionuclides are attached to other molecules, creating various long and confusing names. Examples include 99m-Tc-sestamibi (MIBI, brand name Cardiolite) and 99m-Tc-tetrofosmin (brand name Myoview). The distribution of the radionuclides in the heart is imaged using two main technologies: single photon emission computed tomography (SPECT) and positron emission tomography (PET).

As you can imagine, patients and physicians have a hard time understanding nuclear stress tests. The appropriate stress and radionuclide/imaging techniques are considered on a patient-by-patient basis. Cardiologists who specialize in nuclear imaging studies work closely with primary physicians to select the best test for the patient.

Nuclear imaging provides information that exercise ECGs and stress echocardiograms do not. Regional blood flow is directly assessed in nuclear imaging, and certain nuclear imaging tests can also assess ventricular function (ejection fraction).

Fixed and Reversible Heart Defects

Nuclear imaging tests provide a great deal of information about blood flow to the heart and heart muscle function. In the reports from nuclear imaging studies, perfusion (blood flow) is often described as normal or as having a "defect." The defect can be either fixed or reversible. Also, the amount of area involved in the blood flow defect is sometimes graded as small, of moderate size, or large. A fixed defect refers to an area of the heart that does not get good blood flow under rest or stressed conditions; the defect on the two scans is fixed, meaning it doesn't change with stress. This defect is most often a scar, and the heart artery supplying that area has been completely blocked due to a prior heart attack. A reversible defect refers to a region of the heart that gets good blood supply at rest but not with stress.

The distinction between fixed and reversible blood flow defects is important. There is generally no benefit to opening the artery with a fixed blood flow defect because the heart muscle that it supplies will not recover—it is scar tissue now. A reversible defect identifies heart muscle that is at risk, meaning it is supplied by an artery that is narrowed to the point that the heart muscle it supplies is starved for blood under stress conditions. Opening the artery supplying that region is sometimes beneficial in preventing a future heart attack or improving symptoms of angina.

Viability Study

On occasion, your cardiologist might suspect that what appears to be a fixed defect on a nuclear imaging study may not truly be scar tissue. In those instances, a special viability study can be performed. A viability study uses the same techniques as the stress test but takes images at a later point in time. Late uptake of the radiotracer suggests that the region of the heart in question might actually be viable or alive. If that is the case, revascularization with either angioplasty or coronary artery bypass might be beneficial (see appendix IV).

The cardiologist has to consider all of this information when deciding on a treatment plan. The size and degree of reversibility of blood flow problems, the patient's symptoms, the heart function under rest and stress, other concurrent health conditions—all of these affect the treatment plan.

Nuclear Imaging Safety

Nuclear imaging studies are safe—the radionuclide that is used has a very short half-life, meaning that after a short period of time, it is no longer radioactive. However, as mentioned earlier, it is important to limit the frequency of radiation-based tests, as the total lifetime dose of radiation could become a concern. The risks associated with these tests are the same as those that come with exercise or chemical stresses (discussed previously).

One caveat to nuclear stress tests: Patients with disease in all of the heart arteries can occasionally have a normal nuclear stress test even though they have severe disease. This occurs because all of the arteries are equally poor at dilating in response to vasodilators. So, when adenosine or dipyridamole is used to stress the heart, there is no difference in blood flow between the rest and stress images. This is one occasion when the results of a stress test can be negative even though the CAD is severe.

Study details: Depending on the type of nuclear study your doctor recommends, the test details will vary. Some nuclear studies last less than one hour, whereas others involve taking images over a longer period of time. The differences in test length are related to how long the radionuclide lasts in the circulation. Also, if viability testing is required, a set of late images will be collected. The technician will inject the radionuclide and then images will be collected using a camera or scanner. This process will be repeated after the stress, whether chemical or exercise. If a chemical stress is used, the patient might experience effects of the chemical such as a fast heart rate or flushing. Nuclear stress tests are easily tolerated procedures.

Contraindications: Stress testing is usually not performed in the midst of a heart attack. Other contraindications are related to the chemical used as the stress (as discussed earlier).

ECHOCARDIOGRAM

The echocardiogram (also referred to as an "echo") provides detailed images of the heart using ultrasound technology, the same used for fetal images during prenatal exams. The ultrasound probe generates sound waves that collide with the heart and surrounding structures. The reflection of these sound waves is received by the ultrasound probe and interpreted into one- or two-dimensional images. Dense structures reflect sound waves differently than less dense structures, allowing the echo machine to construct images based on tissue density. Additionally, this technology can be used to measure velocities of heart structures and blood.

Measuring Blood Turbulence

Echocardiograms are frequently used to quantify the severity of heart valve problems that cause turbulent blood flow in the heart. The turbulence can be seen on the echo's images as changes in the speed of blood moving through the valves. Of note, the echocardiogram does not directly visualize the heart arteries.

Study details: An echocardiogram is a safe study that is generally tolerated with very little discomfort. The studies typically last less than half an hour. The technician asks the patient to hold his or her breath at various times and roll onto different sides. What little discomfort patients experience is from the ultrasound probe—occasionally, the technician will have to apply pressure to the chest wall with the probe to improve the image resolution.

Indications: The most important use of echocardiography is to confirm the diagnosis of heart disease by a physical exam. In common practice, echocardiograms are frequently used because they can precisely quantify dysfunction of heart muscle and valve disease. The echocardiogram visualizes all of the segments of the heart, allowing localization of areas of scarred muscle or infiltrative diseases of the heart. Very few diseases are diagnosed solely by echocardiographic criteria; however, the echocardiogram is a useful adjunct in the diagnosis of almost every type of heart disease.

Contraindications: There are no real contraindications to this test. Obesity, obstructive lung disease, and mechanical ventilation can limit image quality.

SPECIAL ECHOCARDIOGRAMS

Stress Echocardiogram

Doctors sometimes request echocardiograms with stress images. Looking at the differences between resting and stress images can be informative in two settings. First, if CAD is suspected, occasionally the stress images will show regional wall motion abnormalities—areas of the heart that do not move well when the heart is stressed. The reason for this finding is usually that blood supply to that area is limited, and under stress that area is starved for oxygen and nutrients. This type of stress echocardiogram is usually done using exercise as the stress. The advantage to the stress echocardiogram over the stress ECG is that the echocardiogram can better localize what areas of the heart are receiving limited blood supply.

The second setting in which a stress echocardiogram is used with echocardiography is for the evaluation of obstructive heart diseases or aortic valve problems. Some forms of heart disease cause a blockage that can limit the outflow of the ventricle into the aorta. This can be caused by aortic valve problems or blockages above or below the valve. Hypertrophic cardiomyopathy, a hereditary heart condition, is a good example. In these settings, the stress is provided by dobutamine, an intravenous medication that makes the heart pump harder. The dobutamine echocardiogram can be used to quantify the obstruction under resting and stressed conditions, as occasionally blockages will change with stress. When evaluating aortic valve disease, the stress echocardiogram can be used to help decide whether valve surgery or other treatment modalities might improve the heart muscle function.

Contrast Echocardiogram

An echocardiogram can be done with intravenous contrast agents to improve the evaluation of the heart cavity and blood flow within the heart. Contrast agents are used in two different settings.

The more common contrast echocardiogram is generally referred to as a bubble study, used to investigate communications within the heart. This is done, for instance, in the evaluation of patients who have had a stroke.

Communications between the right and left sides of the heart are relatively common and benign, usually occurring between the right and left atria. For these studies, agitated saline is used as the source of the microbubbles. These microbubbles are very short-lived in the circulation, and in a heart without right-to-left communication, all the bubbles are removed in the lung. If there is communication between the right and left sides of the heart, however, the bubbles can be seen in the left atrium and left ventricle. This is a safe study with no additional precautions.

The second type of contrast echocardiogram uses different contrast agents that can fill the left side of the heart—a contrast agent that is not filtered in the lungs. The commonly used contrast agents use microbubbles that are encapsulated in a shell of protein, carbohydrate or lipid. These contrast agents are frequently used when the noncontrast echocardiogram is of poor quality—for instance, in an obese patient with emphysema.

There is currently an ongoing debate about whether there is any risk to these contrast agents. After a handful of patient deaths, the U.S. Food and Drug Administration has required a warning be placed on these contrast agents, listing adverse cardiopulmonary reactions as possible side effects. The warning suggests that patients with a shunt, heart failure exacerbations, heart attacks, serious arrhythmias, or lung pathology not undergo this type of testing. As with everything in medicine, all testing decisions are a risk-benefit balance. Most physicians feel that when indicated, the contrast echocardiogram is a low-risk procedure that can be performed safely.

Transesophageal Echocardiogram

The surface echocardiogram is best at seeing structures that are near the chest wall, where the ultrasound probe is located. For accurate visualization of deeper structures such as the mitral valve or left atrium, a transesophageal echocardiogram is superior. This test is similar to the routine echocardiogram, but the ultrasound probe is inserted into the esophagus using an endoscopic probe.

This procedure requires some sedation, just like other endoscopy procedures (such as a colonoscopy). There is a very small risk that the patient might swallow fluid into the lungs or that his esophagus might be damaged during the procedure, but these complications are very rare. For the most part, this test is safe in most patients. Common uses for this procedure include evaluation of mitral valve function, investigation of possible infections on the heart valves, and looking for blood clots in the heart.

COMPUTED TOMOGRAPHY (CT)

Computed tomography (a CT, or CAT, scan) is an imaging technique that takes multiple X-rays rotating around the body and then uses a computer to compile these X-rays into detailed three-dimensional images. For cardiac CT, the X-rays are taken at fast speed with multiple two-dimensional slices through the heart.

CAC Score

Two different types of CT scans are used to evaluate heart disease. The first is called the coronary artery calcification (CAC) score. This screening test quantifies how much calcium is present in the coronary (heart) arteries. Calcium deposits correlate with atherosclerosis, and physicians can use the calcium score to predict risk of future cardiovascular events. The more calcium there is, the higher the risk of developing a heart attack or dying. The CAC score is most useful in ruling out CAD, meaning that if no calcification is seen, it is very unlikely that the patient has blockages in the coronary arteries. This test is a relatively low-radiation test.

CT Angiography

The second CT test is called CT angiography. This technology uses an intravenous contrast agent to visualize the filling of the coronary arteries by a CT scan. In some ways, the information this test provides is similar to what can be gained from a heart catheterization, described on pages 308 to 310. The heart arteries and any blockages in them can be specifically pinpointed using three-dimensional computer reconstruction of the images. Additionally, the heart muscle can also be seen well with this test.

The advantage of a CT angiography is that it is non-invasive, meaning it does not involve accessing an artery with a catheter. However, the test is not as definitive as the more invasive catheterization procedure, and unlike the catheterization, there are no treatments that can be done by CT scanning. It also is a relatively high-radiation test, although newer protocols for performing this test are reducing the amount of radiation used.

Drawbacks to CT

There are two downsides to cardiac CT: variability among physicians in their ability to interpret cardiac CT tests, and the high radiation exposure to patients (although new protocols are reducing this). Additionally, many structures other than the heart

WHAT'S NEW:

Cardiovascular Magnetic Resonance (CMR)

People have become familiar with magnetic resonance imaging (MRI) studies that provide images of soft tissues such as joints or the brain. Like other soft tissues, the heart can be imaged in greater detail using MRI techniques than it can using CT scans. CMR is an MRI study of the heart using new technologies that provide high-definition images.

How does it work? CMR provides three-dimensional images of the heart and vascular structures, with no radiation for the patient. It is useful for diagnosing certain heart muscle cell diseases (cardiomyopathies) that distort the three-dimensional structure of the heart, evaluating the pericardium (the soft tissue surrounding the heart) for disease, and accurately imaging the great blood vessels that exit from the heart. Additionally, there is increased use of CMR for evaluating ischemic heart disease.

CMR can be combined with a chemical stress such as dobutamine or adenosine to look for areas of blood flow changes with stress or scarring. Areas of heart muscle that are alive but not working well because of limited blood flow (so-called "hibernating" muscle) are easy to distinguish from dead, scarred muscle cells by using CMR.

Are there any risks? As with all new techniques, expertise in this field is limited. In hospitals with experienced CMR physicians, this technique is gaining popularity. The main considerations are that patients with certain types of metal in their body (e.g., a prosthetic hip) cannot have an MRI study. Also, patients with chronic kidney disease have to be careful with the contrast agent used in MRI studies. There is an association between the contrast agent (gadolidium) and a disabling fibrotic disease called nephrogenic fibrosing dermopathy.

can be seen on CT scans, and these findings often lead to further monitoring or procedures. In an appropriately selected patient, however, cardiac CT has the potential to provide very useful information about CAD without the risks and discomfort associated with cardiac catheterization.

HEART CATHETERIZATION PROCEDURES

A catheterization or cath is a procedure that involves inserting a very long, hollow tube, much like a long intravenous line, into a blood vessel. In common language, cath is used to describe a specific catheterization procedure, namely coronary angiography. In truth, a number of different catheterization procedures are used for different purposes. We will discuss the heart catheterization procedures in this appendix, but keep in mind that occasionally structures other than the heart are catheterized.

Coronary Angiography

The most common catheterization procedure, coronary angiography, is used to visualize the heart arteries. It is the gold standard for diagnosis of CAD. The procedure involves inserting a catheter into an artery in either the groin or the arm and under X-ray visualization selectively injecting dye into the heart arteries. Blockages to the blood flow through the coronary arteries can be seen as defects as the dye fills the artery; in other words, the dye is blocked or forced to flow through a tight narrowing. Some catheterization centers will perform only diagnostic catheterizations, meaning they will not intervene to open any blockages they diagnose. This illustrates the key distinction between coronary angiography (a diagnostic procedure) and percutaneous interventions (PCIs). A PCI can be used to open the blockage

and in the acute setting (as during a heart attack) can be a lifesaving procedure. We describe PCI in appendix IV.

Indications: As discussed earlier, coronary angiography is the gold standard for the diagnosis of CAD. There are really only two purposes of sending a patient to catheterization: diagnosis and treatment. Which patients should undergo a diagnostic coronary angiography is a debated topic, and different physicians will practice differently. There are reasons to refer patients in whom a stress test has revealed a blockage or when the stress test was equivocal or negative. Every test has its limitations, so if the clinical suspicion for CAD is high, sometimes it is best to do the gold-standard test even if a noninvasive stress test did not show any problems. The second indication for angiography is for treatment of blockages. We address this topic in appendix IV.

Limitations: Coronary angiography is an invasive procedure and can have complications. A tear can develop in the arteries when the catheters are being placed, or a plaque in the artery could break off and cause a stroke. Bleeding at the puncture site can also occur, and on very rare occasions, patients can die. Thus, we try to make sure a patient really needs a cardiac catheterization prior to doing the test. The test also involves radiation exposure, which over a lifetime can cause problems.

Coronary angiography demonstrates abnormalities in the large arteries at the surface of the heart. Sometimes a patient's symptoms are due to blockages in blood flow to the heart, but angiography will not reveal a blockage. Some patients can have microvascular disease, meaning disease limited to the smaller-caliber vessels that are not seen well on angiography. Also, some patients have coronary artery spasms that can come and go. In this condition, the coronary arteries are not blocked by atherosclerotic plaques or blood clots but rather a transient pinching of the artery caused by hormonal or neurologic changes is the cause. This is a very serious condition that can be missed if no symptoms are present at the time of angiography.

It is also important to mention that angiography can reveal narrowing in the coronary artery that is of unclear clinical significance. CAD is a chronic medical condition that does not cause problems unless it is complicated by symptoms of angina, heart attack, or heart failure. Blockages can be seen in many individuals who do not experience any of these consequences. Likewise, even in a patient who is experiencing symptoms, it is sometimes unclear which blockages seen on angiography are causing the patient's symptoms.

Left- and Right-Heart Catheterization

For some conditions, a catheter can be inserted into the heart chambers to measure pressures, sample tissue, or directly visualize the heart cavities. Generically, these procedures are known as heart-catheterization procedures.

A right-heart catheterization involves insertion of a catheter into the venous circulation, usually a large vein in the neck or the groin. A balloon is inflated that functions as a floating bubble, pulling the catheter in the direction of blood flow. The catheter is advanced into the right atrium, then into the right ventricle, and finally into the pulmonary artery. At each part of the heart, the pressure can be measured. These measurements can be used to gauge the function of the heart muscle and heart valves.

A left-heart catheterization is done essentially like a coronary angiography. A catheter is inserted into the arterial circulation and then goes against blood flow in the aorta until it reaches the heart. At the heart, the catheter visualizes the coronary arteries (i.e., coronary angiography) or the catheter can be passed across the aortic valve into the left ventricle and pressures can be measured on both sides of the valve.

Ventriculography: Ventriculography involves injection of contrast into the ventricular cavity, much like an angiography procedure. The contrast fills the ventricles and then tracks the blood flow as the heart contracts and pumps blood. Ventriculography is helpful in quantifying heart muscle impairment and valve problems.

Invasive hemodynamic monitoring: Catheters can be used to measure pressures and blood flow through the heart chambers. The most common hemodynamic procedure is called a Swan-Ganz catheterization (named after the doctors who pioneered the procedure), also known as a pulmonary artery catheterization. This procedure gives detailed information regarding the cardiac output (how well the heart is pumping), blood pressures in the heart chambers, resistance to blood flow leaving the heart, and quantification of heart valve problems. This information is used to tailor medical therapy to the individual patient.

Some heart diseases result from stiffening of the heart muscle (restrictive diseases) or the sac (pericardium) surrounding the heart (constrictive diseases). The pattern of blood flow through the heart chambers can often identify these types of problems. To accurately diagnose a restrictive or constrictive heart problem, the cardiologist will occasionally do a right- and left-heart catheterization at the same time. The way that pressure changes vary between the right and left ventricles can diagnose whether the stiffening is a muscle or a pericardial problem.

Heart Biopsy

Biopsies are needed for the diagnosis of some types of heart muscle diseases and for the monitoring of patients after a heart transplant. Biopsies are taken using a right-heart catheterization procedure. The cardiologist uses a small device that essentially takes a bite out of the heart muscle. Ideally, the biopsy is taken from the heart wall that separates the right and left ventricles. When biopsies are needed for diagnosis, it is usually in a setting of severe heart disease, when the cause is not known and treatment options and prognosis might depend on the specific diagnosis. Patients who have received a heart transplant need to have very frequent heart biopsies to monitor for rejection. (Rejection is the process of immune reaction against the foreign heart.) Catching rejection early is important because medicines to blunt the immune response can protect the transplanted heart.

Electrophysiology (EP) Study

Heart rhythm disturbances are usually diagnosed based on the surface ECG and treated successfully with safe oral medications. For some rhythm problems, however, an invasive study is necessary for diagnosis and treatment. An EP study involves catheterization of the heart (usually a right-heart catheterization, rarely a right- and left-heart procedure). The catheters have the ability to stimulate the heart muscles with electrical activity and include recording devices that can measure electrical activity at various locations within the heart. Computers are used to create an electrical map of the heart. The procedure is useful for defining complicated heart rhythm disturbances and can also be used for treatment.

Q. & A. with Dr. Cannon

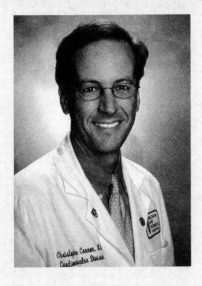

Q. Some tests require X-rays and others inject radiation into the blood. Do I have to worry about radiation?

A. Yes and no. Each test is designed to not give you too much radiation and thus is safe. However, some tests give much more radiation than others. For example, CT scans (of the heart or any part of the body) involve more radiation than simple X-rays. MRI scans and ECG tests give no radiation. It is reasonable to keep track of all the radiation-based tests you have undergone and try not to have unnecessary tests that would increase your total radiation dose.

Q. Do I need to have a yearly stress test to check my risk of a heart attack?

A. No. Stress tests are used mostly to evaluate symptoms that may or may not be heart-related. Routine annual stress tests can sometimes be helpful in certain patients but generally are no longer done regularly. To gauge the risk of heart attack, we look closely at all your risk factors (see chapter 10).

Q. I had a calcium score and it was high. What does that mean?

A. The calcium score looks at how much calcium has built up in the heart arteries. The calcium, however, is not really the problem—it is a marker of cholesterol plaques that are also in the artery. The cholesterol plaques are the dangerous parts; they can rupture and cause a heart attack. The calcium is just mixed in as part of the plaques.

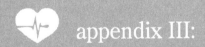 appendix III:

A REFERENCE OF MEDICATIONS THAT TREAT HEART DISEASE AND THEIR SIDE EFFECTS

Over the past fifty years, there has been remarkable progress in the treatment of heart disease. By some measures, these improvements alone are responsible for more than one-third of the increase in life expectancy since 1960. The discovery of new medications and new uses for old medications has been responsible for a large part of this success story. Although significant work remains to be done, the medications available to cardiologists have significantly improved our ability to treat coronary artery disease (CAD), high blood pressure, high cholesterol, and heart failure. As a result, patients can live longer, healthier lives.

ANTIPLATELET MEDICATIONS

Platelets are small cells in the blood that clump together to stop bleeding after an injury. When cholesterol plaques in blood vessels break open, platelets coat the tear and clump together. Unfortunately, when this happens in a vessel that is providing blood to the heart, the result is a heart attack (myocardial infarction [MI]). It makes sense that one of the best ways to stop heart attacks is to prevent platelets from becoming activated. Two medications that are commonly used for this are aspirin and clopidogrel.

Aspirin

How does aspirin work?

Aspirin works by blocking platelet clumping. When platelets are activated, they release several different molecules, including thromboxanes, which activate other platelets. These activated platelets are very sticky and bunch together to form a clot. Aspirin binds to and shuts down a protein (cyclooxygenase or COX) that is needed to produce thromboxane. By blocking the production of thromboxanes, aspirin makes it harder for platelets to form clots and therefore makes it less likely that a heart attack will occur.

When is aspirin used?

Aspirin has a number of different uses, including treating fevers, muscle aches, and pain. For cardiologists, aspirin is most often used to treat CAD and its worst manifestation, heart attacks. Unless there is a specific reason not to, such as an aspirin allergy, all patients having a heart attack—or who are known to have CAD—are given aspirin and should take aspirin every day. In addition, patients who are at higher risk of heart attacks should take a small dose of aspirin everyday because this has been shown to reduce the chances of not only heart attacks but also strokes.

What are some side effects of using aspirin?

Because aspirin works by interfering with blood clotting, taking aspirin means patients are at higher risk of bleeding. In addition, aspirin can be very irritating to the stomach and cause not only upset stomach but also ulcers and stomach bleeding. Kidney damage can also occur if patients take a significant amount of aspirin every day for a long period of time. Because most patients with heart conditions take only small doses of aspirin, they are not likely to suffer kidney damage.

Clopidogrel (Plavix)

How does clopidogrel work?

Similar to aspirin, clopidogrel works by interfering with the ability of platelets to clump together into clots. Instead of blocking the COX protein, clopidogrel attaches to and blocks the adenosine diphosphate (ADP) receptor found on the outside of platelets. Like thromboxane, ADP works by activating platelets and making them stickier. By blocking the ADP receptor, clopidogrel makes it less likely that platelets will become activated and form clots.

When is clopidogrel used?

Clopidogrel does not have the same wide array of uses as aspirin, but it is often used in cardiology patients who are also taking aspirin. As with aspirin, most patients who are having a heart attack get clopidogrel. Exceptions to this are patients who are likely to need coronary artery bypass surgery. Clopidogrel increases the risk of bleeding during bypass surgery and is avoided in patients who need surgery.

Any patient who has had a percutaneous coronary intervention (see appendix IV), especially if a stent has been placed, should take clopidogrel for one year (or longer in many cases) after the procedure. In addition, any patient who should be taking aspirin but cannot because of an allergy or an adverse reaction (e.g., a stomach ulcer) may benefit from clopidogrel. Patients with peripheral artery disease (blockages in the arteries in their legs as opposed to their hearts) and patients who have had strokes or are at high risk of strokes may also benefit from taking clopidogrel.

What are the side effects of clopidogrel?

As expected for a medication that blocks platelets, the biggest downside of using clopidogrel is an increased risk of bleeding, especially bleeding from the stomach. Clopidogrel cannot be used in patients who have an allergy to it or who are currently bleeding from their stomach, intestine, or other organs.

BETA BLOCKERS

Beta blockers include such medications as atenolol, bisoprolol, carvedilol, labetalol, metoprolol, nadolol, pindolol, propranolol, and timolol.

How do beta blockers work?

Beta blockers are medications that attach to and "block" the activation of adrenergic receptors. Adrenergic receptors come in two main forms: alpha and beta. As the name suggests, beta blockers mostly function by binding beta receptors, although some (carvedilol, labetalol) also bind alpha receptors. Adrenergic receptors work within the sympathetic nervous system, a part of the nervous system that helps regulate many involuntary bodily functions. The beta-adrenergic receptors in the heart, when they are activated, cause the heart to beat faster and harder. Alpha receptors are found in blood vessels and when activated cause them to constrict (or narrow). In the short term, this can often be useful. In stressful situations when "your adrenalin starts pumping" and your heart rate and blood pressure go up, the adrenalin rush occurs through activation of adrenergic receptors. Unfortunately, however, when the heart is forced to work faster and harder for a long period of time, it begins to fatigue, much like an overridden horse. Beta blockers help prevent such fatigue by inhibiting the activation of the adrenergic system, which causes the heart to slow down and pump with less force. In most cases, they have the additional beneficial effect of lowering blood pressure.

When are beta blockers used?

Beta blockers are prescribed for the following conditions.

Hypertension: High blood pressure, also known as hypertension, is an extremely common disease. Beta blockers are generally not used as the first option for high blood pressure unless the patient has another condition that can also benefit from beta blocker treatment (e.g., a patient who also has a history of heart attacks or heart failure).

Heart failure: Beta blockers are a cornerstone in the treatment of heart failure. It may be surprising that a medication that causes the heart to beat slower and less forcefully would be useful in patients whose heart cannot pump enough blood. However, multiple studies involving thousands of patients have shown that beta blockers prolong the lives of patients with heart failure. It is believed that by slowing down and relaxing the heart, beta blockers also slow the continuing deterioration of heart function that occurs in almost all patients with heart failure.

CAD/angina: CAD results in blockages in the arteries that supply blood to the heart. When the heart does not get enough blood, patients typically develop a chest pressure or pain called angina. Beta blockers can slow the development of the blockages that cause CAD. By slowing down the heart, they reduce the heart's demand for blood, which reduces the frequency and severity of angina.

MI: Almost all patients who have suffered a heart attack (MI) should take beta blockers. After a heart attack, the heart muscle begins to remodel in response to the damage it has suffered. Beta blockers help limit the remodeling, which can often be detrimental to heart function.

Atrial fibrillation and atrial flutter: Beta blockers, because of their ability to slow down the electrical system of the heart, are often used to control the heart rate of patients with atrial fibrillation or atrial flutter.

What are the side effects of beta blockers?

Taking beta blockers can cause a number of undesirable side effects. Because they slow down the heart's function, they can actually worsen heart failure if used in patients that are not ready to take them. Beta blockers can cause the airways in the lungs to nar-

row. Patients with asthma, emphysema, and chronic bronchitis who already have difficulties with narrowed airways should take beta blockers with caution. Finally, by interfering with the sympathetic nervous system, beta blockers can cause a number of side effects, such as depression, dizziness, fatigue, sexual dysfunction, coldness in the hands and feet, and nightmares.

ACE INHIBITORS (ACE-I) AND ANGIOTENSIN-RECEPTOR BLOCKERS (ARBs)

Angiotensin-converting enzyme (ACE) inhibitors include such medications as Benazepril, Captopril, Enalapril, Fosinopril, Lisinopril, and Ramipril.

Angiotensin-receptor blockers (ARBs) include such medications as Candesartan, Losartan, Irbesartan, Olmesartan, and Valsartan.

How do ACE-I and ARBs work?

One of the main ways the body regulates blood pressures is with the renin-angiotensin hormonal system. When the kidneys sense that the blood pressure is too low, they release a hormone called renin, which works by converting angiotensinogen into angiotensin I. The angiotensin-converting enzyme (or ACE) is a protein found in the lungs that converts angiotensin I into angiotensin II. The effects of angiotensin II include the following:

Vasoconstriction: Blood vessels become narrow, resulting in higher blood pressure.

Aldosterone release: Aldosterone is a hormone made by the adrenal cortex, which causes the kidney to retain more salt and water. As a result, blood pressure increases.

Ventricular remodeling: Angiotensin II can cause the muscle of the heart to remodel itself, which in the long run can result in heart failure.

Renal arteriole constriction: Angiotensin II can cause the blood vessels in the kidney to constrict, which increases the blood pressure inside it. Over an extended period of time, this can lead to kidney failure.

ACE-Is function by blocking the conversion of angiotensin I into angiotensin II, thereby interfering with all of these effects. ARBs work by blocking the binding of angiotensin II to its receptor.

When are ACE-I and ARBs used?

ACE-I and ARBs have overlapping uses, and in general, ACE-Is are preferred. ARBs are used when an ACE-I cannot be used. The following are the primary indications for taking an ACE-I or an ARB:

Hypertension: By causing blood vessels to relax, ACE-Is and ARBs are great medications for lowering blood pressure. They are the preferred medications for hypertension when patients also have a history of heart failure or kidney disease.

Heart failure: ACE-Is and ARBs prevent the progression of heart failure by lowering blood pressure (which reduces the stress on the heart) and by directly preventing ventricular remodeling.

Chronic kidney disease: Patients with kidney disease, especially kidney disease caused by diabetes (diabetic nephropathy), clearly benefit from taking an ACE-I. ACE-Is slow down the progression of kidney damage by lowering blood pressure and more directly, by relaxing the small blood vessels in the kidney.

What are the side effects of ACE-Is and ARBs?

ACE-Is and ARBs have a number of side effects that can limit their use. ACE-Is can cause a chronic cough, which can be persistent and irritating. Often, the cough will go away if patients switch to an ARB. In addition, ACE-Is can cause a sudden swelling of the neck and face, called angioedema. Both ACE-Is and ARBs can actually worsen renal failure. Whenever a patient takes either type of medication, kidney function should be followed closely. Because of their effects on the kidney, ACE-Is and ARBs can cause dangerously high levels of potassium. As with any medication that lowers blood pressure, ACE-Is and ARBs can cause hypotension, which occurs when blood pressure is too low.

CALCIUM-CHANNEL BLOCKERS

There are three classes of calcium-channel blockers:

- Dihydropyridines (Amlodipine, Felodipine, Nicardipine, and Nifedipine)
- Diltiazem
- Verapamil

How do calcium-channel blockers work?

As the name implies, calcium-channel blockers prevent the entry of calcium ions into muscle cells that make up the heart and walls of blood vessels. In the heart, less calcium entering the muscle cells results in less forceful contractions (or decreased cardiac contractility). In medical jargon, this is referred to as a negative inotropic effect. In blood vessels, less calcium results in relaxation of the blood vessel walls and a resultant drop in blood pressure. In addition to their effects on muscle cells, diltiazem and verapamil (but not dihydropyridine) can also slow down the electrical system of the heart (a phenomenon called negative chronotropic effect). By slowing down the conduction of electrical signals through the heart, diltiazem and verapamil can slow the heart rate.

When are calcium-channel blockers used?
Calcium-channel blockers are used to treat the following cardiac conditions:

Hypertension: Calcium-channel blockers lower blood pressure by relaxing the blood vessels in the blood. By relaxing the heart muscles, calcium-channel blockers also reduce the force of heart contractions, which also lowers blood pressure.

Angina: Angina is the chest discomfort or pressure that occurs when the blood supply to the heart does not match the heart's needs. Calcium-channel blockers reduce angina by lowering the heart's need for blood. The amount of blood the heart needs depends on how hard and how fast the heart beats. Calcium-channel blockers can reduce both the speed and the intensity of the heart rate.

Atrial fibrillation and atrial flutter: Diltiazem and verapamil slow down the electrical system of the heart. In situations when the heart is beating too fast (such as atrial fibrillation or atrial flutter) these medications can be useful in lowering the heart rate.

What are some of the side effects of calcium-channel blockers?
All the calcium-channel blockers, because they lower blood pressure, can cause hypotension (excessively low blood pressure). Because they are distinctly different types of molecules, the different classes of calcium-channel blockers can have different side-effect profiles. The dihyrdopyridine class of medications can cause fluid accumulation in the legs (edema). Because they do not slow the heart

rate, taking dihydropyridines can actually result in a faster heart rate as the body tries to compensate for a drop in blood pressure. Dihydropyridines can also cause swelling of the gums (gingival hyperplasia). Because of their effect on the heart's electrical system, diltiazem and verapamil can cause bradycardia (excessively slow heart rate). They are also more likely to cause heart failure than the dihydropyridine medications. Verapamil can give patients severe constipation.

RANOLAZINE

Ranolazine is a new medication used for the treatment of patients with chronic stable angina—the chest pressure or discomfort that occurs when the heart is not getting enough blood.

How does ranolazine work?
The mechanism of action for ranolazine is not exactly understood. It is believed that the medication works by reducing sodium entry into heart muscle cells. As a result, sodium-dependent calcium channels are perturbed, and the muscle cell cannot overload on calcium. (Elevated levels of calcium inside the cell cause muscle cells to contract harder and makes it more difficult for them to relax completely. In this situation, there is an increase in the amount of oxygen [hence blood] required by the muscle cells.) By preventing calcium overload, ranolazine reduces the amount of blood and oxygen that heart muscle cells require and thus reduces angina.

When is ranolazine used?
Ranolazine is used to treat patients with chronic stable angina and generally is used when the angina is not adequately treated by other medications (such as beta blockers, nitrates, and calcium-channel blockers). Unlike the other classes of antiangina medica-

tions, ranolazine does not affect heart rate and blood pressure, so it can be used by patients who have low blood pressure or slow heart rates.

What are some side effects of ranolazine?

Patients on ranolazine may develop what is called QT prolongation on their electrocardiogram (ECG), but recent studoes have not seen this to be dangerous. The other side effects of ranolazine are mild and include nausea, upset stomach, diarrhea, and dizziness.

DIURETICS

Diuretics (often called "water pills") are medications that force the kidney to make more urine and so excrete more water (diuresis). There are several classes of diuretics, including the following:

- Loop diuretics: furosemide, bumetanide, and torsemide
- Thiazide diuretics: hydrochlorothiazide, chlorthalidone, and metolazone
- Potassium-sparing diuretics: spironolactone, eplerenone, amiloride, and triamterene

Diuretics are a broad group of medications with varying effects and distinct uses.

How do diuretics work?

Each class of diuretic works on a different part of the kidney, and therefore produces a different effect.

Loop diuretics: Medications such as furosemide block the ability of the kidney to reabsorb sodium. If the body cannot retain sodium, it cannot retain water. Of all the diuretics, loop diuretics cause the body to eliminate the most sodium and water.

Thiazide diuretics: Thiazide diuretics also cause the kidney to eliminate sodium and water, but because they work at a different location in the kidney (the distal convoluted tubule as opposed to the loop of Henle), they affect urine output less than loop diuretics.

Potassium-sparing diuretics: Loop diuretics and thiazide diuretics cause the body to lose significant amounts of potassium. Potassium-sparing diuretics, as their name implies, do not. For cardiologists, the most important potassium-sparing diuretics are spironolactone and eplrenone. These medications function by binding the receptor for the hormone aldosterone. Normally, aldosterone receptor activation in the kidney causes the kidney to suck in more sodium and water from the urine and dump more potassium into it. Spironolactone and eplrenone block this effect.

When are diuretics used?

The different classes of diuretics have varying uses in patients with heart disease.

Loop diuretics: Patients with heart failure often accumulate excess fluid in their feet (peripheral edema), abdomen (ascites), and lungs (pulmonary edema). The excess fluid comes as the kidney attempts to compensate for the failing heart by retaining more and more salt and water. Loop diuretics, by forcing the kidney to dump sodium and water into the urine, get rid of the excess fluid or prevent its accumulation in the first place. Although they make patients more comfortable and reduce the need for hospitalization, loop diuretics have never been shown to increase the life span of patients with heart failure.

Thiazide diuretics: The primary use for thiazide diuretics is to treat hypertension (high blood pressure). In fact, they are the first-line agent recommended by experts in treating this condition. Unless there is a specific reason a patient cannot take a thiazide diuretic, if he or she needs to be on two or more blood pressure medications one of them should be a thiazide diuretic.

Potassium-sparing diuretics: Spironolactone and eplerenone are used in patients with advanced heart failure. Unlike loop diuretics, they are not used to get rid of excess fluid. Rather, by blocking aldosterone receptors, they slow continued heart function deterioration. For patients with advanced heart failure, taking spironolactone and eplerenone has been shown to increase survival.

What are the side effects of diuretics?

Loop diuretics: Loop diuretics can result in hypovolemia (or dehydration) if they are overused. With increased urination, the body also loses significant amounts of other electrolytes, so there is a risk of dangerously low levels of potassium and magnesium. Patients taking a loop diuretic should have their levels of potassium and other electrolytes in their blood checked regularly.

Thiazide diuretics: As with any medication that reduces blood pressure, there is a risk of lowering blood pressure too far (hypotension). Excessively low levels of potassium and sodium and high levels of calcium can occur while taking thiazide diuretics.

Potassium-sparing diuretics: All potassium-sparing diuretics can cause potassium levels in the body to reach dangerously high levels. In addition, spironolactone and, to a lesser extent, eplerenone can cause a painful enlargement of the breasts, increased body hair, and sexual dysfunction.

LIPID-LOWERING MEDICATIONS

Hyperlipidemia occurs when the levels of lipids (fats) in the blood, such as cholesterol and triglycerides, are elevated. Hyperlipidemia is a significant contributor to CAD. Statins are the primary medication used to treat hyperlipidemia, but they have limitations. For example, they are not effective at lowering triglycerides or at raising the level of HDL. And some patients cannot tolerate statins because of their effect on the liver and muscles. As a result, it is often necessary to prescribe other medications to treat hyperlipidemia. Among these medications are niacin, fibrates, ezetimibe, and bile acid sequestrants.

Statins

HMG-CoA reductase inhibitors (statins) are a group of medications that are used to treat high cholesterol. They include atorvastatin, lovastatin, pravastatin, rosuvastatin, and simvastatin.

How do statin medications work?

Statins work by inhibiting the protein HMG-CoA reductase, which controls the most important step in the production of cholesterol by the liver. When the liver cannot produce more cholesterol, it has to use more of the cholesterol already circulating in the body. As a result, the level of low-density lipoprotein (LDL), the bad cholesterol, in the blood is significantly reduced. Statins are less effective at increasing the level of high-density lipoprotein (HDL), the good cholesterol.

When are statins used?

Statins can significantly reduce the risk of heart attack, stroke, and death. They are indicated for patients who have high levels of cholesterol. Recent studies have shown that patients who have healthy cholesterol levels can benefit from taking statins if they have high levels of C-reactive protein in their blood. It is recommended that most heart attack, stroke, and diabetic patients take statins, unless there is a specific reason not to. Statins have become a mainstay of the treatment for CAD, strokes, heart attacks, and peripheral vascular disease. The current expert guidelines have set target levels of LDL for patients depending on their over all risk of CAD. Patients should take increasing doses of statins and if necessary, take additional lipid-lowering medications (discussed shortly) to reach these targets.

What are some of the side effects of statins?
There are two major risks of taking statins. There is a small risk of an increase in liver enzyme, so patients should have their liver function checked regularly while on a statin medication. Muscle aches can occur but generally are reduced with lower doses or by stopping the medication. Muscles can become inflamed (myositis), and if the inflammation is severe enough, they can break down (rhabdomyolysis). In the most severe cases, rhabdomyolysis can cause sudden kidney failure.

Niacin

Niacin, or nicotinic, acid is actually a vitamin that both lowers the level of LDL and raises the level of HDL. Niacin works by blocking the breakdown of fat molecules in adipose tissue. Niacin is a good medication for patients who have low levels of HDL. There are a number of side effects of niacin that patients often find intolerable, such as flushing, nausea, and itching. Like statins, niacin can also affect the liver.

Fibrates

Fibrates include such medications as gemfibrozil and fenofibrate. By activating the PPAR-alpha receptor in the liver and muscle, fibrates have a number of effects, including decreased amounts of triglyceride and increased levels of HDL. Patients with high triglyceride levels or low HDL levels (both of which often do not respond to statins) can benefit from taking fibrates. Fibrates can increase the risk of gallstones and like statins can cause myopathy (damage to muscles). When used in combination with statins at high doses (which is often necessary), they can increase the risk of muscles breaking down.

Ezetimibe

Ezetimibe binds to and blocks a protein found on the cells that line the intestinal tract that is necessary for the absorption of cholesterol. Because the intestine absorbs less cholesterol, the rest of the body's cells have to draw more cholesterol out of the blood to meet their needs. Ezetimibe has been approved for use, either by itself or in combination with statins, to treat patients with high levels of LDL. Ezetimibe is a well-tolerated drug but, like statins, it may impact the liver and muscle.

Bile Acid Sequestrants

Bile acid sequestrants include medications such as cholestyramine, colestipol, and colesevelam. As the name suggests, bile acid sequestrants bind to bile acids in the intestine. Bile acids are necessary for the absorption of cholesterol from food. The sequestrants are used to treat patients with elevated levels of LDL. Patients generally do not tolerate bile acid sequestrants well because of the number of side effects, which include nausea, vomiting, bloating, and cramping. There is also a risk of liver damage while taking these medications.

ANTIARRHYTHMIA MEDICATIONS

Antiarrhythmics are a group of medications that can suppress abnormally fast heart rhythms (tachycardias) such as atrial fibrillation, atrial flutter, ventricular tachycardia, and ventricular fibrillation. The majority of antiarrhythmic medications should only be prescribed by an electrophysiologist (a cardiologist who specializes in the electrical system of the heart). Antiarrhythmics are usually placed in one of five classes based on their primary effect.

How do antiarrhythmia medications work?

Class I: Class I medications function by interfering with sodium channels. Heart cells become activated when sodium enters the cell through sodium channels. By blocking these channels, Class I agents make the heart less excitable. Class I agents include quinidine, procainamide, disopyramide, lidocaine, mexiletine, flecainide, and propafenone.

Class II: Class II agents are beta blockers (discussed previously). Beta blockers exert their effect by blocking the beta-adrenergic receptors. When the beta-adrenergic receptors in the heart are activated, the heart beats faster. Blocking them slows down the heart.

Class III: Class III agents target potassium channels. After sodium enters and activates the heart cells, potassium deactivates them by leaving the cells through potassium channels. By blocking these channels, Class III medications prolong the deactivation process. While a cell is deactivating, it cannot respond to another activation signal (it is refractory). As a result, it becomes harder to repeatedly activate the heart's electrical system. Class III agents include amiodarone, dofetilide, ibutilide, and sotalol.

Class IV: Class IV agents are the nondihydropyridine calcium-channel blockers verapamil and diltiazem. By blocking calcium channels, they slow the rate of conduction of electrical signals through the atrioventricular node.

Class V: Class V agents include two medications: digoxin and adenosine. Digoxin works by increasing the amount of the signal coming from the portion of the nervous system that tells the heart to slow down (it increases the vagal tone). Adenosine effectively shuts down the atrioventricular node so that tachycardias coming from the top chambers (atria) of the heart cannot affect the more important lower chambers (ventricles) of the heart.

When are antiarrhythmia medications used?

Class I: Because of the risks associated with these medications and the complexity of the situations when they are beneficial, Class I agents are typically prescribed only by an electrophysiologist or cardiologist. They are predominantly used to treat atrial fibrillation (which is a rapid, irregular rate arising from the atria), ventricular tachycardia, and ventricular fibrillation (rapid heart rhythms that originate from the ventricles). Ventricular tachycardia and fibrillation are dangerous rhythms that often require an implantable cardioverter defibrillator. Class I agents can decrease the frequency and duration of these rhythms, but they are generally not lifesaving and in some situations can actually increase the risk of dying.

Class II: We discussed the indications for beta blockers in detail earlier in this appendix.

Class III: The primary indications for class III agents are ventricular tachycardia, ventricular fibrillation, and atrial fibrillation. The most commonly used class III agent is amiodarone. There is some evidence that class III agents are safer than Class I agents. Unfortunately, there are significant side effects when taking amiodarone for an extended period of time.

Class IV: We discuss the indications for calcium-channel blockers on page 317–318.

Class V: Digoxin is used to treat atrial fibrillation, whereas adensosine is used to terminate two specific types of tachycardias, called AVNRT and AVRT.

What are some of the side effects of antiarrhythmia medications?

We discussed the downsides of taking beta blockers and calcium-channel blockers earlier in this appendix. Each specific Class I agent has a unique side effect profile. But as a group, the flip side of their antiarrhythmia effects is proarrhythmia effects. Class I agents can cause some of the very arrhythmias they are supposed to suppress, such as ventricular tachycardia and ventricular fibrillation. As a result, it is vital that patients take these medications only under the close supervision of an electrophysiologist.

Class III agents (especially amiodarone) tend to be less proarrhythmia than Class I agents. Amiodarone has become a commonly used medication for the treatment of arrhythmias. Unfortunately, taking amiodarone for an extended period of time can be damaging to the liver, lungs, and thyroid gland. A new version of amiodarone called dronedarone is currently being reviewed by the U.S. Food and Drug Administration.

Dronedarone is not damaging to the liver, lungs, and thyroid, and has been shown to decrease the risk of heart-related deaths and strokes, as well as the need for hospitalization for patients with atrial fibrillation.

Adenosine is typically used only in the hospital. There is a very small risk of severe bradycardia (slow heart rate) or asystole (when the heart completely stops) after receiving adenosine. We discuss the risks of taking digoxin on page 325.

ANTICOAGULANTS

Anticoagulants, or blood thinners, are medications that make it more difficult for blood to clot. Unlike aspirin and clopidogrel, which block platelets, anticoagulants interfere with the proteins in the blood that are needed for clotting. Although there are a number of different anticoagulants, we will discuss the two most commonly used: warfarin and low molecular weight heparin (LMWH).

How do anticoagulants work?

Warfarin: Warfarin blocks the effects of vitamin K. The liver uses vitamin K in the production of several proteins that are needed to clot blood. By blocking the effect of vitamin K, warfarin interferes with the production of these proteins, and it becomes more difficult for blood to clot.

Heparin/low molecular weight heparin (LMWH): LMWH is a type of injected medication derived from heparin. Heparin is usually made from the intestines of pigs. Heparin and LMWH work by activating a protein called antithrombin III. To keep blood from clotting when it shouldn't, the body has an anticlotting system. Antithrombin III is a key component of this system because it blocks one of the key steps in the clotting cascade. There are several types of LMWH, including dalteparin and enoxaparin. Heparin is injected as an intravenous medication, whereas LMWH can be injected underneath the skin (much like insulin shots).

Direct thrombin inhibitors: One of the final steps in the blood-clotting system is carried out by the protein thrombin. Medications such as bivalirudin and argatroban block the action of thrombin and thus interfere with blood clotting. Bivalirudin is often used to treat patients having a heart attack, whereas argatroban is used to treat patients with blood clots in their legs or lungs who also have an allergy to heparin.

Factor Xa inhibitors: The most commonly used Factor Xa inhibitor is fondaparinux. Like thrombin, Factor Xa is needed for the blood-clotting cascade to work properly. Fondaparinux is most commonly used to prevent blood clots in the legs or lungs after surgery but is also used to treat patients having a heart attack.

When are anticoagulants used?

Warfarin and heparin/LMWH/other anticoagulants have overlapping uses for cardiologists. In general, warfarin is the preferred medication because it is a pill, doctors and patients have more experience with using it, and it is less expensive. The primary reasons to use warfarin are to treat atrial fibrillation, blood clots in the leg (deep vein thrombosis), blood clots in the lungs (pulmonary embolus), and an artificial mechanical heart valve. Warfarin is not used to treat patients having a heart attack. Patients with severe heart failure or with very dilated balloonlike hearts are also at high risk of forming clots in their heart and may benefit from warfarin. In general, heparin/LMWH is used with patients who cannot take warfarin. Patients who are having a heart attack are treated with heparin/LMWH, a direct thrombin inhibitor, or a Factor Xa inhibitor.

What are the side effects of anticoagulant use?

The side effect that causes most concern when using any anticoagulant is bleeding. By interfering with the clotting system, these medications inherently worsen the risk of bleeding and the severity of bleeding. Patients on warfarin need regular blood tests about once every one to two weeks to ensure they are taking the right amount. Patients on warfarin are at slightly increased risk of osteoporosis, and a very small number may develop a severe skin rash called warfarin necrosis. Women who are pregnant or who may become pregnant cannot take warfarin. Patients can be treated with heparin only while in the hospital because they require very frequent blood tests (every six to twenty-four hours). Unlike warfarin and heparin, patients do not need regular blood tests while taking LMWH. There is a risk of low platelet counts while taking heparin/LMWH. Paradoxically, when this occurs there is actually an increased risk of clots forming.

INOTROPES

Inotropes are a broad group of medications that cause the heart muscle to contract with more force. The most commonly used inotropes are catecholamines (dobutamine, dopamine, norepinephrine, epinephrine, and isoproterenol), bipyridines (milrinone and amrinone), and cardiac glycosides (digoxin).

How do inotrope medications work?

Catecholamines: Essentially the opposite of beta blockers, these medications bind to and activate the beta-adrenergic receptors in the heart. When activated, these receptors cause the heart to beat faster and with more force.

Bipyridines: Milrinone (the most commonly used bipyridine) functions as a phosphodiesterase inhibitor. Phosphodiesterase is a protein found inside heart cells, which acts to turn off the signal that comes from activated beta-adrenergic receptors. By turning off phosphodiesterase, milrinone enhances the effect of beta-adrenergic receptors and causes the heart to pump with more force.

Digoxin: In addition to its effects on vagal tone (which slows the heart), digoxin also binds to and blocks the sodium/potassium pump. The sodium/potassium pump normally acts to take sodium out of the cell and put potassium into the cell. When it is blocked, a side effect is that calcium builds up inside the cell. As calcium levels increase, the heart muscle cells contract with more force.

When are inotrope medications used?

Catecholamines are generally used only in the hospital when patients are in severe heart failure. By enhancing the heart's contraction, catecholamines can force the heart to pump the larger volume of blood that the body needs. For a patient in severe heart failure, dobutamine is the most commonly used inotrope. When heart failure reaches the point that blood pressure is dangerously low (cardiogenic shock), patients are often started on dopamine or norepinephrine. All catecholamines can be given only through a large intravenous line. For a small group of patients who have severe heart failure that is not likely to improve, it is possible to be sent home with continuous dobutamine.

Bipyridines (such as milrinone) are used for patients with severe heart failure that can no longer be man-aged with pills (such as digoxin) alone. It can only be given intravenously and requires that the patient be attached to an IV pump twenty-four hours a day. It is preferred over dobutamine for patients outside the hospital. In general, patients who require continuous milrinone treatment should also be evaluated for the feasibility of a heart transplant.

Digoxin is typically taken as a pill. It is indicated for patients with atrial fibrillation or atrial flutter (especially if they also have heart failure). For patients with heart failure, digoxin is used to reduce symptoms (shortness of breath and fatigue) and decrease the need for hospitalization.

What are some of the side effects of inotropes?

Catecholamines: There is an increased risk of dangerously fast heart rhythms (atrial tachycardia, ventricular tachycardia, and ventricular fibrillation) while receiving catecholamines. Because they can only be given intravenously, there is also a risk of infection associated with having a central venous catheter.

Milrinone: Like catecholamines, milrinone increases the risk of dangerous and potentially fatal arrhythmias such as ventricular tachycardia.

Digoxin: The adverse side effects associated with digoxin use depend on how much digoxin is in the body. At high blood levels, the effects include nausea, vomiting, diarrhea, visual disturbances (yellow-green halos), confusion, depression, dizziness, and delirium. Like the other inotropes, digoxin can also cause arrhythmias such as ventricular tachycardia.

NITRATES

Nitrates are a class of medications used to treat angina, the chest pressure or discomfort that occurs when the heart is not getting enough blood. Nitrates come in several different formulations, such as nitroglycerin, isosorbide dinitrate, and isosorbide mononitrate.

How do nitrates work?

Once inside the body, nitrates are converted to nitric oxide, which acts to dilate (open) arteries and veins. By dilating arteries, nitric oxide increases the blood flow in the heart's arteries to the heart muscle. Also, by dilating veins, nitrates reduce the flow of blood returning to the heart, which reduces the workload placed on the heart.

When are nitrates used?

The primary use of nitrates is to treat angina. Angina is the most common symptom of CAD. As the blockages in the arteries to the heart become larger, less and less blood reaches the heart muscle. When there is no longer enough blood to meet the heart's needs, patients develop angina.

Nitrates can be taken under the tongue (as sublingual nitroglycerin) when symptoms of angina develop. Sublingual nitroglycerin is short-acting, with its effect lasting less than five to ten minutes. Nitrates can also be taken as longer-lasting pills to prevent angina from occurring in the first place.

When combined with a blood pressure medication called hydralazine, nitrates can also be used to treat patients with heart failure, especially if they cannot tolerate ACE-inhibitors.

What are some of the side effects of nitrates?

Patients can develop severe headaches (similar to migraines) while taking nitrates. Because of their ability to dilate blood vessels, nitrates can also cause a drop in blood pressure (hypotension) and an increase in heart rate (tachycardia). If taken too frequently, patients can develop tolerance to nitrates.

Nitrates are less effective for treating angina. Nitrates should not be used if Viagra or a related drug has been taken in the previous twenty-four to forty-eight hours.

Q. & A. with Dr. Cannon

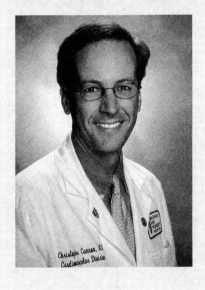

Q. Is aspirin a blood thinner?

A. Not really. In one sense, it is an anti-blood-clot agent, but it is not really a blood thinner. There are two major types of anticlotting drugs: anticoagulants and antiplatelets. Anticoagulants are well described as blood thinners because they decrease the blood's ability to clot; warfarin, the most widely used oral anticoagulant, does this by decreasing the number of clotting factors in the bloodstream. Antiplatelet agents work on the platelets, which are small, irregularly shaped, colorless cells found in blood. Their sticky surface helps form blood clots. Aspirin is an antiplatelet agent and thus is not really a blood thinner.

Q. Do statins (e.g., Lipitor or Crestor) damage the liver?

A. No. Although these agents can change the workings of liver cells and increase the levels of liver enzymes seen in blood tests, no cases of actual damage to the liver have been reported. If you have increased liver enzymes, they do need attention, however, and your doctor will usually recheck and likely reduce the dose of the statin or try a different statin drug, if not another type of lipid-lowering agent. In large studies, the increase in liver enzymes occurs in fewer than 5 percent of patients taking these drugs.

Q. If I take a diuretic for my blood pressure, do I need to eat a banana every day?

A. No, not necessarily. Diuretic medications increase the amount of urine you make and help reduce blood pressure and fluid buildup in congestive heart failure. With the increased urine flow is increased elimination of potassium in the urine. Therefore, you do have to monitor your potassium to ensure that it stays at a stable, normal level. If it is low, your doctor might ask you to take a potassium pill or potentially eat bananas. However, other foods with potassium, such as tomatoes, could help as well. Thus, you don't have to eat "a banana a day," but you will have to check your potassium levels with your doctor.

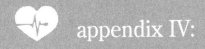 appendix IV:

HEART-SAVING PROCEDURES

Over the past decade, cardiology has advanced significantly. An array of new tools and approaches are now available to cardiologists and cardiac surgeons for the treatment of heart disease. In the following sections, we will discuss the most commonly used procedures. This is not an exhaustive list, but it covers the vast majority of procedures that cardiac patients undergo.

PERCUTANEOUS CORONARY INTERVENTION (PCI)

Percutaneous coronary intervention (PCI), also known as angioplasty, uses a plastic catheter with a balloon at the end to open narrowed arteries in the heart. This procedure is similar to but distinct from coronary angiography, in which a catheter is used to identify blocked arteries in the heart (see appendix II).

Who benefits from PCI?

PCI has been most clearly established as a beneficial procedure for patients having a heart attack. Numerous studies have demonstrated that early intervention with angioplasty and/or coronary artery stenting can be lifesaving during a heart attack. If a patient has a heart attack and arrives at a hospital that has interventional cardiologists who do PCI, early PCI is the treatment of choice.

PCI is also performed in patients with stable coronary artery disease (CAD) who have angina that cannot be treated by medication alone. A stable patient is defined as one whose symptoms are predictable. For example, the patient knows he or she will have chest pain after ten minutes of walking at a normal pace. Patients with chest pain at rest, those whose chest pain is becoming increasingly easier to provoke, or patients in the midst of a heart attack are not considered stable.

PCI with stents is superior to medications for managing the symptoms of severe stable angina, especially if medications have already failed to bring relief to the patient. PCI for these patients will often relieve the angina and limitations on activity associated with severe CAD. However, despite symptom relief, the latest large clinical trials have demonstrated that there is no mortality benefit to stents in this setting. Patients who receive stents for stable CAD, no matter the severity, do not live longer than patients treated only with medications.

It is important to note that not all patients who undergo stress tests (e.g., treadmill tests) need catheterization. In fact, the purpose of the stress test is to separate patients who could benefit from catheterization from those who would not.

Some patients fall in both of the categories mentioned above, but PCI is not always the recommended treatment. Patients with blockages in the left main coronary artery (the biggest artery supplying blood to the heart), patients with blockages in multiple arteries, diabetic patients, and patients with reduced heart function are likely to benefit more from coronary bypass surgery. Recent studies have shown that patients with left main coronary artery blockage can also benefit from PCI if the procedure is performed by a very experienced cardiologist.

What happens during PCI?

PCI is performed under conscious sedation. Patients are given sedatives and pain medications prior to the procedure to help prevent anxiety and discomfort during it. Once the patient is comfortable, a plastic catheter is inserted into the femoral artery in the leg. The catheter is advanced through the blood vessels to the heart, where a contrast dye is injected. This allows the cardiologist to identify the blocked vessels. Once the blockages in the artery are identified, a catheter with a balloon is inserted into the blocked artery. Inflating the balloon pushes cholesterol plaques and blood clots away from the center of the vessel, allowing blood to flow normally. This type of PCI is called balloon angioplasty and was the first catheterization treatment technique developed. It has largely been replaced by stenting.

Stenting

A stent is a small metal mesh that resembles a spring in a ballpoint pen. It is inserted in the coronary artery at sites of blockages to "stent" open the artery. A specialist called an interventional cardiologist uses a balloon to expand the stent at the correct site in the artery. Once expanded, the stent remains open, preventing the blockages from re-forming in the blood vessel. Stenting of blockages provides a more reliable and durable fix than plain balloon angioplasty.

There are different commercially available stents, and the interventional cardiologist may choose the one that is right for the patient and the individual blockages. There are two main types of stents: bare-metal and drug-eluting. The bare-metal stent is simply that: made of bare metal. The drug-eluting stent looks similar to the bare-metal stent but has a chemical coating that releases a drug from the metal backbone. The drug blocks surrounding blood vessel cells from scarring over the stent. This helps prevent the need to reopen the stent in the future.

What are the risks associated with PCI?

PCI is a well-tolerated procedure, and the complications associated with it are infrequent and usually not severe. The most common complication is bleeding and discomfort at the site where the catheter was inserted. This can often be controlled with pain medications and by applying pressure at the site. As with

any invasive procedure, infection both at the site of catheter insertion and in the bloodstream can occur. Rarely, bleeding at the catheterization site can be severe enough to require blood transfusions. Insertion of the catheter in the artery can also cause fistulas (inappropriate connections between the arteries and veins) or pseudoaneurysms (out-pouchings of the wall of the artery). Occasionally, PCI creates a small tear, or dissection, in the coronary artery. Usually, the tear is small and heals by itself. If the tear is severe, it requires immediate treatment, either with another stent placed over the tear or rarely, with urgent bypass surgery (we discuss the details of coronary bypass surgery later in this appendix).

Chest pain after PCI can occur. It is usually caused by small tears in the arteries of the heart, small pieces of cholesterol plaques or blood clots which embolize (or flow down the artery) to a smaller artery and cause a blockage, or vasospasms (spasms of the muscles of the artery wall). The chest pain is usually not severe and does not cause any significant damage to the heart muscles. Patients rarely have significant heart damage due to PCI.

PCI is a proven treatment that saves lives in heart attack patients and relieves the chest discomfort and limitations on activity caused by angina. Its overall success is limited by one of two phenomena:

Restenosis is a slow narrowing of the artery that can occur within months of angioplasty. If the restenosis is severe enough, angina symptoms can come back, and patients may require repeat PCI. Certain conditions also make it more likely that restenosis will occur, including diabetes, high blood pressure, and high cholesterol. It is important, therefore, that these conditions be treated appropriately. Continued smoking will also make restenosis more likely; for this reason, it is vital that smoking cessation be a high priority. The main advantage of stents over balloon angioplasty is in preventing restenosis. Furthermore, drug-eluting stents work better at preventing restenosis than bare-metal stents.

Stent thrombosis: In a small group of patients, the stent can become 100 percent blocked due to blood clots. This can occur anytime, from immediately after the stent is placed in the artery to years after the procedure. Most often, it occurs within thirty days of the procedure.

Stent thrombosis will cause a myocardial infarction (MI) and must be treated as an emergency. The risk of stent thrombosis can be reduced by taking aspirin indefinitely and clopidogrel for one year or longer after stent placement. If you have a drug-eluting stent, the current expert guidelines recommend that patients do not stop taking clopidogrel for at least one year.

Care after PCI

It is important to realize that PCI does not replace the need for medical treatment of CAD. The procedure should be considered as an addition to medicines and lifestyle changes that are proven lifesavers for patients with CAD. Regular exercise, weight loss, and quitting smoking are as important after PCI as they were before. Medical treatments for high blood pressure and high cholesterol must also be continued. If PCI is performed with stent placement, it is vital to take aspirin indefinitely and clopidogrel for at least one year to prevent stent thrombosis. Patients with stents should never stop taking aspirin and clopidogrel without specific instruction from a cardiologist.

CORONARY ARTERY BYPASS GRAFT (CABG)

Who needs a CABG?

CABG is an invasive method for treating coronary heart disease (CHD). CHD is a condition whereby the arteries supplying blood to the heart are blocked by the accumulation of cholesterol, calcium, and blood clots. PCI is the alternative invasive method discussed earlier. Both approaches are used in situations when medical therapy alone is not enough.

Patients with blockages in multiple arteries or with a blockage in the left main artery (the biggest and most important artery supplying blood to the heart) will likely benefit more from CABG than from PCI. If the patient's heart shows reduced pumping function (as measured by stress tests or echocardiography), the patient is also likely to benefit from CABG. If stable angina is severe enough to be intolerable or severely limits a patient's activity despite appropriate medical therapy, CABG is considered.

What is CABG?

CABG is surgery in which a vein or artery from another location in the body is removed and reattached to the blood vessels feeding the heart to bypass a blockage. The surgery is performed under general anesthesia while the patient is unconscious due to medications, with a breathing tube in place. An incision is made in the front of the chest and the sternum (breastbone) is cut to open the chest wall and allow access to the heart. This incision is called a median sternotomy. To attach the bypass vessels to the heart safely, the heart must usually be stopped. This can be done with relative safety because the patient is attached to a cardiopulmonary bypass machine, which functions as an artificial heart and lung. Blood is channeled from the body into the cardiopulmonary machine, where it is oxygenated and returned to the body. While the patient is on bypass, the bypass vessels are attached (grafted) to the aorta and to the coronary (heart) artery beyond the blockage. This allows blood to flow from the aorta to the coronary artery and bypass the blockage. If there are multiple blockages, multiple bypass vessels are grafted to the aorta and coronary arteries. Once the bypass vessels have been attached, the patient is removed from the cardiopulmonary machine and the heart is restarted.

New techniques have been developed that allow for off-pump surgery during which the surgeon operates on a beating heart. This approach is more difficult, cannot always be utilized depending on the location of the blockages, and requires a skilled surgeon. It does, however, prevent some of the complications that arise from being on the cardiopulmonary machine. Another novel approach is called minimally invasive surgery. As opposed to the eight-inch scar of a traditional CABG, the incisions with minimally invasive surgery are only two to three inches long. As a result, there is less bleeding, a lower risk of infection, and a faster recovery.

An important component of CABG surgery is the choice of bypass vessel. Three types of blood vessels are commonly used:

Left internal mammary artery (LIMA): The LIMA is an artery that runs along the inside of the chest wall. It has several advantages over saphenous veins (discussed shortly). First, it does not need to be fully detached. Instead, only one end is removed and attached to the blocked coronary artery after the blockage. Because the LIMA is an artery (as opposed to a vein), it is far less likely to lose its function over time. LIMAs can be expected to last for twenty years.

Right internal mammary artery (RIMA): The RIMA has all the advantages of the LIMA. However, it is used less often than the LIMA because it is located on the right side of the chest wall and so is farther away from the heart's arteries.

Saphenous vein: The saphenous vein is located in the leg and removed (harvested) prior to opening the chest wall. The saphenous vein is easy to harvest, with minimal effect on the leg from which it is removed. Unfortunately, saphenous vein grafts very frequently become blocked after surgery. Typically, they last five to ten years.

Radial artery: The radial artery is located in the forearm and, like the LIMA, is an artery and not a vein. As a result, it is effective for a longer time (although not as long as LIMAs). Unlike the LIMA, the radial artery must be fully removed from the arm and reattached to both the aorta and the blocked coronary artery.

Because CABG is more invasive than PCI, the postoperative recovery is more difficult. The patient typically requires one to three days of care in an intensive care unit where he or she can be more closely monitored for signs of complications. If there are no complications, the patient is often transferred to a regular hospital floor for an additional two to three days. Typically, patients are in the hospital for four to six days after CABG. Unlike PCI, patients usually require four to five weeks of recovery time before returning to work. Patients also require more intensive postsurgical physical therapy. Full recovery often does not occur for several months after surgery.

What are the risks of CABG?
CABG is a significant surgery that requires more time and effort for recovery than PCI. As a conse-

quence, the risks of complications that result in significant illness or even death are higher with CABG than with PCI. The benefit of CABG is in the long run; coronary disease that has been treated with CABG remains treated for a longer time than when treated with PCI.

Numerous complications are associated with CABG, including those that can occur with any significant surgery. These include infection, bleeding, and heart attack (MI). We will focus here on some of the complications that are relatively unique to open-heart surgery:

Atrial fibrillation and other arrhythmias: Atrial fibrillation is very common after CABG surgery and occurs in up to 40 percent of patients. Patients have a fast, irregular heart rate when they are in atrial fibrillation. This rhythm does not usually last very long and can be easily treated with medications that slow the heart rate. However, occasionally patients remain in atrial fibrillation for several weeks or longer after CABG. Bradycardia (slow heart rate), ventricular tachycardia, and ventricular fibrillation (a dangerous rhythm that requires a patient to be "shocked" back to a normal rhythm) can also occur but far less commonly than with atrial fibrillation.

Pericarditis: The pericardium is a sac that surrounds the heart. Because CABG surgery requires manipulation of arteries located in the pericardium, pericarditis, which is an inflammation of the pericardium, often occurs. Pericarditis results in chest discomfort that can be treated with pain medication such as ibuprofen. Pericarditis can also result in accumulation of fluid in the pericardium. If a large volume of fluid accumulates, the patient may have to return to the operating room for drainage of the fluid.

Stroke: Patients undergoing CABG are at increased risk of stroke because of several different factors. Heart attack patients in general are at increased risk of stroke, but the CABG procedure itself and being placed on a cardiopulmonary bypass machine increase this risk. Developing atrial fibrillation increases the risk even further. CABG patients can have both ischemic strokes (blockages in the arteries going to the brain) and hemorrhagic strokes (bleeding in the brain).

Complication of cardiopulmonary bypass machine: The cardiopulmonary bypass machine is a lifesaving device, which allows for a number of operations in addition to CABG that would not be possible otherwise. An unfortunate consequence of its use is short-term and long-term cognitive damage (such as memory loss) that is often more pronounced in the elderly.

Care after CABG

As with PCI, CABG is not a replacement for the medical management and lifestyle modification typically used to treat CAD. Patients should continue to take the medications necessary to control blood pressure, lower cholesterol levels, and treat diabetes. Patients should also continue with a regular exercise regimen, eat a healthy diet, and stop smoking if they have not already done so. If not, the long-term benefits of an invasive procedure can be largely lost.

PACEMAKERS

Who needs a pacemaker?

The heart, in essence, is a mechanical pump propelling blood throughout the body. To pump regularly and respond to the body's changing demand for blood (e.g., more during exercise, less during sleep), the heart also has an intrinsic electrical system that signals each time it's supposed to beat and carries this signal throughout the heart so that all parts pump in a coordinated manner. The signal to contract usually begins in the part of the heart called the sinoatrial (SA) node. From the SA node, the signal travels through the upper chambers of the heart (atria) to the atrioventricular (AV) node and from there to the lower chambers of the heart or ventricles. The signal is delayed at the AV node to allow for the atria to fully contract and push blood into the ventricles. The electrical impulse is then carried through the ventricles, causing their contraction and the pumping of blood into the body. The ventricles are the main pumping chambers of the heart, making it vital that they contract at a regular, reliable rate.

In many people, this electrical system breaks down or operates in an uncontrolled manner, resulting in heart rates that are too slow (bradycardia) or too fast (tachycardia), or in an unsynchronized fashion (dyssychrony).

Bradycardias are by far the most common reason for a pacemaker implantation, and can occur due to one of two mechanisms. Either the SA node may stop firing at a rate that is sufficient for the body's needs (sinus bradycardia) or the AV node may stop conducting the signal from the atria to the ventricles (atrioventricular block). In both situations, the net effect is that the ventricles do not contract at a rate that is fast enough to meet the body's needs. Patients often feel lightheaded or even pass out when their heart rate is not adequate.

Tachycardias are generally not treated with pacemakers. If a patient has atrial fibrillation (where the atria are firing at a very fast, irregular rate) the heart can start contracting at a rate that is too fast. This condition is usually treated with medications that slow the heart. If medications are not successful or possible, it may be necessary to do an ablation, which intentionally damages part of the AV node. This slows the heart so that the ventricles do not contract in response to the excessive number of signals coming from the atria. As a consequence, however, the patient is given an atrioventricular block.

Some patients have what is known as sick sinus syndrome (SSS), which results in alternating tachycardia (fast heart rate) and bradycardia (slow heart rate). Unfortunately, because the medications for tachycardia almost by definition will worsen the bradycardia, patients with SSS often require pacemakers.

Dyssynchrony is a term used to refer to abnormal beating of the two sides of the heart. This happens when the conduction of the electrical beats is delayed due to heart disease, which is seen in many patients with weakened hearts and low ejection fraction. Instead of the left and right sides of the heart beating in synch, one beats a bit earlier than the other, and then the mechanical pumping is not as strong. Using a special "dual chamber" pacemaker—one that goes to both the left and right sides of the heart—can get the beats back in synch and lead to better pumping of the heart.

Expert panels have devised specific guidelines that spell out the situations in which it is recommended that a patient receive a pacemaker. A patient's personal cardiologist is in the best position to determine whether he is likely to benefit from a pacemaker.

What is a pacemaker?

A pacemaker is a small electronic device that is usually implanted under the skin in the chest. It comprises two key components: the pulse generator and the leads.

(1) The pulse generator contains the computer that determines at what rate the pacemaker will signal the heart to beat. It also contains the battery that provides the energy needed to generate the electrical signals sent to the heart.

(2) The leads are flexible wires that extend from the pulse generator to the heart and carry the electrical signal to the heart. In almost all modern pacemakers, they also carry information about the heart's activity back to the pulse generator. In this way, the computer inside the pulse generator can monitor what the heart is doing and respond to it appropriately. Depending on the type of pacemaker, up to three leads can go from the pulse generator to the heart.

Pacemakers come in three main types: single-chamber, dual-chamber, and biventricular, depending on the number of leads. Single-chamber pacemakers have a single lead going to either the right atrium or the right ventricle. Dual-chamber pacemakers have two leads, one going to the right atrium and the other to the right ventricle. Biventricular pacemakers have an additional third lead going to the left ventricle. Biventricular pacemakers are used only in patients with heart failure. Each of these pacemakers can be programmed to monitor not only the heart's activity but also the body's activity and adjust to make sure the heart rate matches the body's needs.

What are the risks of getting a pacemaker?

The major risks of getting a pacemaker are associated with their implantation and, when necessary, their removal. As with any invasive procedure, there is a risk of bleeding and infection. During implantation, a "pocket" or space is made under the skin of the chest wall where the pulse generator is placed. This pocket can get infected, and bleeding can occur into the pocket, necessitating removal of the pacemaker. Also during implantation, the leads are advanced through veins in the body to the heart where they are screwed into the muscle of the heart. During lead implantation, a hole can form in the wall of the heart, resulting in bleeding into the sac around the heart. Over the long term, leads placed in the heart can break or stop functioning properly, and therefore must be removed. Removal of pacemaker leads is a more complicated procedure, with notably higher risks of bleeding and damage to the walls of the heart than implantation.

Care after Getting a Pacemaker

Regular follow-up by a cardiologist or an electrophysiologist (a highly trained cardiologist who specializes in the electric system of the heart) is required for any patient with a pacemaker. These follow-ups are to ensure that the pacemaker is functioning properly and that the pacemaker's battery has enough energy reserve. In more modern pacemakers, it is possible to get tele-checkups. Patients are provided with a special phone that can "interrogate" the pacemaker. During an interrogation, information about the pacemaker's function, the patient's own heart function, and battery power reserves is downloaded and sent to the electrophysiologist taking care of the patient.

Patients are often concerned about the limitations on activity imposed by pacemakers and the possible interference with pacemaker function from a variety of electronic equipment. It is important to realize that there are few true limitations on people who have pacemakers. Household appliances do not pose a risk to patients with pacemakers. Certain medical procedures can interfere with pacemaker function (e.g., magnetic resonance imaging [MRI] or radiation therapy for cancer), and prior to undergoing any test or procedure, patients should ensure that their health care provider is aware of the pacemaker.

IMPLANTABLE CARDIOVERTER DEFIBRILLATOR (ICD)

What is an ICD?

ICDs are electrical devices that monitor the heart's activity for dangerous rhythms and if necessary, provide an electrical shock to the heart to restore a normal rhythm. ICDs are in many ways similar to pacemakers. In fact, many ICDs used now also can function as pacemakers. Like a pacemaker, an ICD contains a pulse generator placed in a pocket under the skin of the chest. The pulse generator has the ICD's battery and computer. Leads extend through the large veins in the chest from the pulse generator to the muscle of the heart. These leads carry electrical energy from the ICD to the heart and return information collected about the heart's activity back to the ICD.

ICDs monitor the heart for dangerous heart rhythms such as ventricular tachycardia and ventricular fibrillations. If these rhythms are sensed, the ICD will attempt to return the heart to a normal rhythm in one of three ways:

Antitachycardia pacing: The initial response of the ICD is usually antitachycardia pacing, during which the ICD provides a rapid sequence of low-energy electrical signals to the heart (much like a pacemaker). In many situations, these signals override the ar-

rhythmia and return the heart to a normal rhythm. Antitachycardia pacing is not painful and in the vast majority of cases is not felt by the patient.

Cardioversion/defibrillation: If antitachycardia pacing fails or is not appropriate, the ICD will provide a high-energy shock to the heart. Whether the shock is a cardioversion or a defibrillation depends on the particular arrhythmia the ICD is trying to treat (for the patient there is essentially no difference). If the patient is awake when the ICD attempts a cardioversion/defibrillation, the shock is quite painful.

Because patients who need ICDs also often need pacemakers, ICDs can be present in the context of any of the different types of pacemakers discussed earlier (single-chamber, dual-chamber, or biventricular).

Who needs an ICD?

Patients at risk of sudden cardiac death have been shown to benefit from ICDs. Sudden cardiac death is caused by an abnormal heart rhythm called ventricular fibrillation or ventricular tachycardia. Ventricular fibrillation is almost uniformly lethal unless treated immediately, whereas ventricular tachycardia can range in severity from deadly to barely noticeable.

When a patient develops abnormal rhythms, his heart's electric activity is incapable of directing the heart to contract in a manner sufficient to pump blood to the body and most importantly the brain.

When people are said to "have a heart attack and drop dead," the cause of death is sudden cardiac death. It is important to understand, however, that the general term heart attack does not mean the same thing as sudden cardiac death. A heart attack

(MI) is only one of many causes of sudden cardiac death. ICDs are used to prevent sudden cardiac death, not MI.

One of the most common causes of ventricular tachycardia and ventricular fibrillation is ischemia (when the heart is not getting enough blood). A number of other medical conditions place patients at high risk of sudden cardiac death, including cardiomyopathy (damage to the heart muscle) and heart failure. A smaller number of patients, despite having hearts that are structurally normal, are at high risk of ventricular fibrillation and ventricular tachycardia because they have inherited genes that interfere with the normal function of the electrical system of the heart.

The indications for ICD placement fall under two broad categories:

Primary prevention: The risk of sudden cardiac death is high enough with certain medical conditions to justify the placement of an ICD despite the absence of any recorded episodes of ventricular tachycardia or ventricular fibrillation. This is called primary prevention. The patients who qualify for primary prevention generally have significant reduction of their heart function (heart failure).

Secondary prevention: After patients have had an episode of ventricular tachycardia or ventricular fibrillation (which they have survived), an ICD is placed for secondary prevention. Because they have already had an episode of arrhythmia, such patients are clearly identifiable as being at high risk of having future episodes.

Expert panels have created guidelines that provide recommendations as to who might benefit from an ICD. Given the complexity of deciding whether someone qualifies for an ICD and potential downsides of having one, the best person, as always, to guide a patient is his or her own cardiologist.

What are the risks of an ICD?

The risks of placing and (if necessary) removing an ICD are very similar to the risks in placement and removal of pacemakers. In addition, having an ICD carries risks that are unique. It is important to realize that ICDs are proven lifesavers. In properly selected patients, those who get ICDs live longer than those who do not. The computer programs of modern ICDs can often differentiate between dangerous rhythms such as ventricular tachycardia or fibrillation and rhythms that are not dangerous such as atrial fibrillation. Unfortunately, they are not perfect. As a result, ICDs can often interpret heart rhythms which are not dangerous as being dangerous and inappropriately shock the patient. In addition, over time, leads can fail. As they fail, they may start interpreting the heart's activity incorrectly, again resulting in shocks that are inappropriate. Because inappropriate shocks almost always occur when a patient is awake, they are painful. Many patients can develop severe anxiety about possible ICD shocks. In fact, post-traumatic stress disorder has been identified in many of these patients. ICDs are proven lifesavers, but they have clear risks associated with them. It is vital to ensure that the benefits outweigh the risks before implanting one.

Care after Getting an ICD

Patients with ICDs, like patients with pacemakers, need regular, close follow-ups with an electrophysiologist. During these checkups, the electrophysiologist evaluates the ICD to ensure that it is functioning properly and has enough battery power, and reviews the information the ICD has recorded about the patient's heart function. As with modern pacemakers, this interrogation of the ICD can be done over special telephones, which allow the ICD to be checked from the patient's home. Based on the information collected from the ICD, the electrophysiologist can adjust the ICD's computer program to better match the patient's particular condition. Beyond regular visits, if your ICD fires you should contact your cardiologist immediately.

Having an ICD places essentially the same limitations on activity as having a pacemaker. These limitations are generally minor (e.g., patients with these devices cannot get MRIs). As with pacemakers, prior to any medical procedure or test the health care provider should be made aware that the patient has an ICD.

ARRHYTHMIA ABLATION

Who needs arrhythmia ablation?

Arrhythmia ablation is a procedure that is used to treat patients with tachycardia. As discussed previously, the heart is, in essence, a mechanical pump that is controlled by an internal electrical system that tells it when to pump. The SA node is a specialized part of the heart that normally generates the electrical signal for each heartbeat. In a number of conditions, the heart beats at a faster rate than is required because an electrical signal is inappropriately generated elsewhere in the heart. If this electrical signal is firing at a rate faster than the SA node, it can override the SA node and cause the heart to beat faster than what is needed or desired. This condition is called tachycardia. A patient might have a tachycardia for a number of different reasons.

Atrial fibrillation is the most common arrhythmia (abnormal heart rhythm). It is caused by many small electrical circuits in the top chambers of the heart (atrium) that fire concurrently at a very fast and erratic rate. As a result, the heart pumps at a fast and irregular rate. This condition is usually treated by medications that either keep the heart from going into atrial fibrillation or if it does, keep it from going too fast. For some patients, medications fail and ablation may become necessary.

Atrial flutter is in many ways similar to atrial fibrillation, but instead of many small electrical circuits in the atrium, one large electrical circuit is firing at a fast but regular rate. Because there is only one electrical circuit, ablation of atrial flutter is often much easier and more successful than ablation of atrial fibrillation. As a result, ablation is often the first treatment for atrial flutter, as opposed to those patients with atrial fibrillation who undergo ablation only when medical therapy has failed.

AV nodal reentrant tachycardia is an arrhythmia caused by an electrical circuit that is localized to the AV node. The AV node is the location of the electrical connection between the atria of the heart and the ventricles of the heart. The AV node normally functions to slow the signals coming from the atrium to the ventricle. During AV nodal reentrant tachycardia, instead of slowing down the atrial signal, the AV node generates a rapid electrical signal of its own, causing the ventricles (which are the main blood pumping parts of the heart) to contract at too fast a rate.

Wolff-Parkinson-White syndrome occurs when a bypass tract allows electrical signals to bypass the AV node and go directly to the ventricles. As a result, the normal delay between atrial pumping and ventricular pumping is lost. Although this is usually well tolerated by itself, having a bypass tract makes it more likely that the heart will go into other fast rhythms, which can be uncomfortable and potentially dangerous to patients.

Ventricular tachycardia is a dangerous heart rhythm. It most often occurs in patients with heart failure or prior heart attacks and occurs because of an electrical circuit that fires at a fast rate from within the ventricles. Patients with ventricular tachycardias most often have ICDs implanted. As discussed earlier, ICDs can shock patients out of ventricular tachycardia. However, being repeatedly shocked by an ICD is traumatic, and patients often require ablation to lessen the frequency of ICD shocks. In addition, some patients develop ventricular tachycardias that are too slow to trigger their ICD but are still uncomfortable or intolerable.

Determining whether ablation is appropriate for you is almost always a complex decision and should be made in discussion with your cardiologist and an electrophysiologist.

What is arrhythmia ablation?
Arrhythmia ablation is a procedure during which catheters are inserted into the large veins in the body (usually the groin) and advanced to the heart. From inside the heart, the electrophysiologist can "map" the electrical system of the heart and identify the location from which the arrhythmia is generated. Once the source of arrhythmia is identified, it is ablated by one of two methods. With radiofrequency ablation, high-frequency electrical signals are used to permanently damage the area of tissue in the heart from which the arrhythmia is generated. Alternatively, the area of tissue may be ablated by freezing it (cryoablation).

What are the risks of arrhythmia ablation?
As with any invasive procedure, there is a risk of bleeding and infection after arrhythmia ablation. As with PCI, complications can arise at the site of catheter insertion in the groin (bleeding, pseudoaneurysm, arteriovenous fistula, and loss of blood flow to the legs). These complications are rare and can most often be treated easily. Some complications are relatively unique to arrhythmia ablation:

Heart block: Because arrhythmia ablations involve not only inserting catheters into the heart but also intentionally damaging heart tissue, it is possible to damage the normal electrical system of the heart. In situations where the arrhythmia being ablated is near the AV node, patients may develop heart block, which is a failure of signals from the atria to reach the ventricles. In such a situation, temporary and sometimes permanent pacemakers are required.

Pulmonary embolus and stroke: Damaging the tissue inside the heart during an ablation makes it more likely that blood clots will form at those sites. If the ablation is in the right side of the heart, blood clots can travel to the lungs, causing a pulmonary embolism. If the ablation is in the left side of the heart, blood clots can travel to the brain, causing a stroke.

Perforation: Because ablation involves intentionally damaging the heart muscle, there is a risk of excessive damage resulting in a hole in the heart wall (perforation).

Care after Arrhythmia Ablation
Arrhythmia ablation is a complex procedure that requires close follow-up with an electrophysiologist to ensure that the ablation has worked, that the old arrhythmia has not resurfaced, and that new ones have not developed. In addition, patients who undergo ablation most often have other significant heart prob-

lems requiring multiple medications, and therefore need close follow-up with a general cardiologist.

REPAIR OF VALVULAR HEART DISEASE

How do the valves work?

The heart is a mechanical pump that propels blood around the body in one direction. Blood returning from the body enters the heart into the right atrium. From the right atrium, blood goes into the right ventricle, where it is pumped into the lungs. After picking up oxygen in the lungs, blood returns to the left atrium and from there enters the left ventricle. As the largest of the four chambers of the heart, the left ventricle is responsible for pumping blood to the body (excluding the lungs). To ensure that blood does, in fact, go in one direction, the heart has valves. Valves have two main functions. They must open easily and widely when blood is being pumped forward, and they must close completely afterward so that blood does not flow backward. There are four valves in the heart:

- The tricuspid valve ensures that blood does not get pumped back from the right ventricle into the right atrium.
- The pulmonary valve prevents blood pumped into the lungs by the right ventricle from flowing back into the right ventricle.
- The mitral valve is between the left atrium and left ventricle and prevents blood from going backward from the left ventricle into the left atrium.
- The aortic valve ensures that blood pumped into the body by the left ventricle does not flow backward.

Valves can become dysfunctional in one of two ways. Stenotic valves prevent easy forward flow of blood because they have become so rigid that they are difficult to open. Insufficient valves fail to prevent backward flow of blood because they cannot close properly. Any of the valves of the heart can become dysfunctional in either fashion, but valvular heart disease most commonly affects the aortic and mitral valves.

Aortic Valve

Stenosis: The most common problem with patients with aortic valve disease is stenosis. Aortic valve stenosis most often develops because of aging, but it can also occur after rheumatic heart disease or due to congenital abnormalities in the structure of the aortic valve (congenital abnormalities are those that someone is born with).

A stenotic aortic valve places a significant amount of pressure on the left ventricle, which now has to pump very hard to get blood out to the body. As a result, patients begin to develop chest pain (angina), pass out (syncope), or become short of breath more easily (heart failure). Patients with stenotic aortic valves require surgery once they have these symptoms or if they are already undergoing open-heart surgery for another reason (e.g., a CABG). In addition, certain patients without any symptoms who are not otherwise undergoing heart surgery may still need to have a stenotic aortic valve fixed because the stenosis *is* so severe that it is only a matter of time before they develop symptoms or their left ventricle begins to fail.

Insufficiency: Aortic valve insufficiency (or aortic regurgitation) is the opposite problem from aortic stenosis. The aortic valve does not close properly after the left ventricle beats and blood flows backward into the left ventricle. As a result, the left ventricle is placed under stress, as it needs to pump more blood to meet the body's needs (to make up for the blood that is flowing backward).

Aortic insufficiency has a number of different causes, including congenital abnormalities in the structure of the aortic valve, high blood pressure, aortic aneurysm (which occurs when the large blood vessel connected to the left ventricle becomes dilated), or an infection of the aortic valve. The repair of an insufficient aortic valve becomes necessary once there is evidence on an echocardiogram (see appendix II) that the left ventricle is beginning to fail. In addition, if a patient with aortic insufficiency is undergoing heart surgery for another reason, the aortic valve is repaired so as to avoid a repeat surgery in the future.

Mitral Valve

Stenosis: Mitral valve stenosis is usually caused by either rheumatic heart disease or a congenital structural abnormality. Mitral valve stenosis makes it difficult for blood to flow from the left atrium to the left ventricle. As a result, pressure inside the left atrium increases over time. The increased pressure causes the left atrium to dilate (get bigger) and makes it far more likely that atrial fibrillation (an abnormal fast and irregular heart rhythm) will develop. The combination of left atrial dilatation and atrial fibrillation means patients are more likely to develop blood clots in the left atrium. In addition, the increased pressure in the left atrium can back up not only into the lungs, but also go all the way to the right side of the heart. If not treated, the result can be heart failure.

Insufficiency: Mitral valve insufficiency is usually called mitral valve regurgitation. It can be caused by a number of processes, including CAD, heart attacks, rheumatic heart disease, congenital heart disease, and/or infection of the mitral valve (endocarditis).

As a result of mitral regurgitation, when the left ventricle beats, not all of the blood flows forward to the body. To make sure the body's needs are met, the left ventricle has to pump more blood. Over time, the increased work this places on the left ventricle can cause heart failure. In addition, the blood that flows backward places more stress on the left atrium. Over time, the left atrium becomes dilated, and the risk of atrial fibrillation increases. Once patients start developing symptoms, such as shortness of breath, or there is evidence by echocardiogram (see appendix II) that the left ventricle is beginning to fail, repair or replacement of the mitral valve becomes necessary. Likewise, if a patient is about to undergo heart surgery for another reason, the mitral valve is repaired or replaced to prevent a repeat surgery in the future.

Stenosis of heart valves generally develops slowly over time. Insufficiency of a heart valve also can develop slowly over time or can occur suddenly (after a heart attack or because of an infection). When valve insufficiency occurs suddenly, it is often a medical emergency, and surgery is required right away.

How is valvular heart disease treated?
Heart valve dysfunction can be treated in one of two ways. The valve can be repaired or it can be replaced. If the aortic valve is diseased, it is almost always replaced. The mitral valve can be either repaired or replaced, depending on the specific clinical situation.

Valvuloplasty: Valvuloplasty is an approach used to repair stenotic valves. A catheter is inserted into a large blood vessel in the body (usually in the groin) and wires are advanced from there to the heart valve that is diseased. A deflated balloon is placed inside the valve opening. When the balloon is rapidly inflated, it cracks open the stenotic valve.

Valvuloplasty is a good approach to treat mitral valve stenosis because it is not invasive (i.e., it does not require open-heart surgery) and there is a good chance that it will be successful. For stenotic aortic valves, valvuloplasty is less useful because aortic valves tend to become stenotic again within six months and there is a good chance that aortic insufficiency will develop. As a result, valvuloplasty is used only as a "bridge" so that patients can get past whatever medical condition is temporarily preventing surgical replacement of the aortic valve.

Valve repair: Mitral valve insufficiency (or regurgitation) can be repaired with open-heart surgery. During valve repair, the surgeon will reshape the valve to prevent or reduce the backward flow of blood. If the valves are too big, the repair may include removal of excess tissue, tightening the rim around the valve (annuloplasty), or replacement of valve chords to better anchor the valve.

Valve repair carries all the risks of large invasive surgery, including many of the same risks associated with valve replacement surgery (discussed shortly) and CABG (discussed previously).

Recent developments allow mitral valve repair to be performed with only a small incision, as opposed to a full open-heart surgery. This approach is less invasive but also much more difficult. In certain patients, mitral valve repair can be accomplished percutaneously with catheters inserted in the groin and advanced to the heart (much like the PCIs discussed earlier). Percutaneous mitral valve repair is less invasive than open-heart surgery, and as a result, it is less likely to result in serious complications. Unfortunately, it cannot be used in most patients who need a mitral valve repair.

Although the aortic valve can also be repaired if necessary, it is far more common to replace an aortic valve than to repair it.

Valve replacement: Valve replacement requires open-heart surgery and is often done in conjunction with CABG. In fact, prior to valve replacement or repair, patients always undergo coronary angiography (see appendix II) to determine whether there is also a need for bypass surgery. Valve replacement surgery is done under general anesthesia and requires that the chest wall be opened (like in bypass surgery). Once the chest wall is opened, the heart must be stopped, and the patient is placed on a cardiopulmonary bypass machine that functions as an artificial heart and lung. Blood is channeled from the body into the cardiopulmonary machine where it is oxygenated and returned to the body. The surgeon then removes the damaged heart valve and replaces it with one of two types of artificial valves.

Bioprosthetic: Bioprosthetic valves are made from natural tissue. Most often, they are valves taken from a pig heart. Because they are not made from artificial material, bioprosthetic valves are far less likely to cause blood clots. As a result, patients often do not need to take warfarin (a blood thinner) after valve replacement surgery. On the other hand, because they are not made of metal, bioprosthetic valves are more likely to break down over time.

Mechanical: Mechanical valves come in a variety of shapes, but all are made of artificial material. Because of the strength of this material, they tend to last for a very long time. Unfortunately, the artificial material also makes it very likely that blood clots will form on them. To prevent blood clots, patients with mechanical valves are required to take warfarin for the rest of their lives.

In deciding between a mechanical or bioprosthetic valve, it is necessary to weigh the risks of lifelong warfarin therapy against the benefits of having a valve that most likely will not have to be replaced. If a patient cannot or will not take warfarin, the only choice is a bioprosthetic valve. For older patients, bioprosthetic valves are also preferred, because most likely the patient will pass away from other causes before the valve fails. For younger patients, mechanical valves are generally preferred so that a repeat surgery is not needed in the future.

Valve replacement surgery, like bypass surgery, is a large invasive procedure that requires at least several days in the hospital. Patients are at risk of bleeding, infections, and many of the same complications that occur with bypass surgery (discussed earlier).

Care after a Valve Repair/Replacement

Patients who have undergone valve repair or replacement need close follow-up with their cardiologist to ensure that the valves continue to function appropriately and that new valve dysfunction or heart failure is not developing. In addition, all patients with mechanical heart valves, as well as some patients with bioprosthetic heart valves, need to take blood thinners (warfarin). To make sure the level of blood thinning is adequate but not excessive, frequent INR (blood clotting) checks are needed (see appendix III). Bioprosthetic and mechanical valves are also more likely to become infected (endocarditis). If a replacement valve becomes infected, it is almost always necessary to replace it again. To avoid this, patients who have replaced valves must be careful to take antibiotics before any medical procedure, even simple dental procedures.

HEART TRANSPLANTATION

Heart transplantation is a complicated procedure that requires a significant amount of planning and testing in advance of the surgery and intensive treatment afterward. It is the only definitive long-term treatment currently available for end-stage heart failure. End-stage heart failure occurs when the heart can no longer pump enough blood to meet the body's basic needs despite maximal medical treatment. Because of the limited number of donor hearts available (approximately 2,000 per year), heart transplantation is an option for only a small number of the millions of patients suffering from heart failure.

Who is eligible for a heart transplant?

Prior to transplantation, patients undergo an intensive evaluation to ensure that they do not suffer from other significant medical problems (e.g., severe lung, liver, or kidney disease) that might make them ineligible for transplantation. The most common reason for being ineligible for transplantation is pulmonary hypertension, which is elevated blood pressure in the blood vessels of the heart. Other common causes of exclusion are active infection and a cancer diagnosis. If patients qualify for transplantation, they are added to a list of patients also awaiting a donor organ. Ranking on the list is determined by a combination of time on the list and severity of illness.

Care after a Heart Transplant

Heart transplant surgery is a complicated procedure performed at a relatively small number of medical centers. The surgery often requires intensive care afterward to recover from the operation and the complications associated with it. Patients require intensive immunosuppressive medications after a transplant, which makes them susceptible to infections. Almost 85 percent of transplant patients are alive one year after a heart transplant, significantly better than those patients who need a transplant but do not receive one. The most common causes of death early after transplant are acute rejection (when the body of the patient does not accept the donor heart) and infections, which are more severe because of immunosuppressive medications that help to prevent rejection. In the long term, death is usually caused by CAD in the transplanted heart. Secondarily, because of the immunosuppressive medications that patients must take for years after transplantation, they are at increased risk of developing cancers such as lymphoma.

Heart transplantation is an amazing lifesaving operation that is limited by the rarity of donor hearts. Because the demand for donor hearts is high, patients in need of transplantation are required to undergo intensive evaluation and are followed by highly trained experts in major medical centers. For more information concerning heart transplantation, See the United Network of Organ Sharing website, www.transplantliving.org.

ADVANCED CARDIOVASCULAR LIFE SUPPORT

Advanced Cardiovascular Life Support (ACLS) is not one specific procedure, but rather a set of procedures and medications used to treat patients with sudden cardiac arrest. ACLS is utilized by a team of trained professionals including physicians, nurses, paramedics, respiratory therapists, and pharmacists to resuscitate patients in emergency situations. Whenever ACLS is needed, the most important factor is time. The faster a patient receives ACLS-directed therapies, the more likely she is to live.

Who needs ACLS?

Patients who have suffered sudden cardiac arrest need to be treated according to the ACLS guidelines as quickly as possible. Sudden cardiac arrest occurs when the heart stops beating effectively so that it is no longer pumping blood to the body. Sudden cardiac arrest is a medical emergency, and prompt treatment is essential. Minutes matter because the longer the body (and most importantly, the brain) goes without blood, the less likely it is that the patient can be resuscitated. Although sudden cardiac arrest is the most common scenario in which ACLS is applied, ACLS can also be used in other emergency situations, such as when a patient is unable to breathe or has lost a significant amount of blood.

There are a number of causes of sudden cardiac death and the most common fall into three broad categories:

- **Arrhythmia:** An arrhythmia occurs when the electrical activity of the heart is abnormal. As a result, the electrical signals directing the heart can be generated to beat quickly (tachycardia), slowly (bradycardia), or in the worst case, in a completely disorganized fashion (ventricular fibrillation). In these situations, the heart's mechanical pumping function (the actual squeezing of the heart muscle) is compromised, and the heart is unable to pump enough blood to the body and the brain.

  Arrhythmias can arise for a variety of reasons. Most commonly, they occur because the heart muscle is not getting enough blood (ischemia) as a result of CAD or a heart attack (MI). Other causes include diseased heart muscle (cardiomyopathy), valvular heart disease (such as aortic stenosis), or a direct dysfunction in the heart's electric system. It is important to note that not all arrhythmias require an ACLS response. Although patients with ventricular fibrillation always require resuscitations, those with bradycardia or tachycardia are often able to maintain blood pressures sufficient enough to meet their body's and brain's needs. In these stable patients, treating their arrhythmia, although still important, is not an immediate emergency requiring ACLS.

- **Pulseless electrical activity (PEA):** PEA occurs when the electrical system of the heart is functioning appropriately as measured on an EKG but the heart is not pumping blood, and as a result there is no pulse. PEA can be caused by a number of conditions, including a heart attack, large blood clots in the lung (pulmonary embolism), severe electrolyte abnormalities (e.g., very high blood levels of potassium), cardiac tamponade (when blood leaks into the sac around the heart and as a result compresses the heart like a vise), hypoxia (not enough oxygen), hypothermia (very low body temperature), and severe hemorrhage (blood loss).

- **Asystole:** Asystole occurs when there is a complete absence of both electrical activity and heart muscle pumping. Asystole, like PEA, is the end result of a number of different processes including hypoxia and heart electric system dysfunction. Most often, asystole occurs when another cause of sudden cardiac death is not treated quickly enough, and the heart's function degenerates completely. As a result, patients in asystole are rarely resuscitated successfully.

What is ACLS?

ACLS is a set of guidelines directing how patients with sudden cardiac arrest should be treated. A team of highly trained professionals including physicians, nurses, paramedics, pharmacists, and respiratory therapists utilize ACLS protocols to treat patients with sudden cardiac arrest quickly and appropriately. Although identifying the cause of sudden cardiac arrest and treating it appropriately is important, the initial and central focus of ACLS is cardiopulmonary resuscitation (CPR) and getting the heart beating effectively again. (See appendix I.)

- **CPR:** When discussing ACLS, the part that most everyone recognizes is CPR (see Appendix I). The most important component of CPR is chest compressions (pressing down on the chest to force blood flow through the heart). A number of studies have shown that vigorous chest compressions are probably the single most important factor in resuscitating a patient with sudden cardiac arrest. The second component of CPR is ventilation (blowing air into the lungs of the patient). Although most people think of mouth-to-mouth breathing, ventilation is now almost always done with a mask. The importance of not letting anything (except for defibrillation) interfere with effective CPR cannot be overstated.

- **Rhythm analysis and defibrillation:** While CPR is performed, the next step in ACLS is to determine the heart rhythm of the patient. If the patient is in ventricular fibrillation or in tachycardia, immediate defibrillation is vital. Defibrillation is the use of an electric shock, administered through a device placed on the chest, to restart the heart in a normal rhythm. It is often referred to as "shocking" the patient.

If the patient is in a shockable rhythm, timely defibrillation, in conjunction with effective CPR, is vital. For patients with bradycardia, instead of defibrillation, the external devices are used to provide a lower-energy electric shock to cause the heart to beat faster (much like a pacemaker). If immediate defibrillation does not work, a variety of medications are given to the patient that can make it more likely that defibrillation will be successful.

- **PEA/asystole:** Unlike arrhythmias, PEA and asystole cannot be treated with defibrillation or external pacing. The focus of treating PEA and asystole (in addition to effective CPR) is determining and treating the cause. Patients with PEA or asystole are often given large amounts of intravenous fluids, medications such as epinephrine and vasopressin (which normally cause blood pressure to increase), and atropine (which causes the heart rate to increase). The goal, when treating PEA and asystole, is to identify a treatable cause and administrate effective CPR until the patient regains a pulse or develops a heart rhythm that can be shocked.

Unfortunately, patients who have sudden cardiac arrest, especially outside a hospital, generally do not do well. It is estimated that less than one in twenty patients who have a cardiac arrest outside a hospital survive. As a result, it is important to realize when continued CPR- and ACLS-directed therapy is futile and should be stopped. If resuscitation efforts have lasted more than thirty minutes, if there was a long delay between cardiac arrest and the start of resuscitation, or if the initial cause of the arrest was asystole, the patient is unlikely to survive, and resuscitation should probably be stopped.

Care after ACLS

The care of patients after successful resuscitation from sudden cardiac arrest can be divided into three broad categories:

Induced hypothermia: Of all organs, the brain is most susceptible to loss of blood flow and oxygen. Within five minutes of cardiac arrest, the brain cells will begin to die in significant numbers. As a result, patients who are resuscitated after sudden cardiac arrest often suffer significant irreversible brain damage. The only therapy that has been shown to minimize brain damage in cardiac arrest patients (other than prompt successful resuscitation) is induced hypothermia.

During induced hypothermia, body temperature is intentionally reduced by four or five degrees. To be effective, hypothermia has to be induced within six hours of cardiac arrest and maintained for twenty-four hours. Several studies have shown that induced hypothermia can significantly reduce the risk and severity of brain damage and can increase the chances that the patient will live. Because induced hypothermia requires close monitoring, it can be done only within intensive care units by specially trained staff.

Treatment of the underlying cause: Finding and treating the cause of sudden cardiac arrest is vital in preventing a repeat event. Sudden cardiac arrest can be the result of a number of conditions and each one has a specific treatment. If the cause was an MI (heart attack), the patient should undergo PCI to open the blocked arteries in the heart. If the cause was an arrhythmia caused by dysfunction of the heart's electric system or damaged heart muscle (cardiomyopathy), the patient will likely benefit from an ICD. Patients who have a cardiac arrest due to bradycardia often receive a pacemaker.

Goals of care: A neurologist should evaluate all patients who have been resuscitated from cardiac arrest to determine the severity and reversibility of the brain damage they have likely suffered. For many patients, even though their heart is restarted, they have suffered a significant amount of brain damage. Patients can be left with a range of deficits, from having mild memory loss to being in a vegetative state. In the worst case, patients can have suffered brain death (no brain activity is present), even though their heart keeps beating. Families and physicians should have a frank discussion about the patient's prognosis and how he or she would want to be treated after such a tragic event.

Sudden cardiac arrest is the most urgent medical emergency. Rescuing a patient who has suffered a sudden cardiac arrest is the closest that medicine can come to bringing someone back to life. The chance of surviving such an event is low and the chance of surviving the event without significant brain damage is even lower.

The ACLS guidelines and efforts that have been put in place to train health care providers and hospitals in the proper delivery of ACLS-directed therapy have improved patient survival. Induced hypothermia has enhanced our ability to reduce brain damage after cardiac arrest. Still, the best way to treat patients at risk is to identify them before an event, treat the underlying disease, and reduce the chances that they will ever need ACLS.

Q. & A. with Dr. Cannon

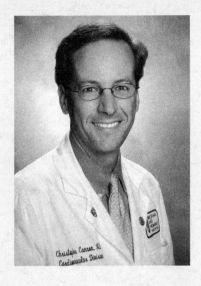

Q. If I need to have an angioplasty and stenting, how long do I have to stay in the hospital?

A. Generally, an angioplasty and stenting procedure requires a twenty-four-hour hospital stay. Usually, if you come in the morning for a cardiac catheterization (to take the pictures of the arteries), the doctors will talk to you about the result, and if a stent is needed, they will do it right away. Then, you are watched overnight to make sure you are stable, and you are discharged in the morning.

Q. How long after a stent can I go back to work?

A. It depends a bit on your overall heart condition. For the stenting procedure itself, you usually need to take at least two to three days off so that the incision site can heal. Your doctor will talk to you about any other limitations based on your heart condition.

Q. My eighty-year-old father just had bypass surgery. They want to discharge him from the hospital and send him to a cardiac rehabilitation hospital for a week or so. Is that advisable, or should he stay at the main hospital?

A. It is likely that he'll go to the rehab hospital. If he has made it through the surgery and is generally stable, most elderly patients need some extra time to regain their strength. A regular tertiary care hospital is not as well suited as a rehabilitation hospital for that next phase of recovery. Generally, patients will stay at the rehab for a week or so after bypass surgery and then will be sent home to complete their full recovery.

GLOSSARY OF CARDIOLOGY TERMS

ablation The removal, isolation, or destruction of cardiac tissue or conduction pathways involved in arrhythmias

acute coronary syndrome (ACS) An umbrella term used to describe patients having a heart attack or worsening chest pain that comes from a lack of blood supply to the heart

Advanced Cardiovascular Life Support (ACLS) A set of guidelines directing how patients with sudden cardiac arrest should be treated

aneurysm An abnormal bulge or ballooning in the wall of an artery

angina Chest pain due to an inadequate supply of oxygen to the heart muscle

angiography An X-ray examination of the coronary arteries using a catheter inserted into a main artery and then passed through blood vessels until it reaches the coronary arteries

angiotensin-converting enzyme inhibitors (ACE inhibitors) Medications that are used primarily in the treatment of hypertension and congestive heart failure

angiotensin-receptor blockers (ARBs) Medications that lower blood pressure and the force with which the heart has to pump

ankle/brachial index (ABI) A test that compares the blood pressure in the arms and legs, to evaluate for blockages in the arteries to the legs

antiarrhythmic drugs A group of pharmaceuticals that are used to suppress fast rhythms of the heart

anticoagulants Blood-thinning medicines that decrease the blood's ability to clot

amiodarone (Cordarone) A Class III antiarrhythmic drug which has multiple actions within the heart, generally decreasing the risk of arrhythmias

antiplatelet agents Medicines that act on platelets, decreasing their ability to clump together and form a clot

aorta The artery carrying oxygen-rich blood from the heart to all the limbs and organs except the lungs

aortic regurgitation (aortic insufficiency) The inability of the aortic valve to properly prevent the backflow of blood from the aorta into the left ventricle

aortic stenosis The stiffening and lack of movement of the leaflets of the aortic valve

aortic valve A valve composed of three leaflets attached to the wall of the aorta, which act as envelopes

arrest (cardiac) Cessation of the heart's normal rhythmic electrical and/or mechanical activity

arrhythmia An abnormal or absent heart rhythm

arrhythmia ablation A procedure used to treat tachycardia in which catheters are inserted into the large veins in the body (usually the groin) and advanced to the heart

arteriography A medical imaging technique used to visualize the inside of blood vessels and organs of the body

arteriovenous malformation (AVM) A congenital abnormal connection between an artery and a vein, which may burst and cause bleeding

atherosclerosis A disease in which plaque builds up on the insides of arteries

atria The plural of atrium

atrial fibrillation (AF) A very fast, disorganized heart rhythm in the atria (the most common arrhythmia)

atrial flutter (AFL) A fast, organized atrial heart rhythm

atrial septal defect (ASD) A heart defect in which the left and right atria are not properly separated

atrial tachycardia (AT) A rapid heart rate that starts in the atria

atrioventricular (AV) node A junction that conducts electrical impulses from the atria to the ventricles of the heart

atrioventricular nodal reentrant tachycardia (AVNRT) An abnormal heart rhythm caused by an electrical circuit that is localized to the atrioventricular node (AV node)

atrioventricular (AV) synchrony The normal action of the heart in which the atria contract and then, after a brief delay, the ventricles contract

atrium An upper chamber of the heart

autologous Cells, tissues, or proteins that are reimplanted into the same person they are drawn from

automated external defibrillator (AED) A device that shocks the heart back to a normal rhythm

beta blocker A blood pressure medication that thwarts the stimulation of specific receptors in the heart called beta receptors

bradycardia (bradyarrhythmia) A slow heart rate; commonly defined as fewer than sixty beats per minute

calcium-channel blocker A blood pressure medication that prevents the muscle cells of the heart and the arteries from having too much calcium inside them

calcium score Use of computed tomography (CT) to check for the buildup of calcium in plaque on the walls of coronary arteries

cardiac arrest The sudden loss of the heart's ability to pump blood, usually caused by irregularities in the electrical impulses of the heart

cardiomyopathy A disease in which the heart muscle becomes inflamed and function is compromised

cardiopulmonary resuscitation (CPR) A procedure used when a patient's heart stops beating and breathing stops—it involves compressions of the chest or electrical shocks along with rescue breathing

cardioversion Delivering an electrical shock to the heart to rapidly return an abnormal heart rhythm back to normal

cardiovascular magnetic resonance (CMR) A magnetic resonance imaging (MRI) study of the heart, using new techniques that allow high-definition images to be collected

carotid ultrasonography Use of sound to detect narrowing or clotting in the carotid arteries and the flow of blood through them

catheterization A procedure that involves inserting a very long, hollow tube into a blood vessel

Coronary Heart Disease (CHD) Narrowing of the small blood vessels that supply the heart with blood and oxygen

Class I antiarrhythmic drugs Medications that slow conduction in all parts of the heart by depressing fast sodium channels

Class II antiarrhythmic drugs Beta blockers that exert their effect by blocking the beta-adrenergic receptors, which slows down the heart

Class III antiarrhythmic drugs Drugs that target potassium channels

clip ligation Clamping off an aneurysm using a metal clip

coil embolization A minimally invasive treatment for aneurysms and other blood vessel malformations

computed tomography (CT, or CAT scans) An imaging technique that takes multiple X-rays rotating around the body and then uses a computer to compile them into detailed, three-dimensional images

congenital heart disease (CHD) A problem wth the heart's structure and function due to abnormal development in the womb

coronary arteries Arteries that supply the heart muscle

coronary artery bypass graft (CABG) Surgery Surgery in which a vein or artery from another location in the body is removed and reattached to the blood vessels feeding the heart to bypass a blockage

CT angiogram A device that uses X-rays to make detailed pictures of blood vessels

defibrillation Restoring a normal heart rhythm by delivering a high-energy electric shock to cardiac tissue

diabetes (diabetes mellitus) A chronic disease in which the body's ability to use or produce insulin is impaired

diastole The time period when the heart is in a state of relaxation and dilatation (expansion)

diastolic blood pressure The bottom number in a blood pressure reading—it represents the pressure when the heart muscle is relaxed between beats

digitalis (digoxin) A medicine used to treat congestive heart failure (CHF) and heart rhythm problems (arrhythmias)

dilation/dilatation The condition of being enlarged or dilated

diltiazem A medication used to control blood pressure, which also blocks calcium ion channels in the heart

DNA (deoxyribonucleic acid) The hereditary material in humans and almost all other organisms

dislipidemia Elevation of blood cholesterol, low-density lipoprotein (LDL), and/or triglycerides, or a low high-density lipoprotein level (HDL)

dissection A tear in the wall of an aorta that causes blood to flow between and force apart the layers of its wall

dissecting aneurysm A condition in which the layers of an artery separate or are torn, causing blood to flow between them—dissecting aneurysms usually happen in the aorta.

diuretic A drug that lowers blood pressure by promoting fluid loss and increased urine production

dual-chamber pacemaker A pacemaker with two leads (one in the atrium and one in the ventricle) to allow pacing and/or sensing in both chambers of the heart to artificially restore the natural contraction sequence of the heart

echocardiogram A test that uses sound waves to check heart function and to detect blood clots inside the heart

ejection fraction A measure of the output of the heart with each heartbeat

electrocardiogram (ECG of EKG) A printout from an electrocardiography machine, which measures and records the electrical activity of the heart

electrolytes Salts that carry an electric charge in blood and other body fluids

electrophysiology (EP) study The use of programmed stimulation protocols to assess the electrical activity of the heart to diagnose arrhythmias

embolic stroke A stroke that occurs when a blood clot forms at another location and travels through the vessels to the brain

embolism (emboli, plural) A blockage (or blockages) in a blood vessel due to a blood clot or other foreign matter moving through the bloodstream

endocarditis An infection inside the heart, usually on the heart valves

endovascular intervention A surgical procedure in which a catheter containing medications or miniature instruments is inserted through the skin into a blood vessel for the treatment of vascular disease

exercise stress testing (ECG) An ECG records the activity of the heart while the patient walks on a treadmill (or sometimes a drug is used to make the heart beat faster)

Flecainide One of the Class I antiarrhythmic drugs—it blocks the sodium channels in the heart.

fibrillation A chaotic and unsynchronized quivering of the myocardium during which no effective pumping occurs—fibrillation may occur in the atria or the ventricles.

genome All of the DNA that an individual possesses

heart block A condition in which electrical impulses are not conducted in the normal fashion from the atria to the ventricles

hemodynamic The forces involved in circulating blood through the cardiovascular system—the heart adapts its hemodynamic performance to the needs of the body, increasing its output of blood when muscles are working, and decreasing output when the body is at rest.

heart failure Inability of the heart to keep up with the demands on it—this can be due to the heart being weak (systolic heart failure) or too thick (diastolic heart failure).

hemorrhagic stroke A "bleeding" stroke, due to a leak or rupture in a blood vessel

hematopoietic stem cells (HSCs) Stem cells that can develop into all blood-cell types

Holter monitoring A technique for the continuous recording of electrocardiographic (ECG) signals—this is usually done for twenty-four to forty-eight hours with a small device the size of an iPod.

hyperlipidemia Elevated levels of lipids (fats) in the blood, such as cholesterol and triglycerides

implantable cardioverter defibrillator (ICD) An implanted device used to treat abnormal, fast heart rhythms

infarct A localized area of tissue that is dying or dead due to loss of a blood supply or thrombosis

inferior vena xcava The large vein that carries deoxygenated blood from the lower half of the body into the right atrium of the heart

inotropes Medications that cause the heart muscle to contract with more force

inferior vena cava filter (IVC filter) A medical device that is implanted into the inferior vena cava to prevent pulmonary emboli (PEs)

internal cardiac defibrillator (ICD) An implanted device that recognizes certain types of abnormal heart rhythms and corrects them

ischemia Insufficient blood flow to tissue due to a blockage in the arteries

ischemic stroke A stroke caused by a blockage in a blood vessel carrying blood to the brain

left ventricular dysfunction A heart condition in which the heart cannot maintain normal cardiac output due to weakness of the left ventricle

left ventricular assist device (LVAD) An electrical pump that assist the heart

lipid A fat—cholesterol and Triglycerides are lipids

magnetic resonance angiography (MRA) A test that uses a powerful magnet and radio waves to produce a detailed, three-dimensional view of the arteries

MERCI retriever A tiny corkscrew-shaped device that wraps around blood clots and traps them

MIBI test (similar to thallium test) A stress test in which a small amount of radioactive material is injected into the blood stream, which enable a camera to show how the blood is flowing to all parts of the heart muscle

mitral regurgitation (MR) The abnormal leaking of blood through the mitral valve, from the left ventricle into the left atrium of the heart

mitral stenosis A disease characterized by poor movement of the flaps of the mitral valve, which doesn't allow blood to flow from the left atrium to the left ventricle

mitral valve A heart valve that controls the flow between the left atrium and the left ventricle—it is composed of two leaflets.

myocardial infarction (MI) Death of a portion of the heart muscle tissue due to a blockage or interruption in the supply of blood to the heart muscle

myocarditis Acute infections of the heart muscle.

myocardium The middle and the thickest layer of the heart wall—it is composed of cardiac muscle.

nitrates (nitro, nitroglycerin) A class of medications that widen (dilate) blood vessels, allowing more room for blood to get past blockages

nucleotide The basic building block of nucleic acids, such as DNA

pacemaker A small device implanted in the chest or abdomen, which uses electrical pulses to help control abnormal heart rhythms

patent ductus arteriosus (PDA) A condition in which a blood vessel called the ductus arteriosus fails to close after birth—the condition causes abnormal blood flow between the aorta and pulmonary artery.

penumbra system A clot-retrieval device that uses suction to grab blood clots in larger vessels of the brain in a safe manner for treatment of acute ischemic stroke

peripheral vascular disease (also, peripheral artery disease) Diseases of blood vessels outside the heart and brain (e.g., the aorta or legs)

percutaneous coronary intervention (PCI, angioplasty) A procedure that uses a plastic catheter with a balloon at the end to open narrowed arteries in the heart—stents are often used as well.

perfusion The passage of fluid such as blood through the heart or other parts of the body

platelets Irregularly shaped, colorless cells found in blood—their sticky surface helps form clots to stop bleeding.

pluripotent A cell that can develop into all cell types (such as heart or kidney cells) except for extra embryonic tissue

polymorphisms A common variation or mutation in DNA

premature atrial contraction (PAC) A contraction in the atrium which occurs earlier than the next expected normal sinus beat

premature ventricular contraction (PVC or VPD) A contraction in the ventricle that occurs earlier than the next expected normal sinus or escape rhythm beat

plaque A deposit of fatty material on the inner lining of an arterial wall

pulmonary arteries Arteries that serve the lungs

pulmonary embolism A condition that occurs when one or more arteries in your lungs become blocked

pulmonary valve A valve that lies between the right ventricle and the pulmonary artery and has three cusps

red blood cell (RBC) Blood cell that contains the protein hemoglobin, which enables it to carry oxygen and carbon dioxide—hemoglobin gives the cells their red color.

remodeling A procss of structural deterioration of the left ventricle

septum The heart tissue that separates the left and right sides of the heart

sinoatrial (SA, sinus) node The heart's natural pacemaker, located in the right atrium—electrical impulses originate here and travel through the heart, causing it to beat.

stable angina The most common form of angina, in which symptoms have stayed the same for months

statins A group of medications used to treat high cholesterol

stem cell A cell that has the ability to continuously divide and develop into other types of cells and/or tissues

stenosis An abnormal narrowing in a blood vessel or other tubular organ or structure

sudden cardiac death (SCD) Death due to cardiac causes within one hour of the onset of symptoms with no prior warning, usually caused by ventricular fibrillation

superior vena cava The large vein that carries deoxygenated blood from the upper half of the body to the heart's right atrium

supraventricular tachycardia (SVT) A tachycardia originating from above the ventricles

syncope Fainting, loss of consciousness, or dizziness

systole The rhythmic contraction of the heart, especially of the ventricles, which pushes blood through the aorta and pulmonary artery after each dilation or diastole

tachycardia (tachyarrhythmia) Rapid beating of either or both chambers of the heart, usually defined as a rate of more than 100 beats per minute

tetralogy of Fallot A congenital heart defect that changes the normal flow of blood through the heart

thallium test (similar to MIBI test) A stress test in which a small amount of radioactive material is injected into the blood stream, which enables a camera to show how the blood is flowing to all parts of the heart muscle

titrate The process of determining the concentration of a substance in a solution

transesophageal echocardiogram (TEE) A special ultrasound test that uses sound waves to take pictures of the heart—the study is done by passing a special tube down the throat into the esophagus or food pipe.

transposition of the great arteries (TGA) The reversal of the major vessels leaving each ventricle

thrombotic stroke A stroke caused by a clot forming around areas of a blood vessel wall damaged by atherosclerotic plaques

thrombosis The formation of a blood clot (thrombus) inside a blood vessel, blocking the flow of blood through the circulatory system

transdifferentiation A process where a non-stem cell transforms into a different type of cell, or when an already differentiated stem cell creates another type of cell

tricuspid stenosis Narrowing of the tricuspid valve, most commonly caused by rheumatic fever

tricuspid regurgitation Abnormal backflow through the tricuspid valve

tricuspid valve A valve with three leaflets, located between the right atrium and the right ventricle

unspecialized stem cells Stem cells are unspecialized until signaled to develop into specific cells such as heart, nerve, or skin cells

unstable angina Angina symptoms that are spiraling out of control

valve replacement surgery An open-heart surgery to replace diseased valves

valvular heart disease Any disease process involving one or more of the valves of the heart

valvuloplasty A surgery to repair stenotic valves—a similar procedure can also be done with catheters

ventilation-perfusion lung scan (V/Q scan) A test that utilizes radioactive material to determine how well oxygen and blood are flowing to all areas of the lungs

ventricle One of the two lower chambers of the heart

ventricular assist device (VAD) A device that is used to partially or completely replace the function of a failing heart

ventricular fibrillation (VF) Very fast, chaotic, quivering heart contractions, which start in the ventricles

ventricular septal defect (VSD) The incomplete
formation of the muscle that separates the left and
right ventricles

ventricular tachycardia (VT) A rapid heart rate
that starts in the ventricles

Verapamil A medication used to control blood
pressure, which also blocks calcium ion channels in
the heart

warfarin (Coumadin) An anticoagulant drug that
makes the blood thinner and less likely to form a
clot

white blood cells The cells in blood that help
fight infections—they are also called leukocytes.

Wolff-Parkinson-White Syndrome A condition
that occurs when a bypass tract allows electrical
signals to bypass the atrioventricular node and go
directly to the ventricles

WEB RESOURCES

The American Diabetes Association (ADA)

The American Diabetes Association funds research and provides information and other services to people with diabetes. The ADA publishes a series of free eNewsletters including *Diabetes World*, a weekly publication that provides the latest news and events occurring in the world of diabetes, and *Diabetes Foodsmart*, which offers tips and recipes for people with diabetes.

www.diabetes.org

The American Heart Association (AHA)

The American Heart Association's Heart Attack Risk Calculator helps you learn your risk of having a heart attack over the next ten years. You also can create an action plan to reduce your risk and upload your results into a personal Google Health account.

www.americanheart.org

CardioSmart

CardioSmart is the patient education site of the American College of Cardiology (ACC). It includes the following:

- A *Learn About Heart Disease* portal that provides easy-to-understand descriptions of the most common heart disease conditions, common tests that your doctor may use to help diagnose symptoms, and information on the most common treatment approaches for the management of heart disease
- A library of videos that provide basic background information on a variety of topics, such as *Understanding Risk Factors for Heart Disease* and *Understanding Tests and Procedures* from leading cardiologists on heart disease

- CardioSmart News, which covers the most recent advances in cardiovascular medicine—you can sign up to receive *CardioSmart News* updates by email.

www.cardiosmart.org

- You can also refer to the physician website of the American College of Cardiology.

www.cardiosource.org

Go Red for Women

The American Heart Association's *Go Red for Women* website celebrates the color red and the red dress campaign, which publicizes the need to improve women's heart health. The portal provides the *Go Red Heart Checkup*, which assesses your cardiovascular risk factors and uses the results to provide you with a customized guide to achieve fitness and nutrition goals.

www.goredforwomen.org

HeartHub

HeartHub is the patient information portal of the American Heart Association. It includes the following:

- Heart360, an online wellness center where you can keep track of your blood pressure, cholesterol, and blood sugar levels—you also can enter your exercise levels and your weight, and keep a diary of your medications.
- An extensive video library with titles such as "Understanding Cholesterol Levels" and "Healing from a Heart Attack"

- Question and answers with experts on frequently asked questions about heart disease and stroke
- The latest facts on heart disease and stroke prevention and treatment
- Heart-healthy recipes
- A Heart Attack Risk Calculator to learn about your risk of having a heart attack over the next ten years

www.hearthub.org

The National Heart, Lung, and Blood Institute (NHLBI)

The NHLBI is one of the institutes of the U.S. National Institutes of Health. Its public information portal offers the following:

- An A-to-Z index of information on heart disease and related conditions
- Information and recipes from the low-salt DASH Eating Plan
- Special heart-healthy recipes for African Americans, Latinos, and others

www.nhlbi.nih.gov/health/index.htm

The National Stroke Association (NSA)

The National Stroke Association provides education, services and community-based activities in prevention, treatment, rehabilitation, and recovery from stroke. The NSA publishes a free magazine, *Stroke Smart*. Archived editions are available on its website.

www.stroke.org

Women's Heart Foundation (WHF)

The Women's Heart Foundation is a coalition of executive nurses, community health directors, and others responding to the "crisis" of women's heart disease and the need for prevention programs. The WHF publishes Healthy Hearts Guides, instructional sheets to assist patients and practitioners in the care and management of heart disease. The guides are available in Spanish and English and can be downloaded from the foundation's website.

www.womensheart.org

ABOUT THE AUTHORS

Christopher P. Cannon, M.D., is an associate professor of medicine at Harvard Medical School in the Cardiovascular Division at Brigham and Women's Hospital in Boston. He is a senior investigator of the Thrombolysis in Myocardial Infarction (TIMI) Study Group and over the past two decades has been the principal investigator for ten international clinical trials in the area of heart attacks and prevention. His recent research showed that "lower is better" for cholesterol and changed international guidelines.

Dr. Cannon graduated from Yale College and earned his medical degree from Columbia University College of Physicians and Surgeons in New York. He has been on staff as a cardiologist at Brigham and Women's for nineteen years.

Dr. Cannon has published more than 500 original articles, reviews, editorials, book chapters, and electronic publications in the field of heart attacks and cardiovascular prevention. His research is published in journals including *Journal of the American Medical Association*, *Lancet*, *Journal of the American College of Cardiology*, and the *New England Journal of Medicine*. He is author or editor of six books, including *The Complete Idiot's Guide to the Anti-Inflammation Diet*.

Dr. Cannon is frequently quoted in the press, including *The Wall Street Journal*, the *New York Times*, and the *Washington Post*. He has appeared as a guest on ABC World News, Good Morning America, NBC Nightly News, PBS, and CNBC, among others. He is the editor-in-chief of the American College of Cardiology's website, Cardiosource (www.cardiosource.com), and an editor for the website for patients, www.cardiosmart.org.

He recently was cited as one of the "Best Doctors in Boston" in *Boston Magazine*.

Elizabeth Vierck, M.S., is a well-known writer on aging and health. She has been a consultant and writer for many national health and aging organizations. She has authored and co-authored twenty books, including *Health Smart*, *Chronic Pain for Dummies*, and *The Complete Idiot's Guide to the Anti-Inflammation Diet*. She is the originator and author of *Aging America*, a highly regarded fact book on aging published in many editions by the AARP and the U.S. Senate Special Committee on Aging.

ACKNOWLEDGMENTS

Writing *The New Heart Disease Handbook* was a team effort. We are fortunate to have had the assistance of a crackerjack group of physicians and medical researchers who drafted chapters and worked hard to make the book comprehensive, up-to-date, and accessible. We heartily thank the following writers:

Farhad Abtahian, M.D., Ph.D., Resident, The Brigham and Women's Hospital

Appendix III: A Reference of Medications that Treat Heart Disease and Their Side Effects
Appendix IV: Heart-Saving Procedures

Subroto Acharjee, MBBS, Research Fellow, Division of Cardiology, Beth Israel Deaconess Medical Center

Chapter 7: Stroke
Chapter 9: How to Determine Your Risk
Chapter 10: Living with Heart Disease
Epilogue: Into the Crystal Ball

Amit Kumar, M.D., Assistant Professor, Department of Hospital Medicine, University of Massachusetts Medical School

Chapter 3: Diseases of Other Arteries
Chapter 15: Women and Heart Disease

Benjamin A. Olenchock, M.D., Ph.D., Resident, The Brigham and Women's Hospital

Appendix I: How to Save a Life
Appendix II: A Reference of Tests to Diagnose Heart Disease

Benjamin A. Steinberg, M.D., Resident, Department of Medicine, Johns Hopkins University School of Medicine

Chapter 4: Diseases of the Heart Muscle
Chapter 5: Diseases of the Electrical System
Chapter 6: Structural Heart Disease
Chapter 8: Your Heart: A Guided Tour

We would also like to thank our illustrious and enduring agent, Marilyn Allen, and the staff at Fair Winds Press for their vision, patience, and skillfulness: Will Kiester, Jill Alexander, John Gettings, Laura B. Smith, and Audrey Doyle.

—Christopher P. Cannon, M.D. &
Elizabeth Vierck, M.S.

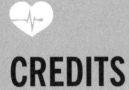

CREDITS

INDEX

Note: Page numbers in italics indicate tables or figures.

Asian Americans, 66, 185

Asians, 185

aspirin, 15, 30, 32, 153, 154, 229, 237, 266, 314, 327

asystole, 346, 347

atenolol (Tenormin), 12, 93, 218

atherosclerosis, 19, 40, 42, 46, 160, 162, 188, 227

atorvastin (Lipitor), 36, 204, 218, 320

atria, 113, 167, 168, *169*, 177, 178–179

atrial clots, *97*

atrial fibrillation, 95, 96, *97*, 98, *99*, 104–105, 109, 316, 318, 322–324, 334

atrial flutter, 106, 316, 318, 322–323

atrial septal defect (ASD), 113, 117, *140*, *141*, 141–142

atrial tachyarrhythmia, 104

atrioventricular (AV) node, 104, 108, 177

atypical symptoms, 262–263, 271, 273, 278

automatic external defibrillators (AEDs), 292, 295, 296, 298

automatic implantable cardioverter defibrillators (AICDs), 270. *See also* implantable cardioverter defibrillators (ICDs)

azithromycin (Zithromax), 118

B

baby aspirin, 30

balloon angioplasty, 15, *17*, 30. *See also* angioplasty

balloon catheters, *31*

beans, 243–244. *See also* legumes

beef, 248

benazepril (Lotensin), 73, 115, 219, 316

beta blockers, 12, 33, 53, 74–75, 87, 218, 228, 315–316, 322

  for arrythmia, 93

  atenolol (Tenormin), 218

  bisoprolol (Zebeta), 218

  carvedilol (Coreg), 218

  labetalol, 315

  metoprolol (Lopressor, Toprol XL), 218, 315

  nadolol, 315

  pindolol, 315

  propranolol, 315

  timolol (Blockadren), 218, 315

bicuspid aortic valves, 117

BiDil, 74

biguanides (Metformin), 231

bile acid sequestrants, 321

bioprosthetic valves, 121, 343–344

biopsy, 310

bipyridines, 324–325

birth control pills, 268

bisoprolol (Zebeta), 12, 93, 218, 315

bivaliriduin, 32

biventricular pacemakers, 336

bleeding, 64

blocked arteries, opening, 29

blood clots. *See* thrombosis

blood flow, 12–13, 167, 179

  restoring, 49–50

  through the heart, *172*

blood glucose. *See* blood sugar

blood pressure, 53, 56, 57. *See also* high blood pressure

  age and, 221

  birth control pills and, 268

  diabetes and, 231–232

  diastolic pressure, 221, *221*

  lowering, 15, 72–73, 216, 217

  measuring, 220–221, *221*

  medications that lower, 15, 72–73

  structural heart disease and, 115–116

  systolic pressure, 221, *221*

  testing for, 219, 232

blood-pressure reducing medications, 15, 72–73

blood sugar, 238

  diabetes and, 230, 231–232

  metabolic syndrome and, 235–237

blood tests, 66, 158

blood thinners. *See* anticoagulants

blood turbulence, 304–305

blood vessels, 12

BMI (body mass index), 248–251, *249*

bradyarrythmia, 104, 108

bradycardia, 335

brain. *See also* stroke

  brain swelling, 154

  stroke and, *160, 161*

bruits, 50

bumetanide (Bumex), 72, 114, 319

buproprion SR (Zyban), 255

bypass surgery. *See* coronary artery bypass surgery

bystolic (Nebivolol), 93

C

CAC score, 306

Caduet, 218

calcium-channel blockers, 12–13, *14*, 34, 94, 116, 216, 218–219, 228, 317–318, 322

  amlodipine (Norvasc), 116, 218, 317

  dihydropyridines, 317

  diltiazem, 317, 322

  felodipine (Plendil), 116, 218, 317

  idradipine (DynaCirc), 218

  nicardipine (Cardene), 116, 219, 317

  nifedipine (Procardia), 116, 317

  nimodipine (Nimotop), 116, 154

  nisoldipine (Sular), 219

  verapamil, 317, 322

calcium ions, *14*

calcium scan, 273

calcium score, 19, 311

calories, 250, 251

cancer, 80

candesartan (Atacand), 73, 115, 220, 316

Cannon, Dr., 24, 44, 68, 87, 109, 147, 163, 190, 200, 210, 223, 238, 259, 278, 289, 298

capillaries, 167

captopril (Capoten), 73, 115, 219, 316

carbohydrates, 229–230, 241

cardiac arrest, 34. *See also* sudden cardiac arrest (SCA)

cardiac catheterization, 15, 30, 34, 81, 122, 272–273, 278, 308–310. *See also* angiography

cardiac defibrillation. *See* defibrillation

cardiac defibrillators. *See* defibrillators

cardiac glycosides, 324–325. *See also* digoxin (digitalis)

cardiac rehabilitation, 36, 192–198, 200

cardiology terms, 351–360

cardiomyopathy, 71, 274–275, 277. *See also* heart failure

cardiopulmonary resuscitation (CPR), 292–295, 298

Cardiovascular Health Study, 245

cardiovascular magnetic resonance (CMR), 307

CardioWest TAH, 288

carotid artery disease, 188

carotid endareterectomy, 154

carotid ultrasonography/Doppler scan test, 158

carotid ultrasound test, 190

carvedilol (Coreg), 12, 74, 93, 218, 315

catecholamines, 324–325

catheter-based ablations, 105

catheterization. *See* cardiac catheterization

caucasians, 66

CHADS2 Score, 96

Chagas disease, 86

chemotherapy, 72, 80

chest compressions, 293, 294–295

chest pain, 9–24, 34–35, 278

chest X-rays (CXR), 56, 66

children

  cholesterol and, *204*, 204

  CPR for, 297

chlorothalidone, 319

chlorothiazide (Diuril), 72, 114

choking, 296

cholesterol, 36, 182–183, 188, 189, 190, 201–210, *209*. *See also* high cholesterol

  adolescents and, 204, *204*

  children and, 204, *204*

  diabetes and, 231–232

  diet and, 202, 241, 246

intravenous inotropes, 75, 77

invasive cardiac catheterization, 122

invasive electrophysiology studies, 98, 100

invasive hemodynamic monitoring, 309

irbesartan (Avapro), 73, 115, 220, 316

iron, 80

ischemia, 40

ischemic heart failure, 80

ischemic stroke, 150, 152–153, 154–155, 159–160, *161*

isolated secundum ASD, 117

isoproterenol, 324

isosorbide dinitrate, 74, 325

isosorbide mononitrate, 325

Isradipine (DynaCirc), 13

J

Japanese Americans, 185

Jarvik 2000 pump, 287

JUPITER study, 206, 267

L

labetalol, 315

lacunar infarction, 162

large-vessel thrombosis, 162

LDL-C (bad cholesterol), 36, 183–184, 188, 189, 202–204, *203*, 208, *209*, 210, 228–229

left anterior descending (LAD) artery, 179

left circumflex (LAC) artery, 179

left-heart catheterization, 309–310

left internal mammary artery (LIMA), 333

left ventricular assist device (LVAD), *76*, 76

leg pain, 47

legumes, 241, 243–244

leukemia, 80

lidocaine, 322

life-saving strategies, 291–298

lifestyle changes, 36, 47, 48, 49, 71, 229, 239–260. *See also* activity; diet; exercise; smoking; stress; weight

life support, 345–348

lipids, 182–183, 228–229, 232, 321. *See also specific lipids*

lisinopril (Prinivil, Zestril), 73, 115, 219, 316

liver enzymes, 205

loop diuretics, 319–320

losartan (Cozaar), 73, 115, 220, 316

lovastatin (Mevacor/generic), 204, 320

low-density lipoproteins (LDL), 228, 243. *See also* LDL-C (bad cholesterol)

low-fat foods, 248

low molecular weigh heparin (LMWH), 323–324

low-sodium diet, 213, 214

lungs, 178–179

lymphomas, 80

M

magnestic resonance angiography (MRA), 51, 56, 159

magnestic resonance imaging (MRI), 56, 62

magnetic resonance imaging (MRI), 51, 59, 158, 159, 307

Marfan syndrome, 57

meat, 248

mechanical valves, 343–344

medical assessment, 194

medications, 153, 280, 313–327. *See also* procedures

    acarbose, 231

    acetazolamide (Diamox), 217

    adenosine, 322

    aldosterone blockers, 36, 72–73, 114, 218, 267

    alendronate (Fosamax), 268

    alpha-glucosidase inhibitors, 231

    amiloride, 319

    amiodarone (cordarone), 94, 322

    amlodipine (Norvasc), 116, 218, 317

    amoxicillin, 118

    amoxicillin/clavulanate (Augmentin), 118

    amrinone, 324

    for angina, 316, 318, 318–319, 325–326

    angiotensin-converting

    enzyme (ACE) inhibitors, 33, 72–73, 87, 115–116, 216, 219, 226, 228, 267, 316–317

    angiotensin-receptor blockers (ARBs), 33, 73–74, 87, 115–116, 216, 220, 228, 316–317 antiarrhythmia medications, 91, 322–323

antibiotics, 116, 117, 118, 147

anticoagulants, 32, 64, 66, 95, 98, 153, 266

anti-ischemic medications, 33–34

antiplatelet medications, 47–48, 49, 153, 314–316

for aortic dissection, 52, 53

for arrythmia, 91, 93, 322–323

aspirin, 32, 153, 229, 266, 314, 327

atenolol (Tenormin), 93, 218

atorvastin (Lipitor), 36, 204, 218, 320

for atrial fibrillation, 316, 318, 322–324

for atrial flutter, 316, 318, 322–323

azithromycin (Zithromax), 118

benazepril (Lotensin), 73, 115, 219, 316

beta blockers, 33, 53, 74–75, 87, 93, 218, 228, 322

BiDil, 74

biguanides (Metformin), 231

bile acid sequestrants, 321

bipyridines, 324–325

bisoprolol (Zebeta), 93, 218

bivaliriduin, 32

for blood clots, 323–324

blood-pressure reducing
    medications, 72–73

blood thinners, 32, 327

bumetanide (Bumex), 72, 114, 319

buproprion SR (Zyban), 255

bystolic (Nebivolol), 93

Caduet, 218

calcium-channel blockers, 116, 154, 216, 218–219,
    228, 317–318, 322

candesartan (Atacand), 73, 115, 220, 316

captopril (Capoten), 73, 115, 219, 316

cardiac glycosides, 324–325. *See also* digoxin
    (digitalis)

carvedilol (Coreg), 74, 93, 218

catecholamines, 324–325

chlorothalidone, 319

chlorothiazide (Diuril), 72, 114

cholesterol absorbtion inhibitors, 206

cholestryamine (Questran, Questran Light), 205

for chronic kidney disease (CKD), 317

cilostazol (Pletal), 49

clindamycin (Cleocin), 118

clofibrate (Abritate, Atromid-S), 205

clopidogrel (Plavix), 32, 49, 153, 266, 314–315

clot busters, 152–153, 266–267

colesevelam (Welchol), 205

colestpol (Colestid), 205

continuous infusion
    medication, 75, 77

for coronary artery disease (CAD), 316, 321

for diabetes, 231

digoxin (digitalis), 75, 94–95, 322, 324–325

dihydropyridines, 317

dilators, 116

diltiazem, 94, 317, 322

disopyramide, 322

diuretics, 71–72, 87, 114, 115, 217–218, 228,
    319–320, 327

dobutamine, 75–76, 77, 324

dofetilide, 322

dopamine, 324

DPP-4 inhibitors, 231

enalapril (Vasotec), 73, 115, 219, 316

for endocarditis, 116, 117, 118

enoxaparin (Lovenex), 64

epinephrine, 324

eplerenone (Inspra), 72, 114, 217, 319

esmolol (Brevibloc), 93

ethnic factors in selecting, 74

ezetimibe (Zetia), 321

felodipine (Plendil), 116, 218, 317

fenofibrate (Tricor, Trilipix), 205

fibrates, 205, 321

fibrinolytic medication, 29, 32

flecainide, 94, 322

fluvastatin (Lescol), 204

fondaparinux, 32

fosinopril (Monopril), 73, 115, 219, 316

multiple SPECT tests, 303

muscle pain, 205

muscle-strengthening activities, 252

muscular dystrophy, 80

myocardial infarction (MI), heart attacks

myocarditis, 85

N

nadolol, 93, 315

nateglinide, 231

National Heart, Lung, and Blood Institute, 29

neuromuscular disorders, 80

niacin (nicotinic acid) (Niaspan), 206–207, 321

nicardipine (Cardene), 13, 116, 219, 317

nicotine gum (Nicoderm/Nicorette and Nicotinell), 255–256

nicotine inhaler (Nicotrol), 256

nicotine lozenges, 256–257

nicotine nasal spray (Nicotrol NS), 256

nicotine patch (Habitrol, Nicoderm CQ, Nicotrol), 256–257

nifedipine (Procardia), 116, 317

nimodipine (Nimotop), 116, 154

nisoldipine (Sular), 13, 219

nitrates, 12, 33–34, 325–326

nitroglycerin, 27, 33–34, 325

noncardiac chest pain, 34–35

nonmodifiable risk factors, 182, 185

non-STEMIs (NSTEMIs), 27, 42

nonsurgical ablation, 91

norepinephrine, 324

Novacor LVAD, 286

nuclear imaging tests, 302–304

nuclear stress test, 271–272

nutritional deficiencies, 80

nuts, 241, 243–244

O

obesity, 184, 235–236, *252*

oils, 241, 242, 243

olmesartan, 316

omega-3 fatty acids, 241, 243, 244–245, 246, 248

omega-6 fatty acids, 243

open repair, 59

oral sulfonylureas, 231

outpatient rehabilitation, 193–194

overweight, *252. See also* weight

oxygen loss, 83–84

P

pacemakers, 77, 79, *99*, 100–101, *102*, 103, 109, 270, 334–336

  biventricular pacemakers, 336

  single-chamber pacemakers, 336

Pacific Islanders, 66

pain, 47, 205

chest pain, 9–24, 34–35, 278

  leg pain, 47

  muscle pain, 205

  women and, 278

panic attacks, 265

patent ductus arteriosus (PDA), 113, 142–143

patent foramen ovale (PFO) device, 156

pediatric cardiology, 146, 147

pentoxifylline (Trental), 49

penumbra system, 156, *157*

percutaneous coronary intervention (PCI), 26, 29, 30, 32, 34, 49–50, 330–332

perforation, 340

pericarditis, 334

peripartum cardiomyopathy, 277

peripheral artery disease (PAD), 46–51, *48*, 68, 188

  age and, 51

  cholesterol and, 47, 50

  diabetes and, 47

  exercise and, 47

  explanation of, 51

  heart attacks and, 47

  hypertension and, 47

  tests to diagnose, 50–51

  treating by restoring blood flow, 49–50

  treating with lifestyle changes, 47, 49

treating with medication, 47–48, 49

women and, 51

PET tests, 301, 303

Pfizer, 218

physical activity, 184, 253. *See also* exercise

lack of, 184

metabolic syndrome and, 236

physical activity counseling, 197–198

returning to normal activity levels, 199

"pill-in-a-pocket" method, 91

pindolol, 315

plant oils, 241, 242

plaque, 19, *20*, 40, 188

plaque rupture, 42

polyunsaturated fats, 242

pork, 248

potassium, 93, 217–218, 219

potassium-sparing diuretics, 319–320

poultry, 241, 244

prasugrel, 33

pravastatin (Pravachol/generic), 204, 320

prediabetes, 232–233, 234–235

pre-excitation, 108

pregnancy, 205, 275–277

aortic dissection and, 57

cardiac abnormalities during, 276

diabetes and, 276–277

heart failure and, 80

high blood pressure and, 276

medications and, 266, 267

peripartum cardiomyopathy, 277

stroke and, 277

preheart attack symptoms, 263

prehypertension, 213

primary hypertension, 221–222

procainamide, 322

procedures, 50, 52, 102, 104, 330–349. *See also* medications; testing

for abdominal aortic aneurysm (AAA), 59, 59–60, 59–60

ablation, 105, 339–340

advanced cardiovascular life support (ACLS), 345–348

angioplasty, *15*, 30, 154–155, 268–269, 349

anticlotting treatments, 30, 32

for aortic dissection, 52, 53

aortic valve replacement, 130, *131*

for arrythmia, 102, 104

arrythmia ablation, 339–340

for atrial septal defect (ASD), 142

balloon angioplasty, 15, *17*, 30

biventricular pacemakers, 336

carotid endareterectomy, 154

catheterization, 15, 30, 34, 137

coronary artery bypass surgery, *16*, 17, 34, *35*, 269, 332–334, 349

defibrillators, 77, 79, 270, 337–339, 337–339. *See also* implantable cardioverter defibrillators (ICDs)

devices, 280, 285–288. *See also specific devices*

embolectomy, 64

endovascular repair, 59, 59–60

endovascular stent graft, *55*, 55

for heart failure, 77, 79, 87

heart transplantation, 77, 79, 344–345

on the heart valves, *119*, *120*, 121

implantable cardioverter defibrillators (ICDs), 270

inferior vena cava, 64, 66

life support, 345–348

nonsurgical ablation, 91

open repair, 59

pacemakers, 77, 79, 87, 89, 270, 334–336

percutaneous coronary intervention (PCI), 26, 29, 30, 34, 49–50, 330–332

for peripheral artery disease (PAD), 49–50

for pulmonary embolism (PE), 64, 66

repair of valvular heart disease, 340–345

stenting, 15, 268–269, 331–332, 349

ventricular fibrillation, 108, 322–323, 337, 338

ventricular septal defect (VSD), 113, 117, 142

ventricular tachycardia, 106, 108, 322–323, 337, 338

ventriculography, 309

verapamil, 94, 317, 322

Viagra, 12

viral infections, 80

vitamins, 80

volitional fatigue, 252

Vytorin, 206

W

waist circumference, 235, 237, 251, *252*

warfarin (Coumadin), 64, 95, 98, 109, 153, 266–267, 323–324

web resources, 29, 93, 104, 113, 121, 189, 215, 230, 235, 296, 361–363

weight, 240, 248–251, *249, 252*

  high blood pressure and, 216

  loosing, 250, 251

  metabolic syndrome and, 235

  rehabilitation and, 195

Western diet, 243

"white coat" high blood pressure, 223

whole-grain foods, 241, 248

Wii, 198

Wilson's disease, 80

Wolff-Parkinson-White Syndrome, *107*, 108

women, 185, 261–278. *See also* pregnancy

  abdominal aortic aneurysm (AAA) and, 61

  alcohol and, 265

  anxiety and, 265

  aortic dissection and, 57

  arrythmia and, 273

  atypical symptoms and, 262–263, 271, 273, 278

  cardiomyopathy and, 274–275

  chest pain and, 278

  of childbearing age, 205. *See also* pregnancy

  coronary artery disease (CAD) and, 273

  depression and, 265

  diabetes and, 277–278

  heart attacks and, 40

  high blood pressure and, 267, 277

  high cholesterol and, 267

  medications for, 266–268

  menopausal hormone therapy and, 267

  peripheral artery disease (PAD) and, 51

  procedures for, 268–270

  risk factors for, 264

  stress and, 265

  stroke and, 159, 273–274, 278

  testing in, 270–273

Women's Health Initiative, 267, 268

Women's Ischemia Syndrome Evaluation, 269

work, 199

X

X-rays, 56, 61, 66, 311

Y

Yusuf, Salim, 243